Fuzzy Logic in Medicine

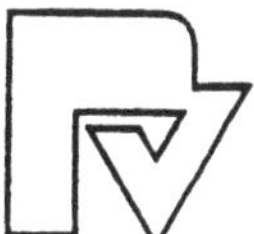

Studies in Fuzziness and Soft Computing

Editor-in-chief
Prof. Janusz Kacprzyk
Systems Research Institute
Polish Academy of Sciences
ul. Newelska 6
01-447 Warsaw, Poland
E-mail: kacprzyk@ibspan.waw.pl
http://www.springer.de/cgi-bin/search_book.pl?series=2941

Further volumes of this series can be found at our homepage.

Vol. 61. D. Driankov and A. Saffiotti (Eds.)
Fuzzy Logic Techniques for Autonomous Vehicle Navigation, 2001
ISBN 3-7908-1341-9

Vol. 62. N. Baba and L.C. Jain (Eds.)
Computational Intelligence in Games, 2001
ISBN 3-7908-1348-6

Vol. 63. O. Castillo and P. Melin
Soft Computing for Control of Non-Linear Dynamical Systems, 2001
ISBN 3-7908-1349-4

Vol. 64. I. Nishizaki and M. Sakawa
Fuzzy and Multiobjective Games for Conflict Resolution, 2001
ISBN 3-7908-1341-9

Vol. 65. E. Orłowska and A. Szalas (Eds.)
Relational Methods for Computer Science Applications, 2001
ISBN 3-7908-1365-6

Vol. 66. R.J. Howlett and L.C. Jain (Eds.)
Radial Basis Function Networks 1, 2001
ISBN 3-7908-1367-2

Vol. 67. R.J. Howlett and L.C. Jain (Eds.)
Radial Basis Function Networks 2, 2001
ISBN 3-7908-1368-0

Vol. 68. A. Kandel, M. Last and H. Bunke (Eds.)
Data Mining and Computational Intelligence, 2001
ISBN 3-7908-1371-0

Vol. 69. A. Piegat
Fuzzy Modeling and Control, 2001
ISBN 3-7908-1385-0

Vol. 70. W. Pedrycz (Ed.)
Granular Computing, 2001
ISBN 3-7908-1387-7

Vol. 71. K. Leiviskä (Ed.)
Industrial Applications of Soft Computing, 2001
ISBN 3-7908-1388-5

Vol. 72. M. Mareš
Fuzzy Cooperative Games, 2001
ISBN 3-7908-1392-3

Vol. 73. Y. Yoshida (Ed.)
Dynamical Aspects in Fuzzy Decision, 2001
ISBN 3-7908-1397-4

Vol. 74. H.-N. Teodorescu, L.C. Jain and A. Kandel (Eds.)
Hardware Implementation of Intelligent Systems, 2001
ISBN 3-7908-1399-0

Vol. 75. V. Loia and S. Sessa (Eds.)
Soft Computing Agents, 2001
ISBN 3-7908-1404-0

Vol. 76. D. Ruan, J. Kacprzyk and M. Fedrizzi (Eds.)
Soft Computing for Risk Evaluation and Management, 2001
ISBN 3-7908-1406-7

Vol. 77. W. Liu
Propositional, Probabilistic and Evidential Reasoning, 2001
ISBN 3-7908-1414-8

Vol. 78. U. Seiffert and L.C. Jain (Eds.)
Self-Organizing Neural Networks, 2001
ISBN 3-7908-1417-2

Vol. 79. A. Osyczka
Evolutionary Algorithms for Single and Multicriteria Design Optimization, 2001
ISBN 3-7908-1418-0

Vol. 80. P. Wong, F. Aminzadeh and M. Nikravesh (Eds.)
Soft Computing for Reservoir Characterization and Modeling, 2002
ISBN 3-7908-1421-0

Vol. 81. V. Dimitrov and V. Korotkich (Eds.)
Fuzzy Logic, 2002
ISBN 3-7908-1425-3

Vol. 82. Ch. Carlsson and R. Fullér
Fuzzy Reasoning in Decision Making and Optimization, 2002
ISBN 3-7908-1428-8

Senén Barro · Roque Marín
Editors

Fuzzy Logic in Medicine

With 100 Figures
and 47 Tables

Springer-Verlag Berlin Heidelberg GmbH

Professor Senén Barro
University of Santiago de Compostela
Department of Electronics and Computer Science
15782 Santiago de Compostela
Spain
senen@dec.usc.es

Professor Roque Marín
University of Murcia
AI and Knowledge Engineering Group
School of Computer Science
Campus de Espinardo
30071 Murcia
Spain
roque@dif.um.es

ISSN 1434-9922
DOI 10.1007/978-3-7908-1804-8

Cataloging-in-Publication Data applied for
Die Deutsche Bibliothek – CIP-Einheitsaufnahme
Fuzzy logic in medicine: with 47 tables / Senén Barro; Roque Marín (ed.). – Heidelberg; New York: Physica-Verl., 2002
(Studies in fuzziness and soft computing; Vol. 83)

Originally published by Physica-Verlag Heidelberg 2002
MyCopy version of the original edition 2002

Hardcover Design: Erich Kirchner, Heidelberg

SPIN 10848743 88/2202-5 4 3 2 1 0 – Printed on acid-free paper
www.springer.com/mycopy

Foreword

To say that Fuzzy Logic in Medicine, or FLM for short, is an important addition to the literature of fuzzy logic and its applications, is an understatement. Edited by two prominent informaticians, Professors S. Barro and R. Marín, it is one of the first books in its field. Between its covers, FLM presents authoritative expositions of a wide spectrum of medical and biological applications of fuzzy logic, ranging from image classification and diagnostics to anaesthesia control and risk assessment of heart diseases.

As the editors note in the preface, recognition of the relevance of fuzzy set theory and fuzzy logic to biological and medical systems has a long history. In this context, particularly worthy of note is the pioneering work of Professor Klaus Peter Adlassnig of the University of Vienna School of Medicine. However, it is only within the past decade that we began to see an accelerating growth in the visibility and importance of publications falling under the rubric of fuzzy logic in medicine and biology - a leading example of which is the Journal of the Biomedical Fuzzy Systems Association in Japan. Why did it take so long for this to happen?

First, a bit of history. My first paper on fuzzy sets, published in 1965, was motivated in large measure by my arrival at the conclusion that mainstream mathematical techniques – aimed as they were, and still are – at the analysis of mechanistic systems, did not provide effective tools for the analysis of biological or, more generally, humanistic systems in which human judgement, perceptions and emotions play an important role. To me, an example of unsuitability of standard tools for mathematical analysis was the work of N. Rashevsky in the 1940s and 1950s. Filled with differential equations, his papers and books dealt with an unrealistic model of biological systems. In a way, his work was pioneering, impressive and worthy of applause. But in the final analysis, it foundered on the hard rocks of Aristotelian logic and crisp set theory.

What became clear to me at that time was that to be able to deal realistically with the intrinsic complexity and imprecision of biological systems it was, and is, necessary to generalize mathematical techniques by introducing the concept of a fuzzy set. This mode of generalization may be described as f-generalization, and it is this mode that underlies many of the applications described in FLM.

In essence, f-generalization may be viewed as a move from two-valued Aristotelian logic – a logic in which nothing is a matter of degree – to fuzzy logic in which everything is a matter of degree. Important though it is, f-

generalization is not sufficient. In a paper published in 1973, a further mode of generalization was introduced. This mode – referred to as $f \cdot g$-generalization – is centered on fuzzy granulation, that is, on partitioning of an object into a collection of fuzzy granules, with a granule being a clump of objects (points) drawn together by undistinguishability, similarity, proximity or functionality. Fuzzy granulation plays a pivotal role in human cognition, reflecting the bounded ability of the human mind to resolve detail and store information. In a sense, fuzzy granulation may be viewed as a human way of achieving data compression.

Fuzzy granulation underlies the basic concepts of a linguistic variable and fuzzy if-then rules. Today, most applications of fuzzy logic, including those described in FLM, employ these concepts in a variety of ways, centering on exploiting the tolerance for imprecision, uncertainty and partial truth to achieve tractability, robustness, low solution cost and better rapport with reality.

In retrospect, what is evident is that introduction of fuzzy granulation was a turning point in the evolution of fuzzy logic. From a historical point of view, what is surprising is that the natural concepts of a linguistic variable and fuzzy if-then rules were not introduced at a much earlier point in the evolution of science.

Insofar as biological systems are concerned, linguistic variables and fuzzy if-then rules serve a key function - they provide a computationally effective way of describing complex and/or ill-defined relationships which do not lend themselves to characterization in the form of differential equations. It is this essential tool that N. Rashevsky did not have.

Applications of linguistic variables and fuzzy if-then rules in the realm of control systems were quick to follow the publication of my 1973 paper. It took much longer for this to happen in the realm of biological and medical systems because such systems are orders of magnitude more complex and less amenable to analysis than mechanistic control systems. $f \cdot g$-generalization opens many more new doors than f-generalization, but some remain closed. What is needed to open these doors is a thrust in a new direction – a direction which is aimed at the development of what may be called the computational theory of perceptions (CTP) and precisiated natural language (PNL). The basis for this statement is the observation that humans have the remarkable capacity to perform a wide variety of physical and mental tasks without any measurements and any computations. In performing such tasks, e.g., driving in city traffic, humans employ perceptions, rather than measurements, of time, distance, speed, direction, intent, likelihood, truth and other attributes of physical and mental objects. Perceptions play a pivotal role in human cognition and, especially, in decision processes on both conscious and subconscious levels. It is this role that makes it so essential to develop a machinery for computation with perceptions, especially in the realms of biologically – and medically – centered systems.

Perceptions are intrinsically imprecise. More specifically, perceptions are f-granular in the sense that (a) the boundaries of perceived classes are unsharp; and (b) the values of perceived attributes are granulated. f-granularity of perceptions places them well beyond the computational capabilities of standard methods of systems analysis.

To develop a machinery for computation with perceptions it is necessary to move beyond $f \cdot g$-generalization by adding what may be called nl-generalization, with nl standing for natural language (NL). The point of departure in this mode of generalization is the assumption that perceptions are described in a natural language; and that the meaning of a proposition drawn from a natural language may be represented as a generalized constraint of the form X isr R, where X is the constrained variable; R is the constraining relation; and r is an indexing variable whose value defines the way in which R constrains X. The collection of combinations, modifications and qualifications of generalized constraints constitutes what is called the Generalized Constraint Language (GCL).

GCL serves as a precisiation language for NL in the sense that a proposition on NL translates into a constraint in GCL which can be dealt with in a computational framework. The subset of NL which consists of propositions which are precisiable through translation into GCL, constitutes what is called precisiated natural language (PNL).

The concept of PNL suggests a new direction in applications of fuzzy logic in medicine and biological systems. In particular, used as a definition language, PNL opens the door to a computationally-oriented way of defining important directions in which applications of fuzzy logic in medicine are likely to evolve. Although FLM does not discuss PNL, it does pave the way for a PLN-based enlargement of the role of natural languages in medicine and biological systems.

The wealth of up-to-date information about fuzzy logic in medicine makes FLM a must reading for anyone who is interested in applications of fuzzy logic in medicine or biological systems. The volume editors, Professors Barro and Marí; the series editor, Professor Kacprzyk; the authors and the publisher, the Springer-Verlag group, have done an outstanding job of producing a work that is certain to have a long-lasting impact in its field. They deserve our thanks and congratulations.

December, 2000 Lotfi A. Zadeh
Berkeley, California

Perceptions are intrinsically imprecise. More specifically, perceptions are f-granular in the sense that (a) the boundaries of perceived classes are unsharp and (b) the values of perceived attributes are granulated. F-granularity of perceptions places them well beyond the computational capabilities of standard methods of systems analysis.

To develop a machinery for computation with perceptions it is necessary to move beyond f.g-generalization by adding what may be called nl-generalization, with nl a mode for natural language (NL). The point of departure in this mode of generalization is the assumption that perceptions are described in a natural language, and that the meaning of a proposition drawn from a natural language may be represented as a generalized constraint of the form X isr R, where X is the constrained variable, R is the constraining relation, and r is an indexed variable whose value defines the way in which [illegible]

Contents

A Call for a Stronger Role for Fuzzy Logic in Medicine

Senén Barro[1] and Roque Marín[2]

[1] Departamento de Electrónica y Computación,
Universidade de Santiago de Compostela
E-15706 Santiago de Compostela, Spain
[2] Departamento de Informática, Inteligencia Artificial y Electrónica
Universidad de Murcia
E-30100 Murcia, Spain

1 Intelligent Systems in Medicine

The presence of intelligent system applications in the medical environment has been undergoing continual growth [45,47] practically since their earliest days. Such is the case of expert systems, which from their appearance, at the end of the 1960s and the start of the 1970s, has had notable influence in the field of medicine. Some of the best known ones are MYCIN [49], dealing with infectious disease, CASNET [31], in the field of ophthalmology, and INTERNIST [39] focused on the vast field of internal medicine.

Intelligent systems aim to achieve a degree of competence close to, or even higher than the human one in those tasks that require special knowledge or ability. To achieve this in medical systems which respond to the adjective intelligent is particularly difficult, amongst other reasons due to the following:

- The complexity of the human body and of the physio-pathological processes that take place in it, presently without comparison amongst artificial systems and processes (the most sophisticated mobile robot or a latest generation nuclear power station are far from the complexity of a living being).
- The enormous quantity of knowledge available on the human being and, which is worse, the still greater lack of knowledge. Although great advances have been made in medical knowledge, which have enabled us, for example, to complement curative actions with preventative ones, and, more recently, with those of a predictive nature, we are still far achieving, even supposing that it is possible, a common direction in medical knowledge, which today is fragmented into a myriad of specialities, diagnostic procedures, therapeutic protocols, etc. To this we have to add the great degree of variability that is shown by different patients, even with the same diagnoses and similar therapeutic actions, and even within the same patient over time.

- In part the nature of the knowledge to be modelled is characteristic of what is usually referred to as "common sense" knowledge, the representation and use of which in reasoning processses has proved much more complicated than expected [47]. Thus it has been necessary to progressively include techniques for managing imprecision and uncertainty, data validation techniques, techniques for dealing with time-dependent information, techniques for representing linguistic variables taken from natural language descriptions of medical knowledge, etc. [35,38,50,52].

- The vast amount of data which it is necessary to handle. In the last few years we have witnessed a spectacular growth in the quantity of data which is acquired, stored and processed in almost all areas of medicine: results of explorations, x-rays, clinical analysis, monitoring of physiological variables, etc. So much so, that the continuing advance in the ability to acquire new signals and parameters that are derived from these has lead to an overload of data and information for medical staff, which, on occasion, may hinder more then help in the decision making process. For example, a number of studies highlight the problems arising from the cognitive overload of medical staff in charge of caring for critical patients.

Faced with these problems, there are certain imbalances that need to be corrected in order to be able to further advance in the design of intelligent systems in medicine. Let us examine some of these, along with the role that Fuzzy Logic (FL) could play in each case [1].

1.1 Knowledge Technologies

In his recent book "What Will Be", Michael Dertouzos [18], director of the laboratory of Computer Science of the MIT, mapped out a future which, according to him, awaits us a few decades from now. In this hypothetical future he places a tourist who suddenly falls ill in Alaska. The patient is introduced into a futuristic medical cabinet in which his multiple physiological variables are measured. In addition, the patient's medical identification card is introduced into the cabinet, and this calls the general practitioner, who lives at the opposite end of the country, who, in turn, asks the technician working the cabinet to take an x-ray of the patient's lung. Under the instruction of the technician, a robotic x-ray system is set into motion in the cabinet, which takes an x-ray of the patient and sends it directly to the radiology expert for interpretation. The analysis is completed with a spyrometer and oxymeter test and, finally, the patient's general practitioner makes the following evaluation: the breathing rate is high, the oxygen level is low and decreasing, and the volume of the expiratory power after a second is abnormally low; the

[1] We employ the term "fuzzy logic" in its widest, but also most usual sense, which basically denotes the fuzzy set theory and all that on which this is based.

patient is suffering from a severe asthma attack, which could turn out to be fatal in less than six hours if he does not receive immediate attention.

If we analyse this hypothetical scenario, we see that it is fundamentally based upon electronic, robotic, computer and telecommunications technologies, and on the breakthroughs that these technologies lend to the design of new sensors that are capable of registering a multitude of variables of a physiological origin in a precise and bloodless manner; on the miniaturisation of systems, which make it possible to produce cards capable of storing a person's complete medical history; on the development of new forms of telecommunications, that permit the virtually instantaneous transmission of enormous quantities of information. The annual growth in storage and computation capacity (between 60 and 70%) and the even faster increase in data transmission speed (approximately 150%) enable us to be optimistic with the realisation, in the not too distant future, of the aforementioned scenario in many of the terms presented.

On the contrary, in the account given above, Dertouzos appears to rule out the possibility of significant breakthroughs regarding the capability for adequately interpreting the state of the patient on the basis of information that is obtained on him in the medical cabinet, for carrying out a reliable diagnosis of the situation and advising on the actions that should be taken. Establishing that the "*the expiratory power after a second is abnormally low*", diagnosing "*a severe asthma attack*" and recommending "*immediate attention*" is something which, in accordance with the account given above, would seem to be solely within the reach of humans, thus conceding little possibility of an important breakthrough in the so-called intelligent systems in the medical domain.

In short, Dertouzos places more emphasis on the predictable evolution of information and communication technologies than on those that could be denominated Knowledge Technologies (KT), capable of handling the data and the medical knowledge available in order to reach a diagnosis. There is no doubt that the task in this last sense is shown as being especially complicated: a piece of information which is so apparently simple, such as "the oxygen level is low" condenses the wide relative knowledge of the meaning which the precise numerical value of the oxygen level has in the framework or context made up by all those factors which condition its evaluation. Nevertheless, in the light of some of the achievements that have already been made, it seems probable that future breakthroughs will also be significant in this sense. With these breakthroughs Fuzzy Logic will undoubtedly have a relevant role to play, as it is one of the knowledge technologies with the greatest potential, and due to the fact that intelligent medical systems frequently resort to approaches based on anthropo-mimetic models with regards to the acting characteristics of human experts, for which it has been demonstrated that Fuzzy Logic is highly adaptable.

1.2 Common Sense = Common Knowledge + Common Reasoning

There are two principal axes in the configuration of Common Sense (CS): Common Knowledge (CK) and Common Reasoning (CR). The equation for common sense, CS=CK+CR, take the contribution of CK, as the practical knowledge used by individuals in many frequent real-life situations (huge knowledge bases, dependent on the most common experiences, on cultural and social aspects, and even on dogmas of faith, for example) and that of CR, as the practical reasoning applied by individuals in those real-life situations (supported by multiple abilities, strategies and criteria of reasoning, based on logical reasoning, pattern matching, rules of thumb, etc.). Particularly, reasoning in medicine is plagued by aspects belonging to common reasoning, which do not, by any stretch of the imagination, fit into a single model of reasoning. Nevertheless, this is not assumed in the majority of intelligent systems developed for any medical environment. Fuzzy Logic in its wider meaning, as we will go on to refer to, is a very good way of connecting symbols and concepts, to deal with "semantics" for representing and comparing concepts, constraining them, extending them, compressing them, generalising them, particularising them, and so on, as humans do. Fuzzy Set Theory provides us with extremely efficient tools with which to deal with all of them, such as the concept of a generalised constraint, point of departure on the theory of fuzzy information granulation; in the same way that there exist multiple types of restrictions (possibilistic, veristic, probabilistic, etc. [62]), capable of being adjusted to the representation of concepts and to the semantic plurality of the real world and of natural language, there also exist transformation mechanisms for these restrictions, which may be considered in the manner of a repertoire of reasoning processes, which are useful for dealing with common sense.

1.3 Modelling the Softness of the Real World

In general, the presence or not of a pathological situation in a patient cannot be considered as being a simple binary problem; neither does its manifestation have a precise correspondence with perfectly defined values of a series of physiological variables or signals. Operating with artificially precise criteria could lead us to make important errors in the evaluation of a set of signs and symptoms when we are in frontier regions between values that are clearly abnormal and those that are not.

At the same time, modelling the real world in a non-soft manner also means losing valuable information about the location of their elements in the discernment classes, which establishes the knowledge of this world. In a crisp set there are no mechanisms for differentiating the elements which are found close to the frontier as opposed to those which are not, and this is information which is very important in many decision-making processes.

The ever-present notion of "softness" in the world in which we live becomes especially patent in the domain of medicine. Amongst the different causes of this medical "softness", some of the most noteworthy are: the difficulty of obtaining complete information on the state of the patient, imprecision in measurement, errors and inconsistencies in data, problems in adequately classifying borderline cases, the lack of a complete understanding of the underlying mechanisms of illnesses, variability of data from patient to patient, natural diversity, difficulty in establishing precise limits for normal and abnormal values for measurements, wide variations in the manner in which each expert physician practices medicine, inaccuracy and subjectivity that are inherent in the verbal expression of knowledge or data, etc. Szolovits [1995] defined medical practice as an attempt at reducing uncertainty in the clinical state of the patient by means of a process of collecting empirical data on the course of the illness, which is subjected to consideration in terms of precision, accuracy, acceptability, cost and security of the tests and considerations on the effects of the medical operations carried out on the patient.

In summary, we can say that medicine is essentially a domain that is continuous, non-linear, incomplete, uncertain and imprecise, and to which fuzzy logic is exceptionally well suited.

2 Fuzzy Medical Systems

It was pointed out, from its very beginning, that FL had been afforded a principal role in the framework of medicine. By 1969, in the first paper on the possibility of developing applications of fuzzy sets in biomedicine [60], Professor Zadeh had stated that "the complexity of biological systems may force us to alter in radical ways our traditional approaches to the analysis of such systems. Thus we may have to accept as unavoidable a substantial degree of fuzziness in the description of the behaviour of biological systems as well as in their characterisation. This fuzziness, distasteful though it may be, is the price we have to pay for the ineffectiveness of precise mathematical techniques in dealing with systems comprising a very large number of interacting elements or involving a large number of variables in their decision trees". Some time later, Zadeh once again insisted on this: "By relying on the use of linguistic variables and fuzzy algorithms its main applications lie in economics, management science, artificial intelligence, psychology, linguistics, information retrieval, medicine, biology, and other fields in which the dominant role is played by the animate rather than the inanimate behaviour of system constituents" [61].

Practically from its origins, Fuzzy Logic has been playing an ever more prominent role in the medical domain, a role which without doubt has been more marked over the last decade (Figure 1). Nevertheless, the prophesised golden role of FL has still not come to full fruition in this field. Probably there are numerous different reasons for this, at the same time that many of these are applicable to many other approaches, which are also well aimed to the design of intelligent systems in this field. In any case, we believe that some key points can be given for which the need to advance is crucial in order to achieve a greater degree of protagonism for FL in medicine: a) new theoretical contributions are needed, and above all, new methodologies, which are adequate for the specificities of the domain; b) there is a need for design and computational implementation tools. One of causes of the "boom" of fuzzy control has been the availability and increasing sophistication of fuzzy control applications design software; c) we need to approach the design of intelligent systems in medicine from heterogeneous perspectives [11]. A controller may be directed solely by means of FL, but it is almost impossible, and not very interesting to do so, with a patient supervision system, or an image-based diagnostic system, to mention only two examples. In this sense, there are more and more hybrid solutions. By way of example are the papers included in this volume by Chang et al., in which FL and neural networks are co-ordinated, or [48], in which FL is integrated with Case-Based Reasoning and Genetic Algorithms.

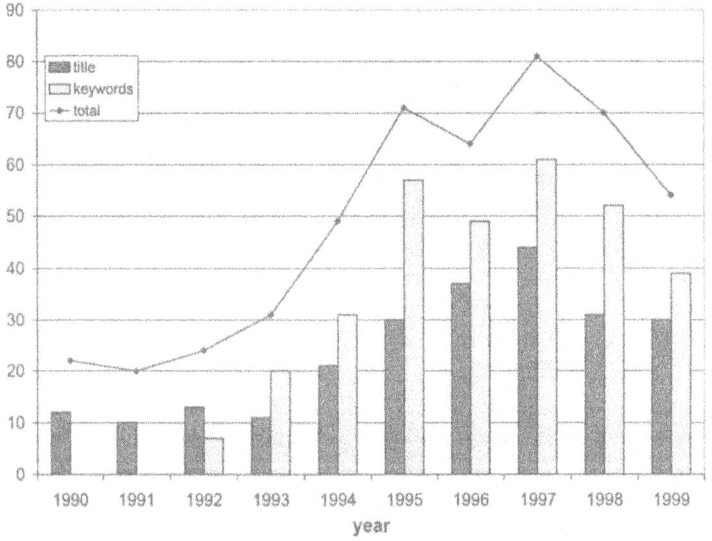

Fig. 1. Evolution in the number of papers on applications of fuzzy logic in medicine quoted in MEDLINE® database. The dark bars show those papers in which "fuzzy" appears in the title; the bright bars indicate those papers in which "fuzzy" figures amongst the key words; finally, the evolution of the total number of papers related with fuzzy logic is shown in solid line (NB. Although this figure is based on that of [53], the results given herein differ considerably from the ones appearing in that study)

In any case, we would be falsifying reality if we reflected a negative vision of the contribution that FL is affording to the design of intelligent systems in medicine, and this volume is a palpable demonstration. Up until now, this contribution has been very important in the number and quality of its applications [2,5,6,26,51], concentrating fundamentally on the one named by [32] the fourth phase of medical AI systems (from about 1987 to the present), where there is an active interest in qualitative reasoning representation, the importance of the temporal framework of the decision process, and the effort to move toward more practical systems that embody decision support for diagnostic or treatment protocols rather than the fully automated decision system; special emphasis is placed on the decision support that such systems can provide in answering queries by the user about diagnostic or treatment protocol choices; but above all, on those problems, such as treatment dosage review, instrumentation monitoring and control, and multimodality imaging, where intelligent systems, whether knowledge- or data-derived, enable us to go beyond the limitations of medical staff. It is precisely on this type of problem that the papers included in this volume principally concentrate.

Since the work of Fujisake in 1971 [23], which is probably the first paper on fuzzy logic in medicine, applications of FL cannot be counted in their hundreds, rather in their thousands, which are to be found in the most diverse medical disciplines, such as cardiology, radiology, preventative medicine, etc., and taking on multiple generic tasks of great interest in all medical domains: diagnosis, monitoring, control, classification, etc. The logical result of this is that we are unable to undertake a relatively exhaustive presentation, not only of these, but also of the classes into which they could be grouped. Simply, and in order to show a selection of the variety of applications that have been approached, we now go on to comment on some of the classes of applications that are related with the different forms of handling fuzzy information and knowledge, and in which the papers comprising this volume can be located. The order followed in their presentation, aims to emphasise the increasing need to model the expert's *modus operandi* as the complexity of the application approached increases, and its level of abstraction grows.

Clustering. Fuzzy clustering is a pattern recognition technique characterised by being a process of unsupervised learning or self-organisation. The objective is to partition a given data (set of objects), into a certain number of natural subgroups (C) in the set. A fuzzy clustering allows us to assign each object a partial or distribution membership to each of the clusters. This is especially interesting in many medical applications, in that the transitions between the subgroups is smooth.

In general, the clustering phase is followed the design process of a classifier which has to enable the classification of new patterns. Taking the classification phase in a wider sense, its objective is to map a space S^n, generated by a set of characteristics $X = \{X_1, ..., X_n\}$, in the set $C = \{C_1, ..., C_m\}$ of discernment classes, it being frequently difficult or inadequate to determine its full ascription to one single class [1,13,19,22]. In the same manner as in the clustering phase, the classification process does not generally operate in general on the basis of classification criteria belonging specifically to the application domain. Paper of Geva and Kerem [24] in this volume is an excellent contribution to this field.

Pattern recognition and signal processing, either unidimensional or multidimensional. There are a number of FL applications which are based on the definition of signal transformation functions, which aim to facilitate the detection of events of interest [15], or the high level description of characteristic patterns on these signals [28]. These types of applications are especially frequent in the case of physiological signals (pressure, in heart cavities and large vessels; electrical activity, as ECG, EMG and EEG; temperature; oxygen levels, ...), and medical images, due, principally, to their notable presence as an element of support in the diagnosis of many of pathologies, the follow up of patients under certain therapeutic actions, the criteria for clinical actuation, the detection of significant events and episodes, etc. In this case FL generally appears in high level stages within the general layout of the processing- interpretation of signals [43], where the integration of knowledge belonging to the application domain is more necessary. Examples in this volume of FL applications on pattern recognition and signal processing are papers of Félix et al. [20], Kobashi et al. [30], and Cheng et al [14].

Monitoring and control. In the same way as in other domains, fuzzy monitoring and fuzzy control have found an important niche in medical applications, being aimed at the monitoring and control of different types of situations: physiological signal monitoring, automatic administration of drugs, breathing apparatus, etc. [37,41,58,59]. First fuzzy mean arterial pressure controller, for example, has been in existence for more than 10 years [57]. Nevertheless, on the contrary to that which is happening in other domains, in which fuzzy control is starting to be a frequent approach to the design of controllers, in medicine there are still no "simple applications" of fuzzy control; the complexity of the domain no doubt makes things very difficult. In any case, the possibility of control by means of knowledge which models the operator (expert) and not the system (patient), is once again being seen to be advantageous in many medical applications. The papers of Jungk et al. [29], Linkens et al. [34], and Zhang et al. [63], included in this volume, belong to this class of applications.

Knowledge-based classification. We use this term to those classifiers in which the classification criteria are laid out explicitly, generally in the form of rules, and it is in this explicit character of the knowledge of the domain that FL can play an especially relevant role, given that the classification knowledge is established by means of an expert knowledge acquisition process, which due to its nature, contains important amounts of subjectivity and imprecision. In this category we include all those applications which involve mapping by way of fuzzy knowledge [8,33]. A classifier may be aimed at very diverse problems: diagnosis malfunction [59], diagnostic classification [16,36], classification of microqualifications in mammography [44], target volume definition for radiotherapy [56], etc. In general a design approach based on fuzzy knowledge is used, which applied on an input pattern obtains in the output the degree of assignation of this pattern to the different classes or categories being worked with. Although this type of classifier has been used in other domains, its presence is especially noteworthy in medical applications. In many cases, the difficulty in obtaining training or design sets with sufficient data and which are representative of the classes to be distinguished, advises against the design of classification systems by way of other types of techniques, at the same time as it makes it interesting to replicate, as far as possible, the classification criteria of human experts. The papers appearing in this volume by Baldwin et al. [7] and Delgado et al. [17] are included in this category, as they are both examples of applications in which knowledge is automatically extracted from databases and not elicited from human experts.

Relation modelling. The manipulation of data and fuzzy relations of very diverse types are inseparable from a number of medical problems, principally diagnostic ones. In this sense the modelling of fuzzy relations has had an important impact in medicine, and there are a large number of studies which can be categorised in this class, [40,46,55]. In these approaches the expert's knowledge is represented as a fuzzy relation between symptoms and diseases; given the fuzzy set A of one patient's symptoms, and the fuzzy relation R between symptoms and diseases, the possible diseases of the patient can be obtained by means of a rule of composition ($B=A^{\circ}R$) (CADIAG-2, a fuzzy expert system for diagnosing rheumatological and pancreatic diseases [3,4], is one of the best known examples). In general, fuzzy relations come from two sources: in some cases they are determined from expert medical documentation (in a diagnosis problem, for example, the rules would show the belief of the expert that determined symptoms are associated with a certain diagnosis), although often the information source is a set of patient's records, a set sufficiently large and representative, that is contains reliable information on the diagnosis and symptoms noticed in the patient. In any case, one disadvantage of this approach based on the use of numerical tabular knowledge, is its inadequacy for affording the explanation of the reasoning and dialogue with the system user.

Within this category, we can also include those applications in which the relations between symptoms and illnesses are not simple matrices, as occurs when the relations are established as constraints that need to be satisfied. This generally involves extending the techniques and methodologies that are characteristic of constraint satisfaction problems to the case in which these constraints are of a fuzzy nature. The paper by Palma et al. [42], included in this volume, is a good example of this.

Expert systems. Although the name fuzzy expert system is usually extended to all knowledge-based fuzzy systems, particularly those in which knowledge is represented in the form of rules [26], we reserve the use of the name expert systems for those systems with a complex knowledge base, where, for example, multiple knowledge representation paradigms and types of reasoning coexist, conflict resolution mechanisms are applied, in order to decide which new piece of knowledge to apply next, etc. In this type of system, nevertheless, there is still no significant presence of FL ([10] and PNEUMON-IA [54] are two of the exceptions). One of the reasons for this relative lack of proposals is the difficulty in maintaining inferences which are sufficiently precise after various levels of the propagation of imprecise information, which is an important drawback in medicine, where it frequent to come across relatively large chains of reasoning (for example in order to obtain responses to diagnostic tasks). Although working with linguistic variables in a symbolic manner can do away with this problem, as occurred with MILORD [25], by doing so, in a certain sense, the very flexibility which characterises FL is lost; hence we think it more opportune to explore other alternatives The paper by Schuster et al. [48], appearing in this volume, can be incorporated into this class.

3 Home Intelligent Medical Systems

The works that are included in this volume and many other applications that have been, and are still being developed, underline the applicability of FL in medicine. Without any doubt, we will witness improvements in already existing applications, as well as the appearance of new application fields in medicine, which have either not yet been explored, or only tenuously so. Amongst these we would venture to point out one that will give rise, probably in the not-too-distant future, to a new range of products in which FL will have an important impact: "Home Intelligent Medical Systems" (HIMSs)[2].

In fact, the market for medical devices used in the home and alternative sites has increased dramatically in the last years [12].

The idea of a HIMS is that of a personal medical assistant. With a more ambitious and general approach, some futuristic visions point to a version of a global medical expert system that "based on what you tell it, the system can triage the cases you can take care of yourself from the ones that require a doctor's care, and the ones that require instant attention" [21]. Nevertheless, we believe that this vision is not a particularly realistic one in a reasonable time scale, due to which we have opted for systems with much more specific tasks. This we illustrate with a very simple example. At present there are already some medical devices for personal use, the sphygmomanometer being perhaps the most well known. Nevertheless its Machine Intelligence Quotient (MIQ) is almost nil. For the layman in medical aspects related with arterial

[2] Although the acronym is similar to OMRON´s health-management system (HMS), the latter is a computer system for aiding large corporations by providing a personal health analysis and proper management plan [27]

pressure, its readings are of little or no value. This value, and hence its MIQ, will only increase notably by "translating part of the medical knowledge of the evaluation of arterial pressure which exists today and which is shared by many individuals related with the field of medicine.

The value of adequate control and evaluation of arterial pressure in unquestionable: hypertension is the leading risk factor of many diseases, such as renal disease or coronary artery disease, amongst others. Nevertheless, what would the interest and tasks of an HIMS- sphygmomanometer be? We will attempt to explain this with an example: If we measure our arterial pressure and we obtain values of 80 mmHg of diastolic pressure and 160 mmHg for systolic pressure, and we use the standard classification table for blood pressure, it can be seen that these readings are normal, due to which we will happily put the sphygmomanometer away until the next time. If however the sphygmomanometer were a HIMS one, which bore in mind our age, weight, height, history of arterial hypertension in our family and many other data of interest, as well as records of previous readings, it could say something along the lines of: "systolic pressure has risen slightly over the last months, and it is a little high. Although the situation is not of grave concern, further tests should be carried out in the near future. If you wish I can programme dates for these tests and give you some advice on how to do them in order that the results be more reliable".

In order to effect this evaluation, it is necessary to be aware of the multiple factors which may specifically influence arterial pressure: anxiety, food intake, tobacco consumption, pain, etc., as well as many others that do so in a more persistent manner: pregnancy, age, obesity, etc. Furthermore, there is a series of established criteria for the treatment of hypertension, which depend on the age of the individual in question, if he or she belongs to a high-risk group or not (those with a family history of hypertension or obesity, who use oral contraceptives, excessive consumption of alcohol, etc.) and many other factors amongst which can of course be found the arterial pressure records themselves (Figure 2). These criteria range from intense monitoring over a period of time to the immediate application of a therapy.

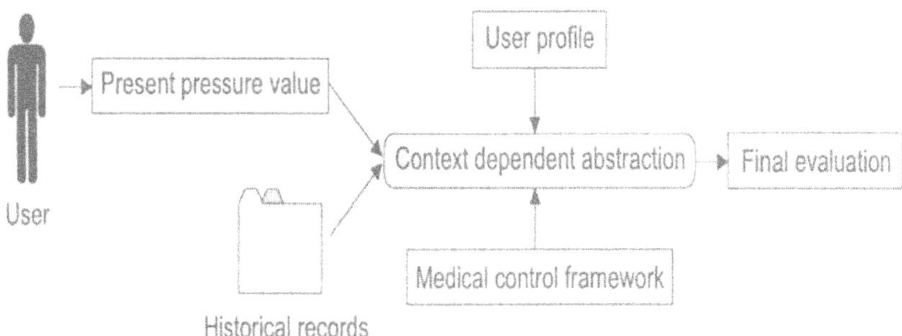

Fig. 2. Basic operational scheme of a HIMS-sphygmomanometer (after [9])

It will be possible to connect the HIMS to a remote medical system, to which it will transfer data, either totally or partially (the user will have control over the level of privacy) and from which it will receive relative modifications to the "medical control framework", through which a physician sets certain user-specific operational steps of the HIMS.

Obviously, one should not think that HIMSs will take the place of the more expert and active role of the physician, but it will be able to play an important complementary role and bring about a more active role for the individual in his or her health care. This is especially important in patients with chronic conditions, for example, as it would help them to assume greater responsibility, it would help to allay their perception of themselves as passive elements in the therapeutic process to which they are submitted, and it would enable the physician to have valuable complementary information. If HIMS come into being, we believe that FL will have an important contribution to them. The reasons are along the same lines as those which were put forward for the more general framework of intelligent medical systems, reinforced by other more specific characteristics, such as the need for HIMSs to be low developmental cost and acquisition devices, they do not have to aim for the optimisation of the diagnosis, being very cautious in their recommendations, will have to be sufficiently flexible in order to be adapted to the different user profiles and medical control frameworks, and the interaction with the user will have to tend towards graphical and natural languages. Furthermore, they will be basically autonomous systems, due to which, although in a narrow field of responsibility, they will have to reach the level of efficiency and eloquence of the physician. However, above all, the HIMSs need to suitably integrate sensor-based levels of processing with those related with the usage and the user, and it is here where FL may have its most crucial role.

We believe that, in the same way that today a large number of electrical appliances are essential in the carrying out of a many domestic tasks, HIMSs will be so in home health care. Once again, FL will serve to reinforce the intelligence of these systems, and we hope that companies in the field of medical instruments and systems see this in the same way as has already happened in the case of fuzzy controllers and electrical appliances.

4 Some Final Remarks

Although FL cannot be considered a panacea for any application domain, there is no doubt that it is fundamental as a theoretical, methodological and design tool in those applications in which crisp, fine-grained information is not available or precise information is costly, as is usual in medicine. As has been pointed out by [62], FL shows its best role when it aims to "exploit the tolerance for imprecision, uncertainty and partial truth to achieve tractability, robustness, low solution costs and better rapport with reality". Thus the application of FL should not just follow along the lines of just generalising the resolution of those medical problems which have already found, or are in the process of finding, a satisfactory solution with a crisp approach, or for those which the treatment of uncertainty and imprecision has been carried out successfully using other approaches.

Paradoxically, advances in the health sciences and information technology have become the more and more complex management of patients; increases in applied knowledge, the number of signals and parameters acquired, and the amount of data and information available, for example, requires the development of more intelligent systems for patient supervision and management, the intelligence of which does not only have to be understood as a measure of their greater complexity, but also as a by-product of the carrying out of higher-level tasks, which up until now were considered as being exclusive to medical and paramedical teams. Until now the significant advances in information and communications, which is also affecting the domain of medicine, has established a strong link between better developments in medical systems and new technological advances. Nevertheless, it is not very probable that this situation be maintained indefinitely, and increasingly we will see the introduction of more intelligence by means of knowledge technologies, or know-ware, the principal motor for solving more complex problems (development of standard ontologies, expert assistance on decision-making, libraries of reusable knowledge, cost-effective clinical protocols, etc.). Machine Intelligence Quotient (MIQ) of medical systems will need to be greatly increased before they can be used as routine systems, from hospitals to the home, and fuzzy logic lead us to systems which have a higher MIQ. It is here where FL is already playing an important role in medical systems, a role that will no doubt grow in importance.

References

1. Acton, P. D., Pilowsky, L. S., Kung, H. F., and Ell, P. J. (1999) Automatic segmentation of dynamic neuroreceptor single-photon emission tomography images using fuzzy clustering. European Journal of Nuclear Medicine, **26**, 581–590.
2. Adlassnig, K. P. (1982) A survey on medical diagnosis and fuzzy subsets. In: Approximate Reasoning in Decision Analysis, Gupta, M. M., and Sanchez, E. (Eds.), North-Holland, 203–217.
3. Adlassnig, K. P., and Kolarz, G. (1982) CADIAG-2: Computer-assisted medical diagnosis using fuzzy subsets. In: Approximate Reasoning in Decision Analysis, Gupta, M.M, and Sanchez, E. (Eds.). North-Holland, New York, 219–247, .
4. Adlassnig, K. P., Kolarz, G., and Scheithauer, W. (1985) Present state of the medical expert system CADIAG-2, Methods of Information in Drug, **24**, 13–20.
5. Akay, M. (1994) Editorial: Applications of Fuzzy Logic. IEEE Eng. in Med. and Biol. Magazine, **13**(5), 665–666.
6. Akay, M., Cohen, M., and Hudson, D. (1997) Fuzzy sets in life sciences. Fuzzy Sets and Systyems, **90**, 219–224.

7. Baldwin, J. F., Hill, C., Ponsan, C. (2001) Mass Assignments Methods for Medical Classification Diagnosis. In: Fuzzy logic in medicine, Barro, S., Marín, R. (Eds.), Studies in Fuzziness and Soft Computing, Physica Verlag.
8. Barro, S., Ruiz, R., and Mira, J. (1990) Fuzzy beats labelling for intelligent arrhythmia monitoring. Computers and Biomedical Research, **23**, 240–258.
9. Barro, S. (1999) Some ideas concerning fuzzy intelligent systems. Mathware and Soft Computing, **6**(2–3), 141–154.
10. Binaghi, E. (1990) A Fuzzy Logic Inference Model for a Rule-Based System in Medical Diagnosis. Expert System, **7**, 134–141.
11. Binaghi, E., Montesano, M. G., Rampini, A., and Cerrani, I. (1996) A hybrid fuzzy expert system shell for automated medical diagnosis. In: Fuzzy Logic and Neural Network Handbook, C.H. Chen (Ed.), McGraw-Hill, Cap. 25, 25.1–25.18.
12. Bowman, B. R., and Schuck, E. (1995) Medical Instruments and Devices Used in the Home. In: The Biomedical Engineering Handbook. J.D. Bronzino (Ed.), CRC Press, 1357–1366.
13. Cabello, D., Barro, S., Salceda, J. M., Ruíz, R., and Mira, J. (1991) Fuzzy K-nearest neighbor classifiers for ventricular arrhythmia detection. Int. J. Biomed. Comput., **27**, 77–93.
14. Cheng, H. D., Hu, Y. G., Wu, C. Y., Hung, D. L. (2001) Mammogram Classification Using Fuzzy Central Moments. In: Fuzzy logic in medicine, Barro, S., Marín, R. (Eds.), Studies in Fuzziness and Soft Computing, Physica Verlag.
15. Czogala, E., Leski, J., Rozentryt, P., and Zembala, M. (1997) Entropy measure of fuzziness in detection of QRS complex in noisy ECG signal. FUZZ-IEEE'97, Barcelona, 853–856.
16. Degani, R., and Bortolan, G. (1987) Fuzzy numbers in computerized electrocardiography. Fuzzy Sets and Systems, **24**, 345–362.
17. Delgado, M., Sánchez, D., Vila, M. A. (2001) Acquisition of Fuzzy Association Rules from Medical Data. In: Fuzzy logic in medicine, Barro, S., Marín, R. (Eds.), Studies in Fuzziness and Soft Computing, Physica Verlag.
18. Dertouzos, M. L. (1997) What Will Be: How the New World of Information Will Change Our Lives. HarperEdge Publishers, New York.
19. Esogbue, A. O., and Elder, R. C. (1983) Measurement and valuation of a fuzzy mathematical model for medical diagnosis. Fuzzy Sets and Systems, **10**, 223–242.
20. Félix, P., Barro, S., Lama, M., Fraga, S., Palacios, F. (2001) A fuzzy model for pattern recognition in the evolution of patients. In: Fuzzy logic in medicine, Barro, S., Marín, R. (Eds.), Studies in Fuzziness and Soft Computing, Physica Verlag.
21. Flower, J. (1994) The other revolution in health care. Wired, **2**, January.
22. Fordon, W. A., and Bezdeck, J. C. (1979) The application of fuzzy set theory to medical diagnosis. In: Advances in Fuzzy Set Theory and Applications, M. M. Gupta, R. K. Ragade, and R. R. Yager (Eds.). North-Holland, 445–461.
23. Fujisake, H. (1971) Proc. Symp. on Fuzziness in Systems and its Processing. Profesional Group of SICE.
24. Geva, A. B., Kerem, D. H. (2001) Fuzzy Clustering in Medicine. In: Fuzzy logic in medicine, Barro, S., Marín, R. (Eds.), Studies in Fuzziness and Soft Computing, Physica Verlag.

25. Godo, L., López de Mántaras, R., and Sierra, C. (1989) MILORD, the architecture and management of linguistically expressed uncertainty. Int. J. of Intelligent Systems, **4**(4), pp. 471–501.
26. Hudson, D. L., and Cohen, M. E. (1994) Fuzzy Logic in Medical Expert Systems. IEEE Eng. in Med. and Biol. Magazine, **13**(5), 693–698.
27. Isaka, S., (1995) Fuzzy Logic Applications at OMRON. In: Industrial Applications of Fuzzy Logic and Intelligent Systems, J. Yen, R. Langari, and L.A. Zadeh (Eds.). IEEE Press, 55–67.
28. Jaulent, M. C., and Degoulet, P. (1994) Diagnosing Renal Artery Lesions with a Fuzzy Logic Model. IEEE Eng. in Med. and Biol. Magazine, **13**(5), 699–704.
29. Jungk, A., Thull, B., Rau, G. (2001) Intelligent alarms for anaesthesia monitoring based on a fuzzy logic approach. In: Fuzzy logic in medicine, Barro, S., Marín, R. (Eds.), Studies in Fuzziness and Soft Computing, Physica Verlag.
30. Kobashi, S., Hata, Hall, L. O. (2001) Fuzzy Information Granulation of Medical Images -Blood Vessel Extraction from 3-D MRA Images-. In: Fuzzy logic in medicine, Barro, S., Marín, R. (Eds.), Studies in Fuzziness and Soft Computing, Physica Verlag.
31. Kulikowski, C., and Weiss, S. M. (1982) Representation of expert knowledge for consultation: the CASNET and EXPERT projects. In: Artificial Intelligence in Medicine, Szolovits, P. (Ed.), Boulder, CO: Westview Press.
32. Kulikowski, C. (1995) History and Development of Artificial Mehods for Medical Decision Making. In: The Biomedical Engineering Handbook. J.D. Bronzino (Ed.), CRC Press, 2681–2698.
33. Kuncheva, L. I. (1994) Fuzzy two-level classifier for high-G analysis. IEEE Eng. Med. & Biol. Mag., **13**(5), 717–722.
34. Linkens, D. A., Abbod, M. F., Backory, J. K. (2001) Awareness Monitoring and Decision-Making for General Anaesthesia. In: Fuzzy logic in medicine, Barro, S., Marín, R. (Eds.), Studies in Fuzziness and Soft Computing, Physica Verlag.
35. Lowe, A., Harrison, M., and Jones, R. (1999) Diagnostic monitoring in anaesthesia using fuzzy trend templates for matching temporal patterns. Artificial Intelligence in Medicine, **16**, 183–199.
36. Marín, R., and Mira, J. (1991) On knowledge-based fuzzy classifiers: A medical case study. Fuzzy Sets and Systems, **44**, 421–430.
37. Mason, D. C., Linkens, D. A., Abbod, M. F., Edwards, N. D., and Reilly, C. S. (1994) Automated Delivery of Muscle Relaxants Using Fuzzy-Logic Control. IEEE Eng. in Med. and Biol. Magazine, **13**(5), 678–686.
38. Miksch, S., Horn, W., Egghart, G., Popow, C., and Paky, F. (1996) Monitoring and Therapy Planning without Effective Data Validation are Ineffective. AAAI Spring Symposium: AI in Medicine: Applications of Current Technologies, AAAI Working Notes, Menlo Park, CA, 119–123.
39. Miller, R. A., Pople, H. E., and Meyers, J. D. (1982) Internist-I, an experimental computer-based diagnostic consultant for general internal medicine. N. Engl. J. Med., **307**.
40. Norris, D., Pilsworth, B. W., and Baldwin, J. F. (1987) Medical diagnosis from patient records. A method using fuzzy discrimination and connectivity analyses. Fuzzy Sets and Systems, **23**, 73–87.
41. Oshita, S., Nakakimura, K., and Sakabe, T. (1994) Hypertension Control During Anesthesia. IEEE Eng. in Med. and Biol. Magazine, **13**(5), 667–670.

42. Palma, J. T., Marín, R., Sánchez, J. L., Palacios, F. (2001) A Model-Based temporal abductive diagnosis meted for an intensive Coronary Care Unit. In: Fuzzy logic in medicine, Barro, S., Marín, R. (Eds.), Studies in Fuzziness and Soft Computing, Physica Verlag.
43. Presedo, J., Vila, J., Barro, S., Palacios, F., Ruíz, R., Taddei, A. and Emdin, M. (1996) Fuzzy modelling of the expert's knowledge in ECG-based ischaemia detection. Fuzzy Sets and Systems, **77**, 63–75.
44. Rifqi, M., Bothorel, S., Bouchon-Meunier, B., and Muller, S. (1997) Similarity and prototype based approach for classification of microcalcifications. Seventh IFSA World Congress, Prague, 123–128.
45. Rogers, E. (1998) AI and the changing face of health care. IEEE Intelligent Systems, Vol. January/February, 20–25.
46. Sanchez, E. (1979) Medical diagnosis and composite fuzzy relations. In: Advances in Fuzzy Set Theory and Applications, M. M. Gupta, R. K. Ragade, and R. R. Yager (Eds.). North-Holland, 437–444.
47. Scherrer, J. (1997) AI technologies: Conditions for further impact. In: Artificial Intelligence in Medicine, E. Keravnou, C. Garbay, R. Baud, and J. Wyatt (Eds.). Lecture Notes in Artificial Intelligence, 1211. Springer, 15–18.
48. Schuster, A., Adamson, K., Bell, D. A. (2001) Fuzzy Logic in a Decision Support System in the Domain of Coronary Heart Disease Risk Assessment. In: Fuzzy logic in medicine, Barro, S., Marín, R. (Eds.), Studies in Fuzziness and Soft Computing, Physica Verlag.
49. Shortliffe, E. H. (1976) Computer-based medical consultations: MYCIN. Elsevier, New York.
50. Steimann, F. (1996) The interpretation of time-varying data with DIAMON-1, Artificial Intelligence in Medicine, **8**(4), 343–357.
51. Steimann, F. (1997) Editorial: Fuzzy set theory in medicine, Artificial Intelligence in Medicine, **11**, 1–7.
52. Szolovits, P. (1995) Uncertainty and decisions in medical informatics. Methods of Information in Medicine, **34**, 111–121.
53. Teodorescu, H. N. L., Kandel, A., and Jain, L. C. (1999) Fuzzy Logic and Neuro-Fuzzy Systems in Medicine and Bio-Medical Engineering: A Historical Perspective. In: Teodorescu, H. N. L., Kandel, A., and Jain, L. C., Eds., Fuzzy and Neuro-Fuzzy Systems in Medicine. CRC-Press, 3–16.
54. Verdaguer, A. Patak, A., Sancho, J. J., Sierra, C., and Sanz, F. (1992) Validation of the Medical Expert System PNEUMON-IA". Computers and Biomedical Research. AMIA, **25**(6), 511–526.
55. Vila, M. A., and Delgado, M. (1983) On medical diagnosis using possibility measures. Fuzzy Sets and Systems, **10**, 211–222.
56. Waschek, T., Levegrün, S., van Kampen, M., Glesner, M., Engenhart-Cabillic, R., and Schlegel, W. (1997) Determination of target volumes for three-dimensional radiotherapy of cancer patients with a fuzzy system. Fuzzy Sets and Systems, **89**, 361–370.
57. Ying, H., Sheppard, L. C., and Tucker, D. M. (1988) Expert-system-based fuzzy control of arterial pressure by drug infusion. Medical Progress through Technology, **13**, 202–215.
58. Ying, H., and Sheppard, L. C. (1994) Regulating Mean Arterial Pressure in Postsurgical Cardiac Patients. IEEE Eng. in Med. and Biol. Magazine, **13**(5), 671–677.

59. Yoshizawa, M., Takeda, H., Yambe, T., and Nitta, S. (1994) Assessing Cardiovascular Dynamics During Ventricular Assistance. IEEE Eng. in Med. and Biol. Magazine, **13**(5), 687–692.
60. Zadeh, L. A. (1969) Biological application of the theory of fuzzy sets and systems. In: Proc. Int. Symp. Biocybernetics of the Central Nervous System, Little, Brown & Co., Boston, 199–212.
61. Zadeh, L. A. (1973) Outline of a new approach to the analysis of complex systems and decision process. IEEE Trans. Systems, Man, and Cybernetics, **3**, 28–44.
62. Zadeh, L. A. (1997) Toward a theory of fuzzy information granulation and its centrality in human reasoning and fuzzy logic. Fuzzy Sets and Systems, **90**(2), 111–127.
63. Zhang, X., Huang, J. W., Roy, R. J. (2001) Depth of Anesthesia Control with Fuzzy Logic. In: Fuzzy logic in medicine, Barro, S., Marín, R. (Eds.), Studies in Fuzziness and Soft Computing, Physica Verlag.

Fuzzy Information Granulation of Medical Images. Blood Vessel Extraction from 3-D MRA Images

S. Kobashi[1], Y. Hata[1] and L.O. Hall[2]

[1] Information Systems Laboratory. Department of Computer Engineering. Himeji Institute of Technology. 2167 Shosha Himeji Hyogo, 671-2201, Japan

[2] Department of Computer Science and Engineering. University of South Florida 4202 East Fowler Avenue, ENB 118, Tampa, Florida, 33620-5399, U.S.A.

E mails: {kobashi, hata}@comp.eng.himeji-tech.ac.jp, hall@csee.usf.edu

1. Introduction

Along with the population of high field magnetic resonance imaging (MRI), MR angiography (MRA) imaging with no contrast is rapidly gaining acceptance as a versatile noninvasive alternative to the conventional MRA with contrast and the CT angiography (CTA). To construct the volume visualizations of the cerebral blood vessels from volumetric MRA images of the brain, maximum intensity projection (MIP) technique has been widely used by many physicians [1]. The MIP image is created by selecting the maximum value along on an optical ray corresponding to each pixel of the image. The technique and the mutations have some advantages. For example, it gives densitometric information of raw images without any parameters needing to be tuned, and its implementation is relatively simple [1][2]. However, it also contains critical limitations. They are that it cannot depict the spatial relationship of overlapping vessels, and large bright structures may disturb region of interests (ROIs) along on optical rays from both directions. Some studies investigated the advantages and the disadvantages of three visualization techniques, i.e. MIP, volume rendering (VR), and surface shaded display (SSD) [3][4]. They concluded that SSD is useful to evaluating overlapping vessels, and it provides a better definition of the aneurysm neck and the morphology of saccular aneurysms. However, SSD is not used widely today because there is no application to automatically segment the blood vessel region. To construct the SSD images, a user must manually segment the blood vessel region for slice by slice, even though it involves time-consuming human interaction that is subject to inter- and intra- operator variation.

Many image segmentation methods based on thresholding, hard/soft clustering, region growing, and so on have been proposed. Although they have been used in many systems, they are not applicable to segmentation of the blood vessel region from the MRA image. The serious problem is that blood vessel voxels cannot be recognized by using only the intensity information because the unnecessary region often connects with the blood vessel region and has similar intensity on the images.

Fuzzy information granulation (fuzzy IG) introduced by Zadeh [5] has been attracting a great deal of attention in soft computing [6]. The concept treats fundamental problems between whole and its parts. Bortolan *et al.* discussed an implementation of fuzzy IG on the representation and reconstruction of numerical and nonnumeric data in fuzzy modeling [7]. In addition, the concept has been applied to medical image segmentation, e.g. threshold-finding for human brain MR image segmentation [8], segmentation of brain portions [9], and so on. They treat medical images as information, and the fuzzy granules are anatomical parts. Their implementations are based on fuzzy matching technique and fuzzy rule based system, respectively.

This chapter presents an implementation of fuzzy IG concept for medical image segmentation problems, and then applies it to segmentation of MRA images. This method consists of volume quantization and fuzzy merging. At first, volume quantization, which is to gather up similar neighboring voxels, generates three-dimensional (3-D) quanta from raw volumetric images. The quanta are elements of fuzzy granule. At the second step, the method forms the fuzzy granules by merging the neighboring quanta selectively. The merging process is iteratively carried out according to fuzzy degrees calculated by comparing each quantum with pre-defined fuzzy models. The fuzzy models written in fuzzy variables represent anatomical knowledge of 3-D time-of-flight (TOF) MRA images of the brain, and they are derived from physician's expertise. The proposed method is applied to blood vessel extraction from 3-D TOF MRA data. The features used to describe expert's knowledge are intensity and 3-D shape of the object. In the experimental results, the reconstructed two-dimensional (2-D), and 3-D images generated using target MIP and SSD are shown. The comparison with the conventional MIP images showed that unclarity regions in conventional images are clearly depicted in the produced images. The qualitative evaluation from a clinical viewpoint was done for the 2-D reconstructed images, and for the 3-D volume rendered images of the obtained blood vessels. The evaluations showed that the method could extract blood vessels from 3-D TOF MRA images, and that the results might be available for diagnosis of the cerebral diseases. These experiments denote that fuzzy IG is applicable to, and suitable for medical image segmentation problems.

2. Material

The image acquisition method used in this study was 3-D TOF angiography with no contrast. TR (repetition time) = 61 msec and TE (echo time) = 3 msec. FOV (field of view) was 120 mm. Matrix was 256 by 256. Thickness of the slice was 0.8 mm. The images are acquired from axial plane. Raw MRA images are shown in Figure 1. Each of the volume data is composed of about 100 separated volumetric slices. Voxel size was $0.47 \times 0.47 \times 0.80$ mm^3. The sliced images were reconstructed to 3-D voxels of the human brain consisted of $256 \times 256 \times$ (the number of slices). The intensity of all intracranial structure ranged between 0 and 4096.

The brain anatomy on MRA image is shown in Figure 2. In this image, the blood vessels are appeared as rather light gray. The tissues contained in such images are the air, bone, skin, muscle, cerebrospinal fluid (CSF), white matter (WM), gray matter (GM), blood vessel, and fat. Figure 3 shows the MIP images.

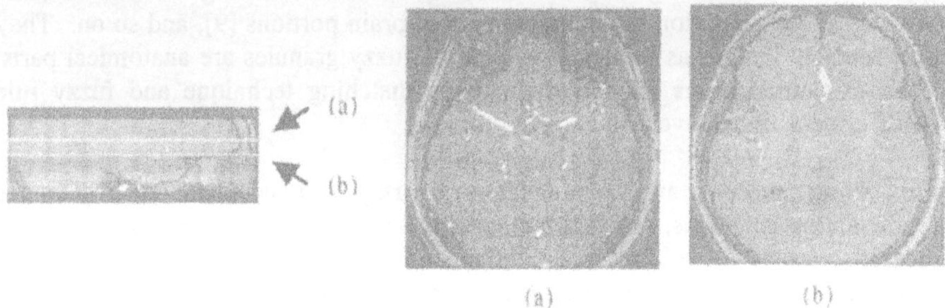

Figure 1. Raw MRA images of the brain. Left: sagittal plane. (a) and (b): axial plane images at the white line in sagittal image.

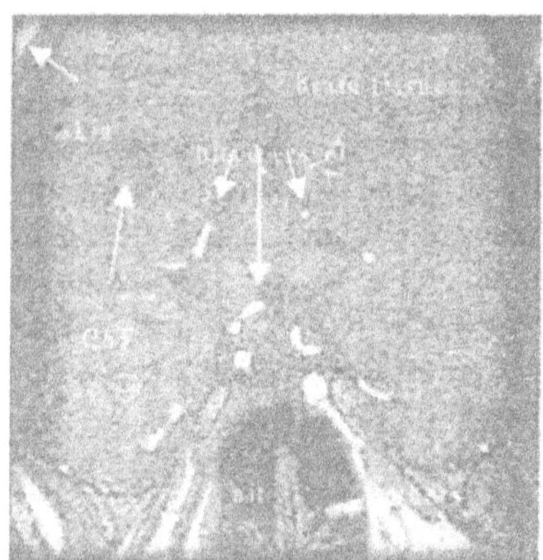

Figure 2. Brain anatomy on MRA image.

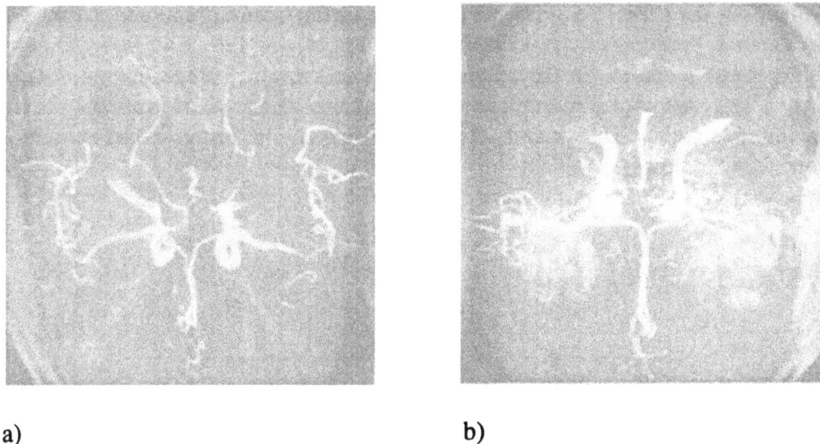

a) b)

Figure 3. MIP images: (a) View from the top of the head. (b) View from the front of the head.

3. Fuzzy Information Granulation on Medical Image Segmentation

Fuzzy information granularity is the concept introduced by Zadeh [5]. The concept considers that information consists of fuzzy granules, and a granule is a clump of elements. Moreover, each element called "quantum" in this chapter is composed of points. The concept then defines fuzzy IG is to derive fuzzy granules from information. For example, fuzzy granules of a human head are the nose, forehead, hair, cheeks, etc. In the case of human head information, fuzzy IG is to derive such parts from the information. The concept of fuzzy IG is more general than image segmentation, decomposition, clustering, and so on, because it can apply various information such as database, image, and sound.

This chapter shows a novel implementation of fuzzy IG concept, which is illustrated in Figure 4. By gathering up similar points, called quantization, a quantum is defined as a clump of points. The generated quantum is associated with a set of features derived from relationship of composed points. In the case of image processing, we can regard a raw image as information, and a clump of pixels (or voxels) as a quantum. By quantizing the image, we can estimate the features such as the shape and intensity distribution. Moreover, experts handling the information might have some knowledge of the information. We describe such knowledge according to features of quantum. Because the knowledge obtained from experts often includes imprecision and uncertainty, fuzzy variables is suitable for describing the knowledge. For example, the knowledge of the human eye is that the feature is the shape, and the fuzzy linguistic is round or square. Furthermore, by merging quanta with specific feature values, we can obtain different quanta with different feature values. It is decided to merge them by comparing the state of quanta with the state of the quantum merged them. We duplicate such processes by representing the state of quantum with fuzzy degrees for knowledge models. In the result of iterative merging, some quanta will be retained. They are granules that are principal components of information. In the following, this chapter shows an application of fuzzy IG to blood vessel extraction from MRA volume data.

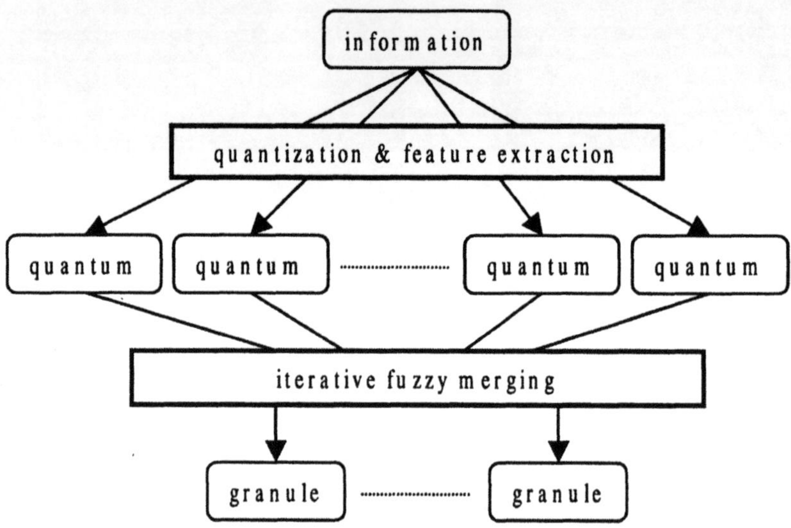

Figure 4. An implementation of fuzzy information granulation concept.

According to fuzzy IG concept, MRA volume data is regarded as fuzzy information, and anatomical parts such as the blood vessel and fat are regarded as fuzzy granules. This introduces that granulating MRA volume data would extract blood vessels from MRA volume data. According to the procedures discussed above, it consists of two parts:

1. Volume quantization and feature extraction
2. Iterative fuzzy merging.

The first part shown in Section 4, which is to segment whole MRA volume data into quanta, is performed with 3-D watershed segmentation [10]. Each quantum is represented with three spatial and densitometric features: "vascularity", "narrowness", and "histogram consistency". The second part shown in Section .5 gathers up similar quanta by indistinguishability, similarity, or functionality. This process is done with evaluating fuzzy degrees for pre-defined fuzzy models, which represents anatomical knowledge of the MRA images. Figure 5 illustrates an example of fuzzy IG of a 2-D image. By quantizing the image shown in Figure 5 (a), five quanta are obtained (Figure 5 (b)). In the result of iterative merging, two granules are retained as shown in Figure 5 (c). Then, each granule is classified into the belonging class by evaluating the degrees for knowledge models.

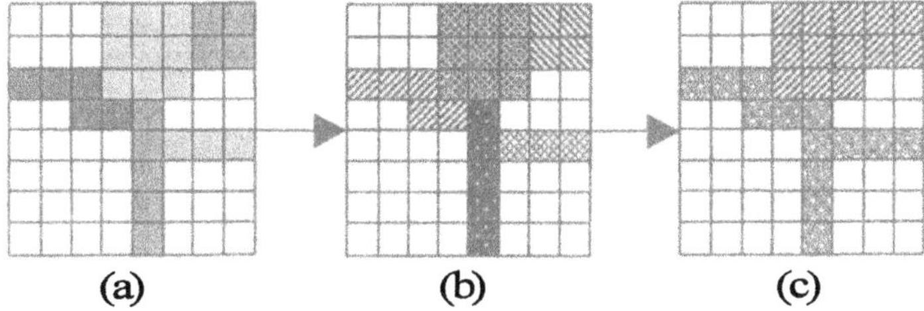

Figure 5. Example of fuzzy IG on image segmentation

4. Volume Quantization and Feature Extraction

By gathering similar neighboring voxels, called volume quantization, we can estimate the 3-D spatial features of an object. The volume quantization is performed with the watershed segmentation technique [10]. The technique consists of three steps:

1. Remove background,
2. Detection of ultimate eroded points (UEPs), and
3. Dilation from each UEPs according to the intensity and the Euclidean distance.

First, the background region is suppressed by using thresholding and noise reduction techniques. Thresholding is to set the voxel whose intensity is less than a threshold to zero. Noise reduction is to eliminate the primitives with small size (the number of voxels < 10 in our experiment) and no connection to other ones. The techniques have been discussed in many literatures (e.g. see [10]). Thus, 3-D watershed segmentation is applied to the 3-D volume data composed of gray level images where the intensity of the background voxel is set to zero.

Secondly, the method finds 3-D local maximum points on the 3-D volume data, and they are saved as a 3-D volume data. The UEPs, namely the local maximum points, would be found in both the blood vessel and fat regions. This shows that if there is an intensity valley between the blood vessel and the neighboring fat region, UEPs are set to each region. Therefore, the method can separate touching features that their intensities are partially same, e.g. relationship between the blood vessel and fat regions.

Thirdly, dilation is done from each UEP as if water drops from the top of mountain to the valleys. Consequently, the volume data is decomposed into quanta.

Three features, vascularity, narrowness, and histogram consistency estimate the characteristics regarding to both of the 3-D shape and the intensity distribution.

Vascularity

Because the blood vessel is a tube that carries blood, a vertical plane to the principal axis must be like a circle. This feature value, *vascularity*, estimates the degree of likeness to the 3-D shape of a vascular. Consider a primitive as shown in Figure 6. In this figure, $\vec{P}$ is the principal axis, and $\vec{S}_m$ is the 2-D object on a vertical plane to the axis. The 3-D principal axis and the vertical planes are calculated by using the methods (e.g., described in Ref. [11]). We define *vascularity*, A_v, as the mean value of the circularity (Ref. [10]) of $\vec{S}_m$, formed as

$$A_v = \int_m \frac{4\pi S_m}{L_m^{\ 2} M} dm ,$$

where L_m and S_m is the perimeter and area of the object $\vec{S}_m$, respectively, and M is the full length of the quantum for the direction of the principal axis.

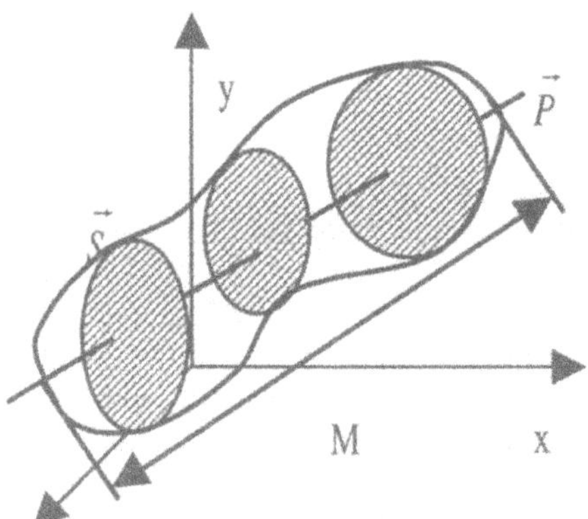

Figure 6. 3-D shape of a primitive

Narrowness

As the quantum is long and narrow, the 3-D shape resembles to the blood vessel. We estimate this feature by calculating *narrowness*, A_n, formed as

$$A_n = \frac{V}{S^{3/2}} ,$$

where the number of voxels of the quantum is V, and the mean value of the area of vertical plane is S.

Histogram Consistency

Anatomical parts appeared in medical images must have coherent intensity distributions. Especially, intensity distributions of the blood vessel and fat in MRA volume data are characteristic, i.e., a blood vessel quantum is composed of many high intensity voxels and little low intensity ones, and a fat quantum is composed of many low intensity voxels and little high intensity ones. These characteristics are more clarified by using the histogram of whole volume data. Figure 7 illustrates intensity histograms of the whole volume data, f_W, blood vessel quantum, f_{BV} and fat quantum, f_{FT}. The histograms are normalized so that the highest value is 1.0. The intensity among Th_{low}, which is to suppress background, and Th_{high} (=600 in this study) is ranged between 0 and 1. When the normalized histogram of a quantum of interest is f_C, the *histogram consistency*, A_h, is defined as

$$A_h = \frac{\int x \cdot g_p(x)dx}{\int g_p(x)dx}, \text{ where } g_p(x) = \frac{f_p(x)}{f_w(x)}.$$

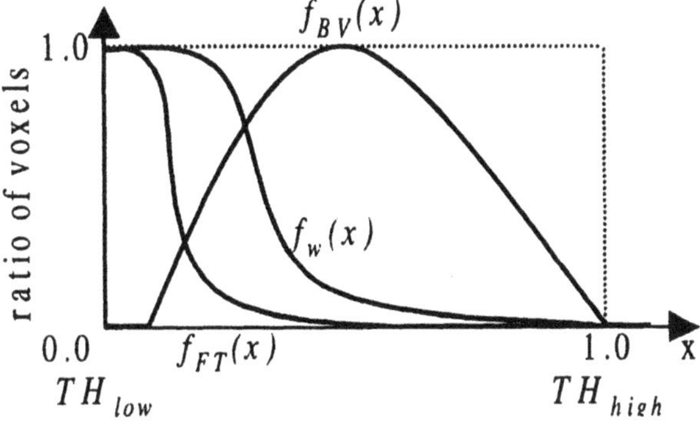

Figure 7. Illustration of intensity histograms

5. Iterative Fuzzy Merging

According to the three features, the anatomical knowledge of MRA image is given by a physician. Table 1 shows the obtained knowledge of the MRA image of the brain. In this table, *L*, *rL*, *rH*, and *H* are fuzzy variables to represent the degree of the feature values. The membership functions are shown in Figure 8. For example, knowledge representation of model C is that "a quantum that the vascularity is rather low, the 3-D feature is long and narrow, and the intensity distribution is rather high is the blood vessel".

Using this table, the degree for each model is calculated by

$$\mu = \min(\frac{\mu_v + \mu_n}{2}, \mu_h)$$

where μ_v (for *vascularity*), μ_n (for *narrowness*) and μ_h (for *histogram consistency*) are calculated by minimum between the feature values and the corresponding membership functions.

Table 1. Knowledge representation of MRA volume data (BV: blood vessel; FT: fat).

Model	Tag	Vascularity	narrowness	histogram consistency
A	BV	*H*	*H*	*H*
B	BV	*RH*	*RH*	*rH*
C	BV	*RL*	*H*	*rH*
D	FT	*RL*	*H*	*rL*
E	FT	*RL*	*RL*	*rL*
F	FT	*L*	*L*	*L*

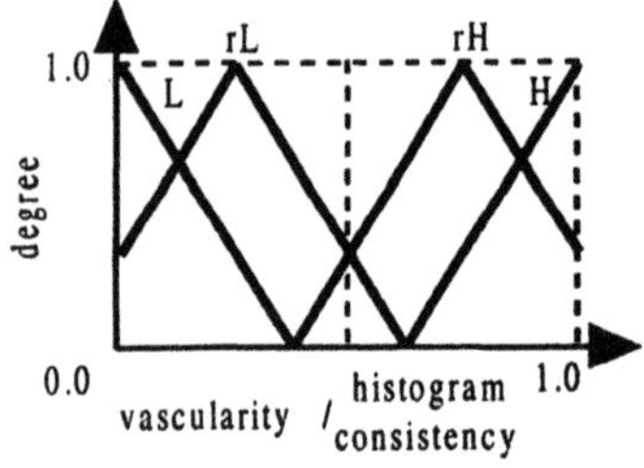

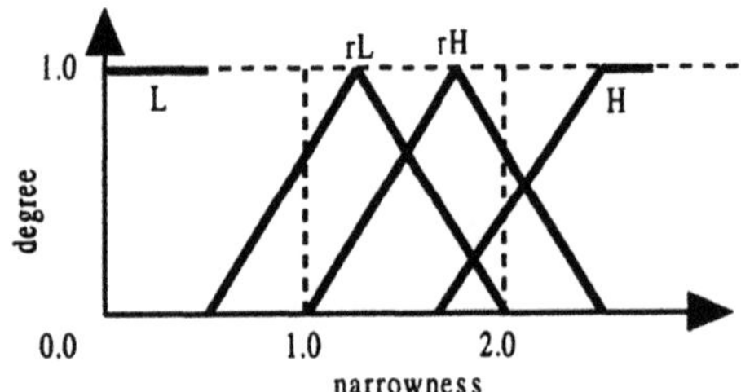

Figure 8. Membership functions

[Example 1] Calculation of fuzzy degrees for knowledge model

Assume two quanta whose feature values are shown in Table 2. For each model, the degrees for each feature and the total degrees are calculated as shown in Table 3. In this case, quantum X belongs to model C (the blood vessel) because the degree for model C is highest of all, and quantum Y belongs to model D (the fat).

Table 2. An example of feature values.

	A_v	A_n	A_h
quantum X	0.86	2.86	0.63
quantum Y	1.00	2.44	0.49

Table 3. An example of fuzzy calculation.

model	quantum X				quantum Y			
	Degree			total degree	degree			total degree
	A_v	A_n	A_h		A_v	A_n	A_h	
A	0.63	1.00	0.01	0.01	1.00	0.92	0.00	0.00
B	0.71	0.00	0.68	0.35	0.33	0.08	0.31	0.21
C	0.00	1.00	0.68	0.50	0.00	0.92	0.36	0.31
D	0.00	1.00	0.00	0.00	0.00	0.00	0.69	0.36
E	0.00	0.00	0.00	0.00	0.00	0.00	0.36	0.00
F	0.00	0.00	0.00	0.00	0.00	0.00	0.00	0.00

[End of Example]

This chapter proposes a new method to merge quanta based on expert's knowledge. Fuzzy logic is used to represent their knowledge. The conceptual diagram is shown in Figure 9. In this figure, quantum A (Q_A) and quantum B (Q_B) are quanta extracted from a scene taken a house. Assume that Q_A looks like "a mountain" whose degree is μ_A, and that Q_B looks like "a window envelop" whose degree is μ_B. Quantum C, Q_C, is obtained by merging Q_A and Q_B, and it looks like "a house" whose degree is μ_C. "Mountain", "window envelop", and "house" are pre-defined knowledge models given by an expert. Their knowledge models are defined by some features such as circularity, perimeter, area, and so on. Under these assumption, when μ_C is higher than both μ_A and μ_B, we would understand that Q_A and Q_B are pieces of Q_C. In this case, for example, when $\mu_A = 0.65$, $\mu_B = 0.75$ and $\mu_C = 0.85$, we can merge Q_A and Q_B to be a quantum that has higher degree.

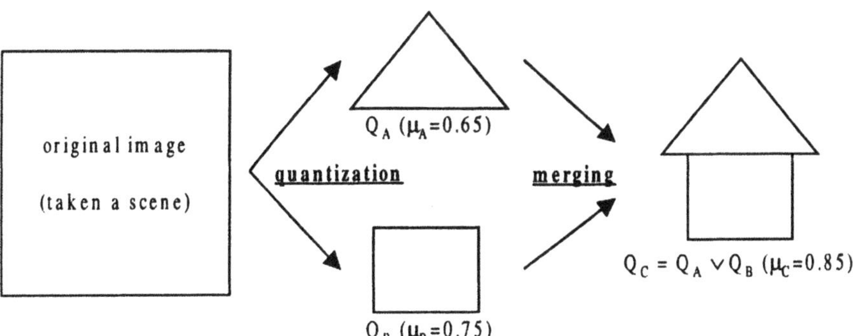

Figure 9. Fuzzy merging scheme

In more specific terms, consider a quantum X and N neighboring quanta Y_1, Y_2, ..., Y_N, which connect with quantum X. Let the quantum X's highest degree is μ_x, the quantum Y_i(i=1, 2, ... N)'s highest degree is $\mu_y(i)$, and merged quantum's highest degree is $\mu_{x,y}(i)$. For every combination of quantum X and quantum Y_i, if $\mu_{x,y}(i) > \mu_x$ and $\mu_{x,y}(i) > \mu_y(i)$, they will be merged. After these processes are done for all quanta, they are merged. The merging processes starts from the quanta whose degrees will be highest one when they are merged.

[Example 2] Fuzzy merging

Assume that two quanta described in **[Example 1]** are connected with each other, and a set of feature values of merged quantum is {0.83, 1.71, 0.60}. The degrees for each model are {0.00, 0.60, 0.00, 0.00, 0.07, 0.00}. In this case, because the highest degree of merged quantum, 0.60, is higher than both of the degree of quantum X for model C, 0.50, and the degree of quantum Y for model D, 0.36, the quanta will be merged.

[End of Example]

The above three processes; (1) estimation of feature values, (2) decision to merge, and (3) merging, are iterated until no quantum is modified. Consequently, some quanta are retained as granules. They are easily classified into the blood vessel or fat by evaluating the degrees for each model.

6. Experimental Results

The method was evaluated on a 3-D TOF MRA data. The volume data was composed of 256 × 256 × 78 voxels. The dimension of the given voxel was 0.47 × 0.47 × 0.8 mm^3. Figure 10 shows the 2-D reconstructed images of experimental results. The 3-D images generated using conventional MIP, target MIP and SSD are shown in Figure 11. The target MIP image is created by applying MIP technique to only segmented region. In this image, the images of each row are generated from same direction. The enlarged image of Figure 11 (a) and (b) are shown in Figure 12. They show that the unclarity regions appeared in conventional images are clearly depicted by applying the proposed method. Then, qualitative evaluations of the performance of the proposed method were done by physicians. They give us comments that are:

1. Narrow vessels, which were not described in the conventional MIP images, could be described.
2. The description of the bifurcation was enough for diagnosis of aneurysms.
3. This method enables to alternate the invasive imaging methods (e.g., angiography, and CT angiography) with MRA.

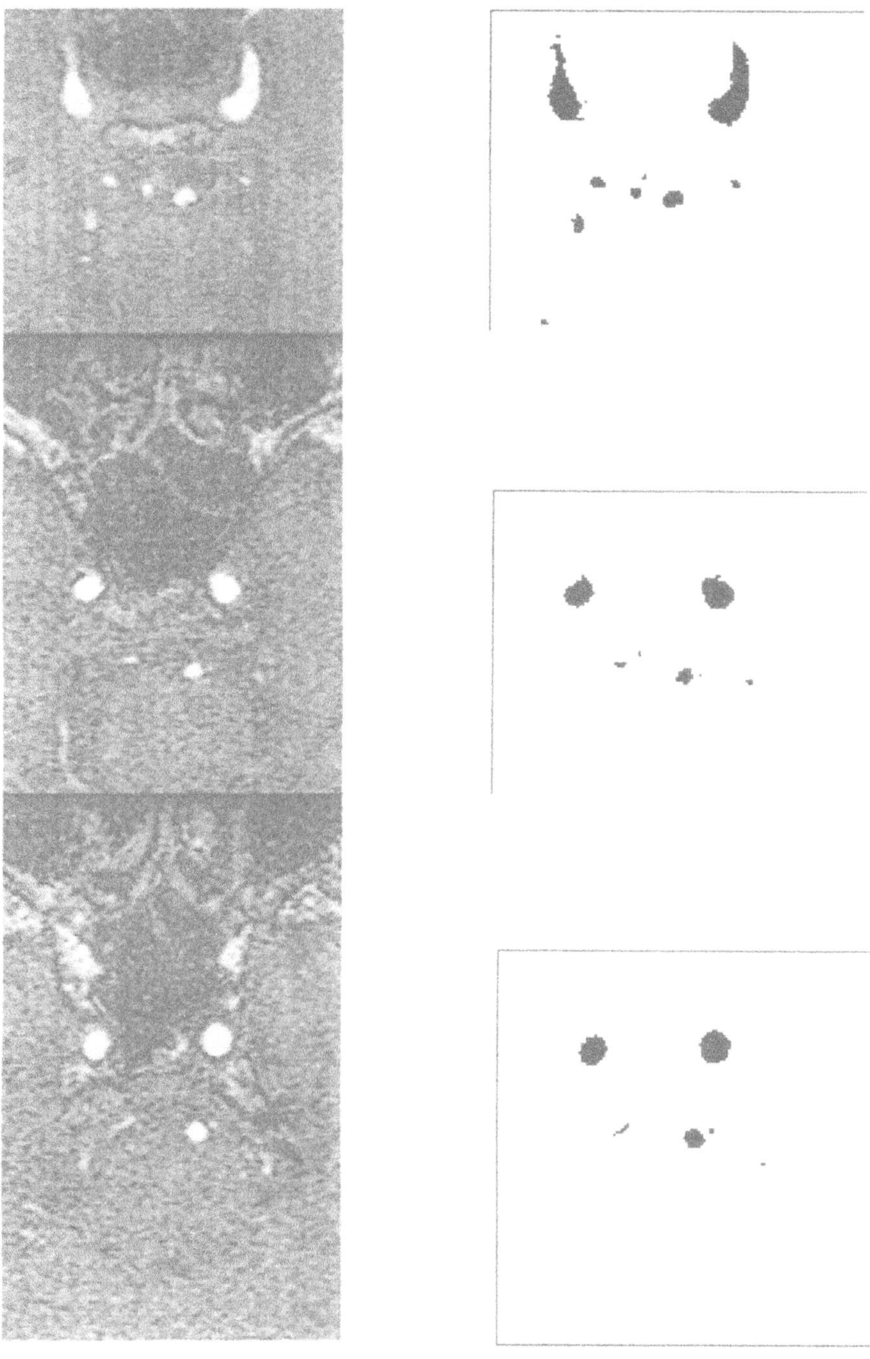

Figure 10. Experimental results on 2-D images: Raw MRA Images (left) and Segmented blood vessels (right).

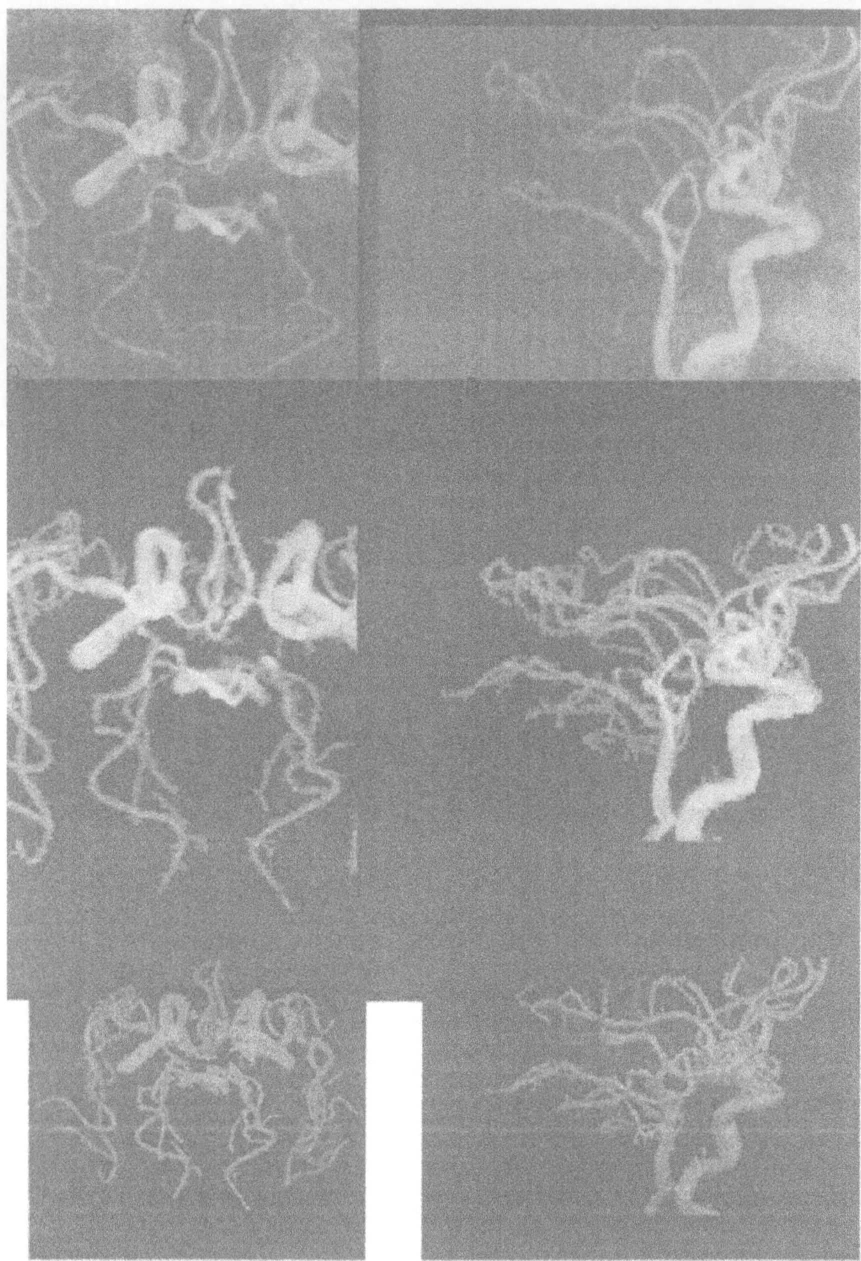

Figure 11. Experimental results (exam #1). Left images are views from inferior of the head. Right images are views from right of the head. (A: anterior, P: posterior, I: inferior, S: superior, L: left, R: right)

The proposed method was also applied to 14 cases. It was achieved in all cases (14/14). Some of them are shown in Figure 13, 14, and 15. CPU time for the segmentation of each case is less than ten minutes on SGI O2 (R10000, 174 MHz, IRIX 6.3, 192 Mbytes).

Figure 12. Enlarged images of part of Figure 11

7. Concluding Remarks

This chapter presents a method for implementing fuzzy IG concept for medical image segmentation. It has been applied to blood vessel extraction from MRA volume data. The method is composed of volume quantization and fuzzy merging. The first part, quantization, detects the 3-D watershed of the gradient magnitude of the raw volume data. Thus, the method is efficient for an image segmentation problem that overlapping of intensity distribution of different objects in an image. Moreover, the second part, fuzzy merging, can be embedded expert's knowledge. These features help to segment the blood vessels with automatically and high accuracy. In order to qualitatively evaluate the segmentation performance, the method was applied to 14 cases. In the 2-D and 3-D images of extracted blood vessels, the unclarity regions in conventional images were clearly depicted in our images. The evaluation from a clinical viewpoint shows that the images are helpful to understand the spatial relationship of the blood vessels and to find aneurysms. These studies denote that fuzzy IG concept is applicable to, and suitable for medical image segmentation problems. Future research will focus on an investigation of effectiveness of proposed method on the MRA volume data with various diseases, and should evaluate the experimental results quantitatively by comparing with the manually segmented results.

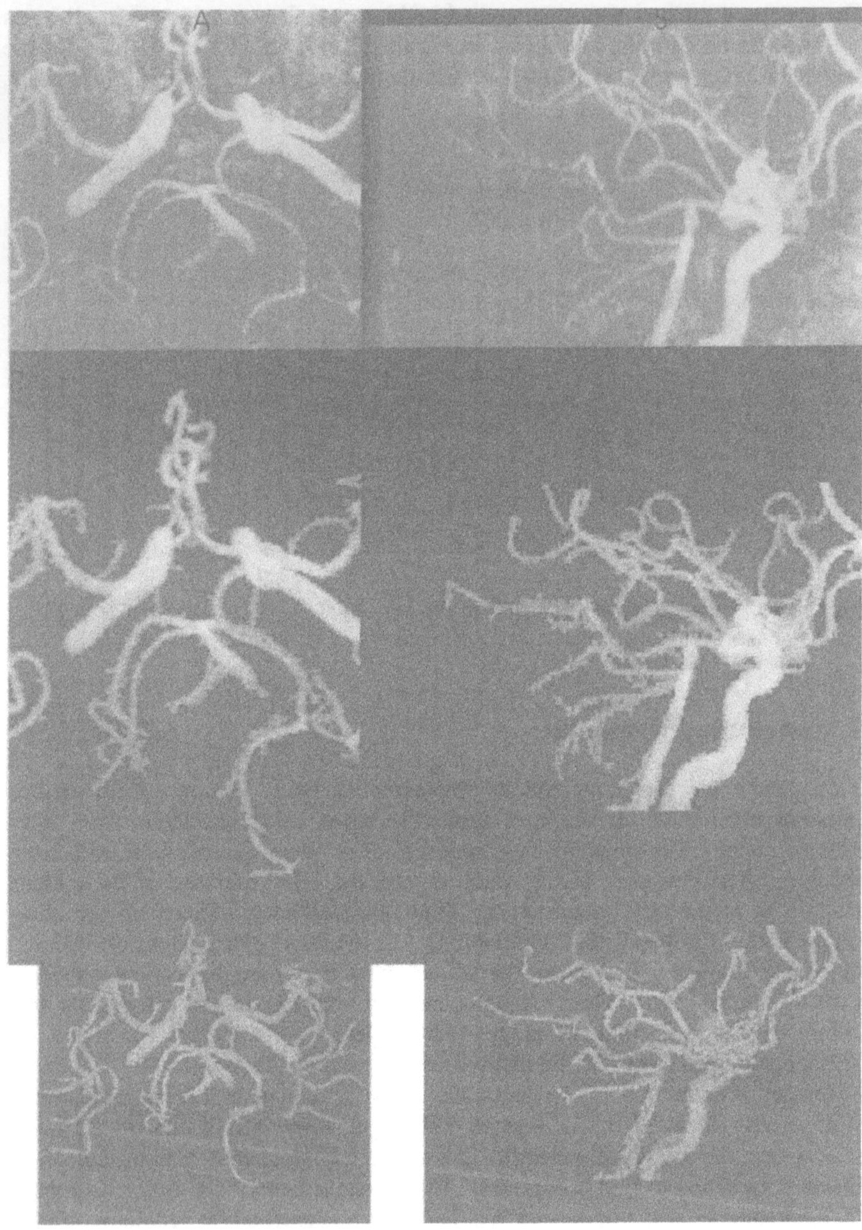

Figure 13. Experimental results (exam #2). Left images are views from inferior of the head. Right images are views from right of the head. (A: anterior, P: posterior, I: inferior, S: superior, L: left, R: right)

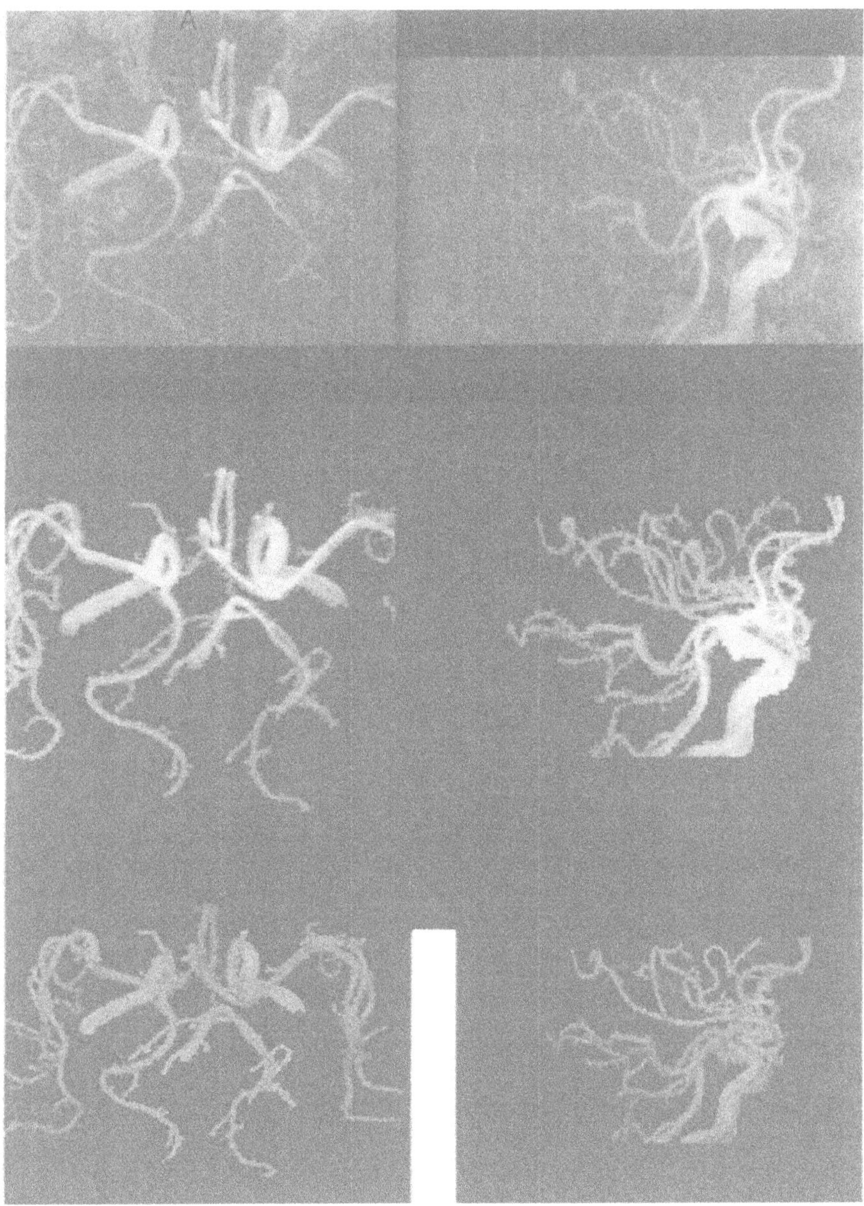

Figure 14. Experimental results (exam #3). Left images are views from inferior of the head. Right images are views from right of the head. (A: anterior, P: posterior, I: inferior, S: superior, L: left, R: right)

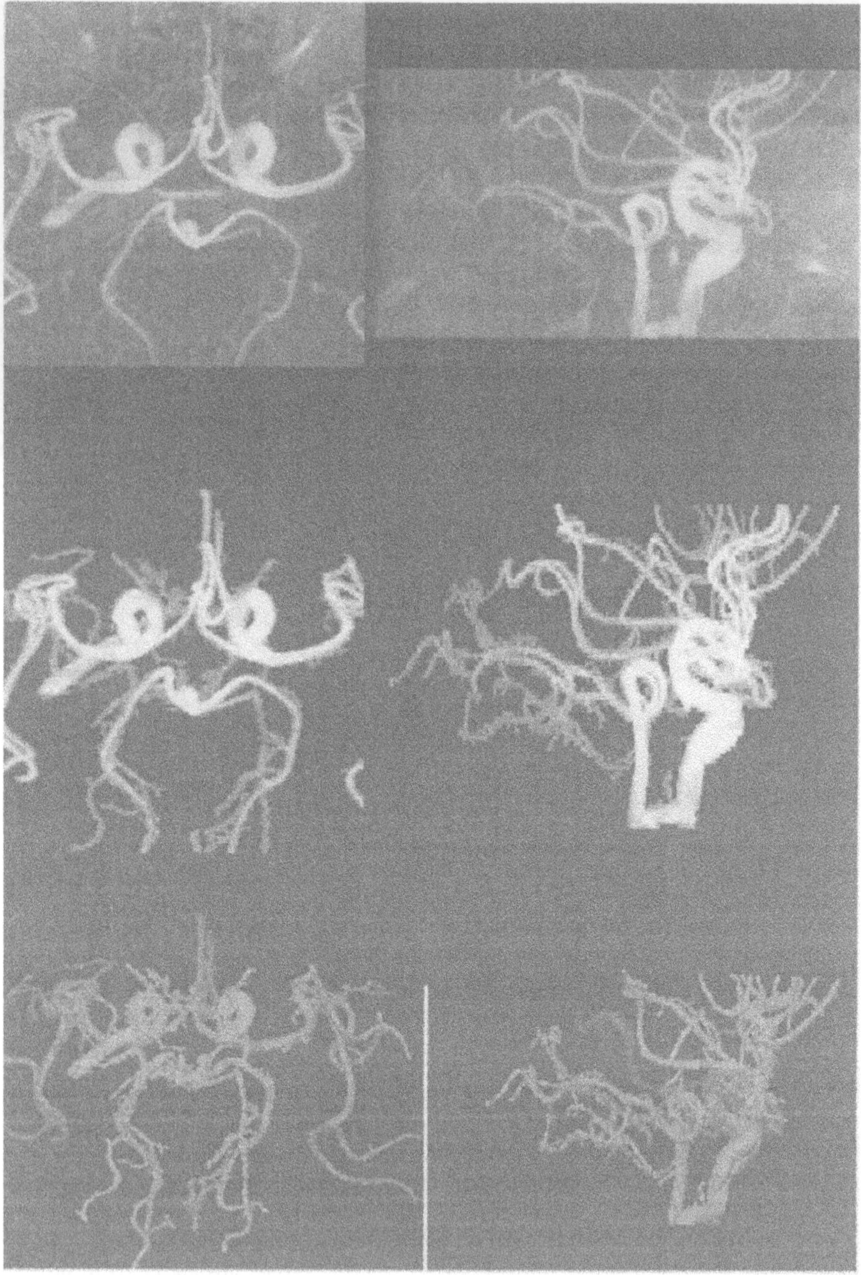

Figure 15. Experimental results (exam #4). Left images are views from inferior of the head. Right images are views from right of the head. (A: anterior, P: posterior, I: inferior, S: superior, L: left, R: right)

In the area of medical image processing, a use of fuzzy logic techniques is appropriate for handling medical images, which are often vague and ambiguity. The benefit is that it can represent a physician's knowledge with fuzzy variables. This chapter introduces fuzzy logic techniques to medical image processing, and shows applications to cerebral blood vessel extraction from MRA images. The methods can be modified to deal with various medical images. For the medical images, a physician's knowledge is represented with fuzzy variables, and then used to desired image processing techniques.

References

[1] G. Laub, "Displays for MR angiography," Magnetic Resonance in Medicine, vol. 14, no. 2, pp. 222-229, May, 1990.

[2] Y. Sato, N. Shiraga, S. Nakajima, S. Tamura and R. Kikinis, "Local maximum intensity projection (LMIP): a new rendering method for vascular visualization," Journal of Computer Assisted Tomography, vol. 22, no. 6, pp. 912-917, 1998.

[3] P. P. Maeder, R. A. Meuli and N. der Tribolet, "Three-dimensional volume rendering for magnetic resonance angiography in the screening and preoperative workup of intracranial aneurysms," Journal of Neurosurg, vol. 85, no. 6, pp. 1050-1055, Dec. 1996.

[4] D. G. Heath, P. A. Soyer, B. S. Kuszyk, D.F. Bliss, P. S. Calhoun, D. A. Bluemke, M. A. Choti and E. K. Fishman, "Three-dimensional spiral CT during arterial portography: comparison of three rendering technique," Radiographics, vol. 15, no. 4, pp. 1001-10011, Jul. 1995.

[5] L. A. Zadeh, "Toward a theory of fuzzy information granulation and its centrality in human reasoning and fuzzy logic," Fuzzy Sets and Systems, vol. 90, no. 2, pp. 111-127, Sep. 1997.

[6] L. A. Zadeh, "Soft computing and fuzzy logic," IEEE Trans. Software, vol. 11, no. 6, pp. 48-56, Nov. 1994.

[7] G. Bortolan and W. Pedrycz, "Reconstruction problem and information granularity," IEEE Trans. Fuzzy Systems, vol. 5, no. 2, pp. 234-248, May 1997.

[8] S. Kobashi, N. Kamiura and Y. Hata, "Fuzzy information granulation on segmentation of human brain MR images," Journal of Japan Society for Fuzzy Theory and Systems, vol. 10, no. 1, pp. 117-125, Feb. 1998.

[9] S. Hirano, N. Kamiura and Y. Hata, "A fuzzy rule based approach to segmentation of the human brain portions," Journal of Japan Society for Fuzzy Theory and Systems, vol. 10, no. 5, pp. 937-946, Oct. 1998.

[10] J. C. Russ, *The image Processing Handbook*, 2nd edition, CRC Press, Inc., 1994.

[11] J. K. Udupa and G. T. Herman, *3D Imaging in Medicine*, CRC Press, Inc., 1991.

Breast Cancer Classification Using Fuzzy Central Moments

H. D. Cheng[1], Y. G. Hu[1], D. L. Hung[2], and C. Y. Wu[1]

[1] Department of Computer Science
Utah State University
Logan, UT 84322-4205, USA

[2] Department of Computer, Information and Systems Engineering
San Jose State University
San Jose, CA 95192-0180, USA

1 Introduction

Breast cancer continues to be one of the most deadly diseases among American women, which is the second leading cause of cancer-related mortality among American women. Currently there are more than 50 million women over the age of 40 at risk of breast cancer and approximately 144,000 new cases of breast cancer are expected each year in the United States. One out of eight women will develop breast cancer at some point during her lifetime in this country [1,2]. Because of the high incidence of breast cancer, any improvement in the process of diagnosing the disease may have a significant impact on saving lives and cutting costs in the health care system. Since the cause of breast cancer remains unknown and the earlier stage tumors can be more easily and less expensively treated, early detection is the key to breast cancer control. Mammography has proven to be the most reliable method and the major diagnosis means for detecting and classifying breast cancer in the early stage. Studies have shown a decrease in both severe breast cancer and mortality in women who undergo regular mammographic screens [3].

To obtain proper treatment in the early stage of breast cancer, it is necessary for a physician to distinguish between benign lesions and the various degrees of malignant lesions from mammography or biopsy images. There are three steps in many mammogram analysis methods [4]:

- Enhancement of features and removal of noise: Mammographic feature enhancement is the first step for mammogram analysis. It is performed by emphasizing image features and suppressing noises so that the image quality can be improved.
- Segmentation (Localization) of suspicious areas: Segmentation is a fundamental step to extract the suspicious areas.
- Classification of suspected areas as normal, benign and malignant tumor areas: Training and testing are conducted.

Lots of researchers have paid attention to the analysis of mammograms. Microcalcifications and masses are the two most important indicators of malignancy in mammograms, and their automated detection is very important for early breast cancer detection. Since masses are often indistinguishable from the surrounding parenchymal tissues, the automated detection of masses is more challenging.

Although computer-aided mammography has been studied over the last two decades, automated interpretation of masses remains very difficult. The major reasons are:

1. masses are with various size, shape and density, therefore, simple matching or detection method will not work;
2. masses may be closely connected to surrounding tissue, and simple segmentation algorithm cannot work well;
3. masses may be low contrast so that the intensity difference between suspicious areas and their surrounding tissues can be quite slim;
4. in some dense tissues, and/or skin thickening, especially in the breasts of younger women, suspicious areas are almost invisible;
5. the fuzzy nature of mammography and breast structure makes traditional methods work poorly.

In this paper, we focus on the mass pattern of the mammogram. As above mentioned difficulties, mammographic feature enhancement is a necessary step for mammogram analysis. It is performed by emphasizing image features and suppressing noise so that the image quality can be improved. In order to obtain higher performance and increase the accuracy of diagnosis, computer image classification plays a very important role. Since mass is one of the primary signs for early breast cancer detection and classification, it is important to develop an efficient method that can classify the mass patterns of the mammograms into normal, benign and malignant in the early stage.

[5] used a nonlinear bilateral subtraction scheme to enhance the features of masses based on the deviation from the symmetry of the right and left breasts. [6] proposed a method to diagnose breast cancer using artificial neural networks in mammography. [7] presented a technique for the detection of tumors. In this method, adaptive thresholding was used to extract regions of interests and a modified Markov random field (MRF) model-based method is utilized for further segmentation. After segmentation, a fuzzy binary decision tree is used to classify the segmented regions. A method using line skeletons and modified Hough transformation is reported in [8] to detect spicules on mammogram. Image enhancement is essential to the success of image classification. An adaptive neighborhood image processing technique is proposed to enhance mammographic features [9]. An adaptive neighborhood-based image processing technique has been reported to enhance the contrast of selected features [10]. A region-based contrast enhancement technique has been presented to improve the contrast of mammographic feature with different size and shape [11]. An adaptive density-weighted contrast enhancement (DWCE) filtering technique has been studied to enhance objects and suppress noise [12]. Several image processing methods for detecting circumscribed masses

are compared by [4]. It concluded that selective median filtering with a 5 × 5 mask is best for feature enhancement and noise removal among the five techniques.

Fuzzy set theory has been successfully applied to many areas, such as control, image processing, pattern recognition, computer vision, medicine, social science, etc. Specifically, it obtains great success in many commercial products, such as intelligent washing machine, vacuum machine, camcorder, air conditioners, etc.

It is generally believed that image processing bears some fuzziness in nature due to the following factors:

- Information loss while mapping 3-D objects into 2-D images;
- Ambiguity and vagueness in some definitions (such as edges, boundaries, regions, textures, etc.)
- Ambiguity and vagueness in interpreting low level image processing results [13-19].

In this paper, we will use fuzzy logic to handle the fuzziness of the mammograms and use fuzzy central moments as the features of the mammograms.

2 Proposed Method

The mass-related features for the lesions are mostly shape and density of the mass patterns. They can be divided into five major categories:

- The existence of the area with abnormal density
- Shape of the area with abnormal density
- Size of the area with abnormal density
- Margin spiculation
- Pattern of density

Each category in the above list contains several detailed features that the radiologists used to grade the images. However, these detailed features do not exceed the scope of the shape and density of the mass patterns.

The proposed algorithm consists of following steps:

1. Find the region of interest (ROI) from the mammograms (In this study, ROIs are located by radiologist, and automated allocating ROIs is out of the scope of this chapter.), then transform the image (ROI) into fuzzy domain and enhance the image using the following algorithm [19]:
   Given an $M \times N$ image X with L different gray levels, and parameters a, b_{opt} and c selected by the above method, the adaptive fuzzy contrast enhancement can be described as follows:
   Step 1. Construct the membership μ_X which measures the fuzziness of an image X:

$$\mu_X(x_{mn}) = S(x_{mn}, a, b_{opt}, c), \quad m = 0, 1, \cdots, M, n = 0, 1, \cdots, N$$

Step 2. For each pixel (m,n) with $\mu_X(x_{mn})$, apply edge gradient operator, such as Laplacian or Sobel operator, and find edge value of the image in fuzzy domain $\delta_{\mu(x_{mn})}$ Here, we use Sobel operator.

Step 3. Compute the mean edge value $E_{\mu(x_{mn})}$, within a window W_{mn} centered on pixel (m,n), using the formula:

$$E_{\mu(x_{mn})} = \sum_{(m,n)\in W_{mn}} (\mu(x_{mn})\delta_{\mu(x_{mn})}) / \sum_{(m,n)\in W_{mn}} \delta_{\mu(x_{mn})}$$

Step 4. Evaluate the contrast related to the membership value $\mu(x_{mn})$,

$$C_{\mu(x_{mn})} = |\mu(x_{mn}) - E_{\mu(x_{mn})}| / |\mu(x_{mn}) + E_{\mu(x_{mn})}|$$

Step 5. Transform the contrast $C_{\mu(x_{mn})}$ to $C'_{\mu(x_{mn})}$

$$C'_{\mu(x_{mn})} = (C_{\mu(x_{mn})})^{\sigma_{mn}}$$

where σ_{mn} is the amplification constant, $0 < \sigma_{mn} < 1$ for enhancement, and $\sigma_{mn} > 1$ for de-enhancement.

Step 6. Obtain the modified membership value $\mu'(x_{mn})$ using the transformed contrast $C'_{\mu(x_{mn})}$:

$$\mu'(x_{mn}) = \\ = \begin{cases} E_{\mu(x_{mn})}(1 - C'_{\mu(x_{mn})}/(1 + C'_{\mu(x_{mn})}), & \text{if } \mu(x_{mn}) \le E_{\mu(x_{mn})} \\ E_{\mu(x_{mn})}(1 + C'_{\mu(x_{mn})}/(1 - C'_{\mu(x_{mn})}), & \text{if } \mu(x_{mn}) > E_{\mu(x_{mn})} \end{cases} \quad (1)$$

Step 7. Defuzzification: transform the modified membership value $\mu'(x_{mn})$ to the gray level by the formula:

$$x'_{mn} = \begin{cases} L_{min} \\ \quad \text{for } \mu'(x_{mn}) = 0 \\ L_{min} + \frac{L_{max}-L_{min}}{c-a}\sqrt{\mu'(x_{mn})(b-a)(c-a)} \\ \quad \text{for } 0 < \mu'(x_{mn}) \le \frac{(b-a)}{(c-a)} \\ L_{min} + \frac{L_{max}-L_{min}}{c-a}(c - a - \sqrt{(1-\mu'(x_{mn}))(c-b)(c-a)}) \\ \quad \text{for } \frac{(b-a)}{(c-a)} < \mu'(x_{mn}) < 1 \\ L_{max} \\ \quad \text{for } \mu'(x_{mn}) = 1 \end{cases} \quad (2)$$

2. Extract the features of the enhanced mammogram image using fuzzy central moments.
3. Input the fuzzy central moments into back-propagation neural networks for training, testing and classification.

2.1 Determine the Brightness Membership Function

We start with the concept of a *fuzzy event* introduced by Zadeh [13]:

Definition Let (R^n, F, P) be a probability space in which F is the σ-field of Borel sets in R^n and P is a probability measure over R^n. Then, a *fuzzy event* in R^n is a fuzzy set A in R^n whose membership function, μ_A ($\mu_A : R^n \rightarrow [0,1]$), is Borel measurable. The *probability* of a fuzzy event A is defined by the Lebesgue-Stieltjes integral:

$$P(A) = \int_{R^n} \mu_A(x) dP \tag{3}$$

Based on this definition, the fuzzy set "brightness of gray levels" can be considered as a fuzzy event. Let's consider an image having L gray levels ranging from r_1 to r_L and a histogram of $h(r_k), k = 1, \ldots, L$. Let the triplet of the probability space be (Ω, F, P), then, for the fuzzy event "brightness of gray levels", $\Omega = \{r_1, r_2, \ldots, r_L\}$, P is the probability measure of the occurrence of gray levels, i.e., $P\{r_k\} = h(r_k)$, and brightness membership function $\mu(r_k) \in F$ denotes the degree of brightness possessed by gray level r_k.

The probability of this fuzzy event can be calculated by Eq. (3), and for discrete case, it can be calculated by:

$$P(bright) = \sum_{r_k \in \Omega} \mu(r_k) P(r_k) \tag{4}$$

The *entropy for the occurrence of the fuzzy event "bright"* can be calculated as:

$$\begin{aligned} H(bright) = & -P(bright) \log(P(bright)) \\ & -(1 - P(bright)) \log(1 - P(bright)) \end{aligned} \tag{5}$$

$H(\cdot)$ $(0 < H(\cdot) < 1)$ measures the fuzzy uncertainty, caused by the inherent variability and/or fuzziness rather than the randomness. Based on the *Maximum Entropy Principle*, we can find a brightness membership function such that its corresponding fuzzy event has the maximum entropy.

The standard S-function can be used as the membership function to represent the degree of brightness of gray levels. It is defined as [14]:

$$\mu(x) = S(x; a, b, c) = \begin{cases} 0 & x \leq a \\ \frac{(x-a)^2}{(b-a)(c-a)} & a \leq x \leq b \\ 1 - \frac{(x-c)^2}{(c-b)(c-a)} & b \leq x \leq c \\ 1 & x \geq c \end{cases} \tag{6}$$

where x is a variable representing a gray level in Ω, and a, b, and c are the parameters determining the shape of the S-function.

Notice that in this definition, b is not necessarily the midpoint of the interval $[a, c]$, and can be any point between a and c.

Assume the image has gray levels from L_{min} to L_{max}. The detailed procedure to determine parameters a and c is described as follows:

1. Compute the histogram $H(g)$.
2. Find the local maxima of the histogram, that is $H_{max}(g_1)$, $H_{max}(g_2)$, ..., $H_{max}(g_k)$.
3. Calculate the average height of the local maxima

$$\overline{H_{max}(g)} = \frac{1}{k}\sum_{i=1}^{k} H_{max}(g_i)$$

4. Keep the peaks which is greater than $\overline{H_{max}(g)}$.
5. Select the first peak $P(g_1)$ and the last peak $P(g_k)$.
6. Determine the gray levels B_1 and B_2, such that the information loss in the range $[L_{min}, B_1]$ and $[B_2, L_{max}]$ equals to f_1, $(0 < f_1 < 1)$, that is,

$$\sum_{g=L_{min}}^{B_1} H(g) = f_1$$

$$\sum_{g=B_2}^{L_{max}} H(g) = f_1$$

7. Determine parameters a and c as given below:
   Let $f2$ = constant, $(f_2 < 1)$, and:
   (a) $a = (1 - f_2)(g_1 - L_{min}) + L_{min}$
   if $(a > B_1)$
   $a = B_1$
   (b) $c = f_2(L_{max} - g_k) + g_k$
   if $(c < B_2)$
   $c = B_2$

In our experiments, f_1 and f_2 are set to 0.01 and 0.5, respectively. According to information theory [21–23], entropy measures the uncertainty of an information system. A larger value of the entropy of a system indicates more information in the system. The selection of parameter b is based on the maximum fuzzy entropy principle. That is, we should compute the fuzzy entropy for each b, $b \in [a+1, c-1]$, and find an optimum value b_{opt} such that

$$H_{max}(X, a, b_{opt}, c) = max\{H(X; a, b, c) | L_{min} \leq a < b < c \leq L_{max}\}$$

After b_{opt} is determined, the S-function is decided which will be used to map the image to fuzzy domain.

2.2 Fuzzy Central Moments

The task of recognizing an object independent of its orientation, position, or size is very important for many applications of pattern recognition, image processing, and computer vision.

Many methods have been proposed to describe and extract the features of digital images [24]. Among them, moment is one of the most popularly used techniques for extracting rotation-scaling-translation-invariant features.

In the early 1960's, [25] discussed moment invariant for two-dimensional pattern recognition based on the methods of algebraic invariants. [26] evaluated a number of moments for pattern recognition, such as regular moments, Legendre moments, Zernike moments, pseudo-Zernike moments, rotational moments, and complex moments. [27] summarized some well-known properties of the zero$_{th}$-order, first-order and second-order moments. It discussed the problems of image reconstruction from the inverse moments, and suggested using the orthogonal moments to recover an image.

The regular or geometric two-dimensional moments of order $(p+q)$ of an area A, for a continuous fuzzified image $\mu(x,y)$, is defined as

$$M_{pq} = \iint_A x^p y^q \mu(x,y)\, dx\, dy \tag{7}$$

where $p, q \in \{0, 1, 2, \ldots\}$.

The moment of a digital image of area A is:

$$M_{pq} = \sum_{(x,y)\in A} x^p y^q \mu(x,y) \tag{8}$$

We can define the fuzzy central moments of a digital image with area A, and these fuzzy central moments are translation invariant:

$$\beta_{pq} = \sum_{(x,y)\in A} (x-\bar{x})^p (y-\bar{y})^q \mu(x,y) \tag{9}$$

where:

$$\bar{x} = \frac{M_{10}}{M_{00}}, \qquad \bar{y} = \frac{M_{01}}{M_{00}}$$

The normalized central moments are:

$$\xi_{pq}(k) = \frac{\beta_{pq}(k)}{max(\beta_{pq}(k))} \tag{10}$$

where $k = 1, \ldots, n$, and n is the number of images.

In this paper, we use fuzzy central moments to extract the features of the mammograms, which are enhanced by the approach in [19], then use a neural network to classify mammograms into normal, benign and malignant.

2.3 Neural Networks

A neural network is a massively parallel distributed processor that has a natural propensity for storing experimental knowledge and making it available for use. It resembles the brain in two respects:

1. Knowledge is acquired by the network through a learning process.
2. Interneuron connection strengths known as synaptic weights are used to store the knowledge[28].

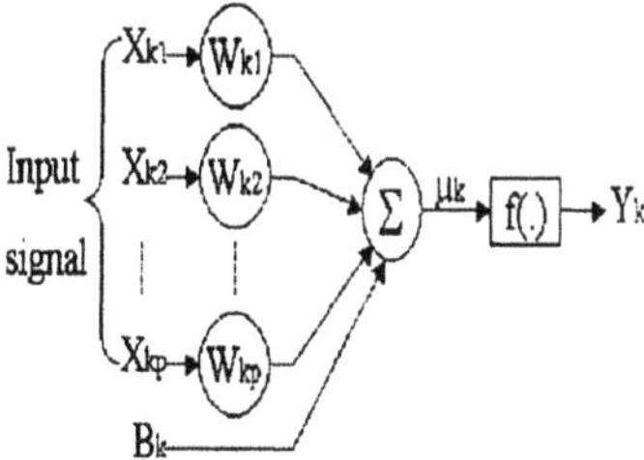

Fig. 1. The model of a neuron

The model of neuron is depicted in Fig. 1.

Neuron can be described as:

$$\mu_k = \sum_{j=1,\dots,p} W_{kj} X_{kj} + B_k \tag{11}$$

and

$$Y_k = f(\mu_k) \tag{12}$$

where X_{k1},X_{k2}, ... ,X_{kp} are the input signals; B_k is the bias; W_{k1},W_{k2},... ,W_{kp} are the synaptic weights of the neuron k; $f(.)$ is the transfer function, and Y_k is the output signal of the neuron k.

There are many different kinds of transfer functions, such as hard limit, symmetrical hard limit, linear, saturating linear, symmetric saturating linear, log-sigmoid, etc. [20]. Here, we use the linear function.

The architecture of a 3-layer network is illustrated in Fig. 2. There are one input layer, one hidden layer, and one output layer.

There are many learning algorithms and they can be categorized into three paradigms: supervised learning, unsupervised learning and reinforcement learning.

In supervised learning, examples are input to a neural network along with the correct outputs. The weights are adjusted to minimize the difference between the calculated output and expected output. Among the algorithms

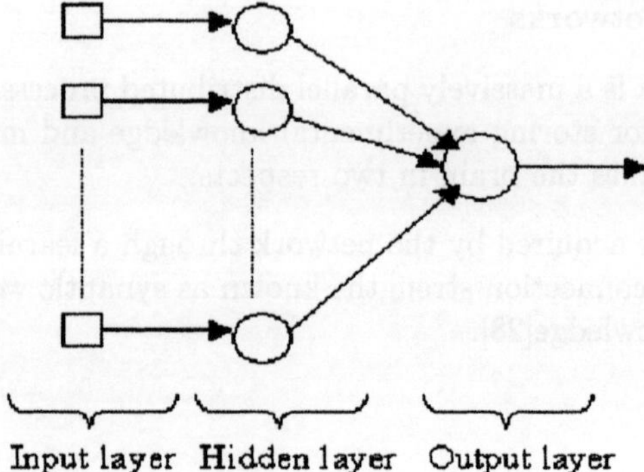

Fig. 2. The architecture of the multi-layer network

of supervised learning, back-propagation algorithm is the most widely used algorithm for multilayer networks.

There are two distinct phases in back-propagation learning:

- the forward phase, and
- backward phase.

In the forward phase, the inputs propagate through the network layer by layer, eventually produce an output at the output layer. The produced output is compared with the expected output, and the differences are then propagated through the network in a backward direction.

In the backward phase, the weights of network are changed to minimize the difference between the produced output and expected output.

Back-propagation learning has successfully solved many difficult problems. Here, we will use back-propagation learning.

3 Experimental Method and Results

To increase the accuracy of classification, we first enhance the mammograms. The original image is shown in Fig. ??(a). The image is very fuzzy, blur, and noisy. This mammogram contains masses with stellate shapes, which are the important indicators of malignancy. Fig. 3 3(b) shows a mammogram after applying the enhancement method in [19].

Fig. 4(a) shows the mass with spiculated margin and architecture distortion, which is another important feature of malignancy. The spiculated features are well enhanced in Fig. 4(b).

Fig. 5(a) shows a different type of mass, which has a well-circumscribed border indicating benign. The main features are considerably improved after

(a)

(b)

Fig. 3. Case 0960542, Size 304 × 280, Malignant. (a) Original Image; (b) Enhanced Image by Approach in [19]

enhancement in Fig. 5(b). By enhancing the mammogram, the features of the mammogram will be more distinquishable and useful for mass detection and classification.

Fig. 6(a) shows another mammogram with mass which is benign. The features are well enhanced in Fig. 6(b).

There are 47 mammograms for this study. Among them, 16 are normal, 19 benign and 12 malignant, and they are preclassified by experienced radiologists. The limited size of the available data set and the need to divide

(a)

(b)

Fig. 4. Case 10479642, Size 277 × 228, Malignant. (a) Original Image; (b) Enhanced Image by Approach in [19]

it into separate training and testing sets constrain the accuracy of both the training and testing of the neural network classifier.

The *leaving-one-out technique*, also called the *jackknife procedure*, is used to solve this problem. In this procedure, one sample from a data set containing n samples is saved for testing. The remaining $n-1$ samples are used to train the neural network. After the neural network is trained, the withheld sample is then tested. This procedure is repeated by leaving out different sample for testing each time until n different classifiers are constructed. Because no samples were used for both training and testing on the same classifier, the

(a)

(b)

Fig. 5. Case 0038863, Size 164 × 128, Benign. (a) Original Image; (b) Enhanced Image by Approach in [19]

estimated error rate is unbiased and is k/n where k is the number of errors [29]. The advantage of this approach is that all n samples are used as the training data and the testing data.

Thus, all n data are efficiently exploited. The final classifier will then be constructed by training the neural network using all n samples. Although there is no remaining sample for testing, the final classifier should have an unbiased error rate at least as low as k/n.

(a)

(b)

Fig. 6. Case 0689939, Size 231 × 195, Benign. (a) Original Image; (b) Enhanced Image by Approach in [19]

In order to increase the accuracy, we use 36 central moments ($p, q = 0, 1, 2, 3, 4, 5$) as the features of the mammograms, and neural networks as classifiers to classify the mammograms into normal, benign and malignant.

The structure of the neural network will consist of three layers and use the back-propagation algorithm. During training phase, for normal mammograms, the desired output is 0, for benign is 1 and for malignant is 2. During testing phase, if the output is 0±0.1, then the mammogram is normal; if the output is 1±0.1, then the mammogram is benign; if the output is 2±0.1, then the mammogram is malignant; otherwise it is undecided. However, there are no undecided cases in this study.

Table 1 lists the corresponding moments of Figs. 3, 4, 5, and 6, respectively. According to the pre-diagnosis by the radiologists, we use the *leaving-one-out* technique to train and test 47 back-propagation neural networks. Two sets of 47 back-propagation neural networks are constructed using different approaches. Both sets of the neural networks consist of an input layer of 37 input nodes and an output layer of one output node. However, the number of the nodes in the hidden layers are different. The first set of the neural networks are constructed using the *cascade* structure. In this structure, by maximizing the correlation between output of the hidden units and the desired output of the network across the training data, the hidden nodes will be increased by one every training cycle. Therefore, the number of the hidden nodes are not fixed. By using this approach, a better classification can be achieved. But when there are a lot of data, it takes longer to train the neural networks.

Using this approach, after two hours of training and testing on a Pentium II 450 PC, the artificial neural networks successfully classify the images into normal, benign and malignant without any misclassification. The final classifier is then obtained by using all 47 data for training.

Table 2 shows a portion of the results from the experiments. Another set of the neural networks have a fix number of nodes in the hidden layer. When the hidden layer consists of ten nodes, a result of only one misclassification can be achieved. Therefore, the error rate is $1/47 \approx 2.13\%$. This structure takes less time to train. Using this structure, it takes one hour to train and test the neural networks.

If we do not enhance the mammograms first, the classification error rate can be as high as 50%. This result shows the importance of enhancing the mammograms and prove that it is hard to classify the mammograms without eliminating the noise.

4 Conclusions

Breast cancer continues to be a significant public health problem in the United States. Mammography has been proven to be the most reliable method and the major diagnosis means for detecting and classifying breast cancer in the early stage. In this paper, we employ fuzzy logic to handle the fuzziness of mammograms, and use the fuzzy central moments as the features of the mass patterns, then we input the fuzzy central moments to neural networks to classify the mammograms as normal, benign and malignant. As the experimental results show a 97% to 100% accuracy, it demonstrates the usefulness of the proposed method for breast cancer control.

Table 1. The Central Moments of Figs. 3, 4, 5 and 6

Order of Moment	Fig. 3	Fig. 4	Fig. 5	Fig. 6
m_{00}	0.332050	0.223881	0.070778	0.169609
m_{01}	0.083918	0.226604	0.079476	0.252004
m_{02}	0.118928	0.047654	0.003548	0.026809
m_{03}	0.004426	0.002873	0.000201	0.004193
m_{04}	0.040590	0.009644	0.000168	0.004000
m_{05}	0.001140	0.000321	0.000006	0.000510
m_{10}	0.223390	0.283986	0.072317	0.094103
m_{11}	-0.026700	-0.000304	-0.000437	0.006924
m_{12}	0.038425	0.010224	0.000421	0.003458
m_{13}	-0.007194	-0.000695	-0.000031	0.000708
m_{14}	0.009482	0.001251	0.000008	0.000306
m_{15}	-0.002313	-0.000195	-0.000002	0.000075
m_{20}	0.108040	0.060637	0.006941	0.032090
m_{21}	0.011396	0.003261	0.000130	0.000350
m_{22}	0.042855	0.014352	0.000387	0.005670
m_{23}	0.011579	0.001777	0.000028	0.001449
m_{24}	0.015619	0.003098	0.000019	0.000906
m_{25}	0.004277	0.000308	0.000002	0.000407
m_{30}	0.074495	0.138212	0.001335	-0.004170
m_{31}	-0.005506	0.000158	-0.000033	0.000910
m_{32}	0.032621	0.026757	0.000059	-0.000368
m_{33}	-0.001469	-0.000101	-0.000002	0.000099
m_{34}	0.005530	0.002442	0.000001	-0.000028
m_{35}	-0.000469	-0.000036	0.000000	0.000011
m_{40}	0.033443	0.016264	0.000633	0.005743
m_{41}	0.002529	0.000593	0.000005	-0.000014
m_{42}	0.013874	0.004018	0.000037	0.001061
m_{43}	0.001397	0.000154	0.000001	0.000079
m_{44}	0.005205	0.000890	0.000002	0.000174
m_{45}	0.001575	0.000071	0.000000	0.000075
m_{50}	0.018793	0.034665	0.000082	-0.001278
m_{51}	-0.001356	0.000119	-0.000003	0.000139
m_{52}	0.026982	0.024310	0.000013	-0.000609
m_{53}	-0.000375	-0.000013	0.000000	0.000015
m_{54}	0.003219	0.001607	0.000000	-0.000031
m_{55}	-0.000122	-0.000008	0.000000	0.000002

Table 2. The Comparison of Partial Results Obtained by Computer and Physicians.

Case	Classified by physicians	Classified by computer
1041211	Benign	Benign
0960394	Benign	Benign
1047964	Malignant	Malignant
0960542	Malignant	Malignant
0960541	Malignant	Malignant
0566401	Benign	Benign
0916227	Benign	Benign
1001676	Malignant	Malignant

References

1. C. C. Boring, T. S. Squires, T. Tong, and S. Montgomery, "Cancer statistics", *CA-A Cancer J. Clinicians*, Vol. 44, pp. 7-26, 1994.
2. E. Marshall, "Search for a kill: Focus shits from fat to hormones", *Sci.*, Vol. 259, pp. 618-621, 1995.
3. I. Andersson and B. F. Sigfusson, "Screening for breast cancer in Malmo: A randomized trial", *Recent Results in Cancer Research*, Vol. 105, pp. 62-66, 1987.
4. S-M Lai, X. Li, and W. F. Bischof, "On techniques for detecting circumscribed masses in mammograms", *IEEE Trans. Med. Imag.*, Vol. 8, No. 4, pp. 337-386, 1989.
5. F. F. Yin, M. L. Giger, K. Doi, C. E. Metz, C. J. Vyborny and R. A. Schmidt, "Computerized detection of masses in digital mammograms: Analysis of bilateral subtraction images", *Medical Physics*, Vol. 18, No. 5, pp. 955-963, Oct. 1991.
6. Y. Wu, M. L. Giger, K. Doi, C. J. Vyborny, R. A. Schmidt, and C. E. Metz, "Artificial neural networks in mammography: Application to decision making in the diagnosis of breast cancer", *Radiology*, Vol. 187, No. 1, pp. 81-87, April 1993.
7. H. D. Li, M. Kallergi, L. P. Clarke, V. K. Jain and R. A. Clark, "Markov random field for tumor detection in digital mammography", *IEEE Trans. Med. Imag.*, Vol. 14, No. 3, pp. 565-576, 1995.
8. H. Kobatake and Y. Yoshinaga, "Detection of spicules on mammogram based on skeleton analysis", *IEEE Trans. Med. Imag.*, Vol. 15, No. 3, pp. 235-245, June 1996.
9. R. Gordon and R. M. Rangayyan, "Feature enhancement of film mammograms using fixed and adaptive neighborhoods", *Applied Optics*, Vol. 23, No. 4, pp. 560-564, 1984.
10. A. P. Dhawan and E. L. Royer, "Mammographic feature enhancement by computerized image processing", *Computer Methods and Programs in Biomedicine*, Vol. 27, pp. 23-35, 1988.

11. W. M. Morrow, R. B. Paranjape, R. M. Rangayyan, and J. E. L. Desautels, "Region-based contrast enhancement of mammograms", *IEEE Trans. Med. Imag.*, Vol. 11, No. 3, pp. 392-406, 1992.
12. N. Petrick, Heanf-Ping Chan, B. Sahiner and D. Wei, "An adaptive density-weighted contrast enhancement filter for mammographic breast mass detection", *IEEE Trans. Med. Imag.*, Vol. 15, No. 1, pp. 59-67, Feb. 1996.
13. L. A. Zadeh, "Probability measures of fuzzy events", *Journal of Mathematical Analysis and Applications*, Vol. 23, pp. 421-427, 1968.
14. James C. Bezdek, "Fuzzy models - what are they, and why?", *IEEE Trans. on Fuzzy Systems*, Vol. 1, No. 1, February 1993.
15. X. Li, Z. Zhao and H. D. Cheng, "Fuzzy entropy threshold approach to breast cancer detection", *Information Sciences, An International Journal, Applications*, Vol. 4, No. 1, 1995.
16. L. Chen, H. D. Cheng and J. Zhang, "Fuzzy subfiber and its application to seismic lithology classification", *Information Sciences, Applications, An International Journal*, Vol. 1, No. 2, March 1994.
17. H. D. Cheng, J. R. Chen and J. Li, "Threshold selection based on fuzzy c-partition entropy approach", *Pattern Recognition*, Vol. 31, No. 7, pp. 857-870, 1998.
18. H. D. Cheng, Y. M. Lui, and R. I. Freimanis, "A novel approach to microcalcification detection using fuzzy logic technique", *IEEE Trans. Med. Imag.*, Vol. 17, No. 3, pp. 442-450, June 1998.
19. H. D. Cheng and H. J. Xu, "A novel fuzzy logic approach to contrast enhancement", *Pattern Recognition*, Vol. 33, No. 5, pp. 809-819, May 2000.
20. M. T. Hagan, H. B. Demuth and M. Beale, *Neural Network Design*, PSW Publishing, 1996.
21. S. K. Pal and D. K. D. Majumder, *Fuzzy Mathematical Approach to Pattern Recognition*, John Wiley & Sons, 1986.
22. S. K. Pal and R. A. King, "Image enhancement using smoothing with fuzzy sets", *IEEE Trans. on System, Man and Cybernetics*, Vol. 11, No. 7, pp. 404-501, July 1981.
23. N. R. Pal and S. K. Pal, "Entropy: A new definition and its applications", *IEEE Trans. Syst., Man Cybernetics*, vol. 21, no. 5, pp. 1260-1270, 1991.
24. R. C. Gonzalez and R. E. Woods, *Digital Image Processing, 3rd Edition.* Addison-Wesley, MA, 1992.
25. M. K. Hu, "Visual pattern recognition by moment invariants", *IRE Trans. on Information Theory*, IT-8, pp. 179-187, Feb. 1962.
26. C. H. Teh and R. T. Chin, "On image analysis by the methods of moments", *IEEE Trans. on Pattern Analysis and Machine Intelligence*, Vol. 10, No. 4, pp. 496-512, July 1988.
27. M. R. Teague, "Image analysis via the general theory of moments", *J. Opt. Soc. Am.*, Vol. 70, No. 8, pp. 920-930, Aug. 1980.
28. S. Haykin, *Neural Networks - A Comprehensive Foundation*, Macmillan College Publishing Company, Inc., 1994.
29. E. Gose, R. Johnsonbaugh, and S. Jost, *Pattern Recognition and Image Analysis*, Prentice Hall, New Jersey, 1996.

Awareness Monitoring and Decision-Making for General Anaesthesia

D.A. Linkens, M.F. Abbod and J.K. Backory

Department of Automatic Control and Systems Engineering
University of Sheffield
Sheffield S1 3JD
United Kingdom
E-mail: {d.linkens, m.f.abbod}@shef.ac.uk

Introduction

The measure went of anaesthetic depth during surgical anaesthesia has always been an inexact science where the experience of the anaesthetist is called upon to provide the control of drug administration. The anaesthetist has to maintain the patient at a suitable level of sedation by carefully controlling several anaesthetic drugs so that the surgical procedure can proceed without causing awareness in the patient. There have been many publications on the subject that have shed much light on the subject and which has as a result improved the control of anaesthetic depth.

Ever since the introduction of muscle relaxants into clinical anaesthesia, there has existed the possibility of not recognising an inadequately anaesthetised patient. Many of the classic signs of light anaesthesia are made unreliable or are ablated by muscle relaxants. Coupled with this, the general tendency to use balanced anaesthetic techniques using several drugs to control each of anaesthesia, analgesia and paralysis to maintain the patient at a lighter level (for safety) of anaesthesia has increased the risk of awareness. There have been reports of incomplete general anaesthesia by patients who were pharmacologically paralysed while under general anaesthesia (Tracy, 1993). Anaesthetists currently use autonomic responses (changes in blood pressure and heart rate, sweating and lacrimation) to determine the depth of anaesthesia (DOA). Unfortunately, these responses are also affected by other drugs such as opioids and anticholinergics, making the responses unreliable. Furthermore, matters have been made more complicated by the introduction of intravenous anaesthetic drugs. Unlike inhalational anaesthetics, the relationship between dose rate and blood level concentration of intravenous agents varies widely between subjects (Thornton et al, 1985), making it inappropriate for monitoring DOA.

The Mid Latency Auditory Evoked Potentials (MLAEP), on the other hand, has been shown to produce graded changes with increasing concentration of anaesthetic drugs and they have also been shown to give the balance between the depression of the nervous system caused by the anaesthetic drugs and arousal caused by surgical stimulation (Thornton and Newton, 1989). There has been since then an extensive investigation on the effects of various inhalational and intravenous anaesthetic agents on the various components of the Auditory Evoked Potentials (AEP). The outcome points to the fact that the MLAEP may effectively be used as an indicator of anaesthetic depth during surgery.

These encouraging results obtained with the use of MLAEP have prompted this study in which the MLAEP are used to produce a reliable indicator of DOA that may be used in the operating theatre. In various studies, the latencies of the characteristic peaks of the MLAEP are obtained after visual inspection, and these are interpreted by an expert to get the DOA. In an automated system, these features have to be automatically extracted; such a feature extraction method using a neural network as a time-series approximation was described and used in (Linkens et al, 1996a). Previous studies (Linkens et al, 1994, 1996b) have also required that the baseline observations be obtained as these are used with the intra-operative observations to calculate the depth of anaesthesia. Baseline observations are often difficult to obtain and they are also highly corrupted by noise and the large EEG signal. It is now known that anaesthetic drugs at the same potency produce similar graded changes in humans; Schwender et al (1994) were able to create MLAEP from individual responses from several patients under the same anaesthetic depth. It was deemed to be feasible to produce a DOA monitor that would not require baseline values. This is investigated here through the use of multiresolution wavelet analysis (MRWA) to extract significant features from the MLAEP (Samar et al, 1995).

This chapter describes an intelligent controller design for anaesthetic depth amenable for use in the operating theatre. The approach taken to developing the system is based on identifying three major components: 1) the monitoring of the DOA from the signal of choice, 2) the modelling of the patient to be used in the controller, and 3) the controller subsystem used to control the anaesthetic drug dosage.

Auditory Evoked Responses

With the modern anaesthetic practice using safer anaesthetic drugs which also obscure the classical signs of awareness, the relevance of monitoring anaesthetic depth has seen a dramatic increase. There are several indicators of anaesthetic depth that have been developed, investigated and used over the years. Their individual limitations have been determined and the use of the MLAEP as a more accurate indicator of anaesthetic depth has been introduced. The AEP is discussed in detail and a review supporting its use in determining DOA is given. The recording of AEP and its pre-processing before it is analysed is discussed as well as the averaging and filtering processes required in its use.

Mid-Latency Auditory Evoked Potential

A monitor of anaesthetic depth during general anaesthesia would be useful for assessing a patient's response to anaesthetic agents and for titrating administration of the agents (Smith et al., 1996). Anaesthetic depth is often defined in terms of a response-to-stimulus test, such as whether or not the patient moves during surgical stimulation or responds to a voice command. Such an anaesthetic depth indicator defines only a dichotomous scale of observed anaesthetic depths having two levels: 'response' and 'no response'. This type of test defines a critical threshold point dividing the continuum of anaesthetic depth into two levels only. This poses a serious question: what should be the strength of the stimulus? Stimuli of different strengths will define different thresholds thereby leading to different interpretations for the same underlying anaesthetic depth.

Instead of the dichotomous scale, a multilevel, or indeed a continuous, scale is much more preferable as this would more reliably indicate the changes in the patient's underlying anaesthetic depth. However, this is extremely difficult using current methods because of the lack of a very good indicator (reflecting the continuous change in the DOA) and also the noise and difficulties associated with such recorded indicators.

Thornton and Newton (1989) proposed the following criteria for a signal to be used as a monitor of anaesthetic depth: 1) show graded changes with anaesthetic concentration, 2) show similar changes for different agents, 3) show appropriate changes with surgical events, 4) indicate awareness or very light anaesthesia. By judging the effects on the MLAEP of general anaesthetic agents against these criteria, it will be possible to determine the effectiveness of using the changes in the MLAEP as an indicator of DOA.

As previously indicated, the review article by Thornton and Newton (1989) and the extensive coverage on whether the MLAEP could be used as a reliable monitor of anaesthetic depth by Thornton (1991) cover much of the discussion related to this topic. Elkfafi (1995) also explains in great detail the subject of AEPs. They all come to the similar conclusion that the MLAEP shows dose dependent changes in a graded manner with anaesthetic concentration. There were similar graded changes with different general anaesthetics, surgical stimulation changed the response by reversing the effects of the anaesthetic drugs, and awareness or light anaesthesia could be identified by a typical 'three-phase' waveform in a particular time window.

The MLAEP are brain responses to auditory stimuli, usually loud clicks through earphones. The AEP which lasts for about 1 second is made up of three parts: the brainstem response which is the first 10 ms of the response, the MLAEP which lasts from 10 to about 50 ms, and the Late Cortical Response which lasts from 50 to 1000 ms. The MLAEP contains three characteristic peaks (Na, Pa and Nb) which have been studied by several investigators. The changes in latencies and amplitudes of these peaks with several anaesthetic drugs (intravenous and inhalational) and with surgical stimuli have been shown to correlate well with observed anaesthetic depth as well as with signs of awareness. Figure 1 shows the characteristic peaks forming the AEP signal.

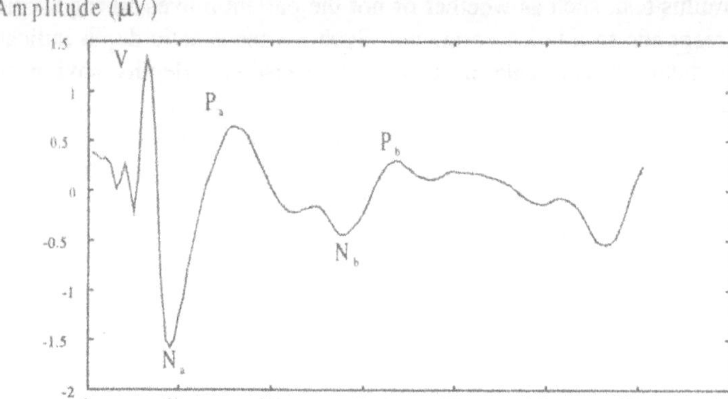

Figure 1: The auditory evoked potential. This figure shows the characteristic peaks forming the AEP. The peaks forming the brainstem response, peaks I-V, are in the first 15 ms of the response.

Acquisition and Extraction of AEPs

MLAEPs are usually recorded non-invasively in the operating theatre using surface electrodes. There are currently several commercially available recording systems on the market. The system used in this research was the one developed at the Northwick Park Hospital and the basic recording system is shown in Figure 2. It comprises an IBM-compatible PC (with an Intel 486 chip) fitted with a Digital Signal Processing (DSP) board for fast signal processing and the signal is sampled at a rate of 1 KHz. A pre-amplifier is used to amplify the responses before they are transmitted to the DSP board where the signal is analogue-filtered and digitised.

Prior to digitisation and extraction of the relevant information, the signal is first analogue filtered (an anti-aliasing band-pass filter with cut-off frequencies 0.1–

400 Hz) in the pre-amplifier box. The filtered signal is then transmitted to the computer where it is sampled at a rate of 1 KHz. The auditory stimulus was a rarefaction click presented to both ears simultaneously at 75 dB above the average hearing threshold at a rate of 6.1224 Hz. The first 120 ms of data, corresponding to 121 data points, after each stimulus presentation was recorded as the AEP signal.

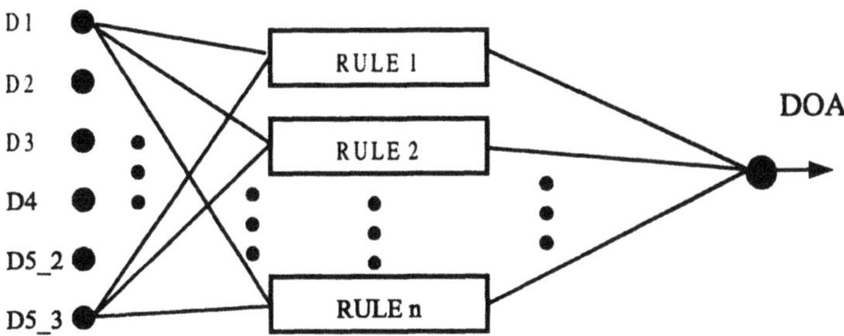

Figure 2: Block diagram of the basic Evoked Response system

The computer also displays the signal during intra-operative recording based on the user's settings. Among the user-settings possible are various high-pass and low-pass filter settings, artefact rejection values and the number of sweeps used to create each average. These are, however, for a visual analysis of the AEPs on-line; here we are interested in a further analysis of the raw signal to obtain an index for the DOA. This raw digital signal is stored, as well as the averages according to the user's settings, onto the hard disk. These, because of their large size, are stored on optical disks for retrieval at a later stage.

The AEP has typical amplitudes of a few microvolts in an awake person while the ongoing Electroencephalogram (EEG) has typical amplitudes of tens of microvolts. Whereas the EEG is an ongoing activity and is seemingly random, the AEP, in contrast, is deterministic: it is time-locked to the stimulus delivered to the ears. The AEP cannot be measured directly from the scalp recordings as they are buried in the ongoing EEG. The signal to noise ratio (with the EEG being the noise, unwanted signal, and the AEP being the signal) of typical recordings is less than -40 dB. It is this small signal to noise ratio that makes waveform estimation and hence signal classification a difficult process.

Due to this very low signal to noise ratio, signal processing techniques have to be used to extract the AEP from the EEG. Since the AEPs are time-locked to the stimuli while the EEG is not, averaging a sufficient number of responses will strengthen the AEP signal while removing the EEG signal. To further enhance the AEP, digital filtering may be used to remove those unwanted frequencies that do not constitute the AEP. A low-pass filter with a cut off of about 100 Hz may be used to remove the electromyogram (EMG). In contrast, in most reported research work on this subject the trend up till now has been to use a high-pass filter with a cut-off of about 20-25 Hz to remove the EEG composed of low frequencies.

Patients and Methods

In this section the clinical setting in which the auditory evoked potentials were measured is described. The patients' demography is detailed and, more importantly, the anaesthetic technique used during the surgical procedures is explained. While the determination of depth of anaesthesia (DOA) to improve on its quality during surgery is important, it is not sufficient by itself. The delivery of the anaesthetic drug that best maintains an adequate level of DOA is also required so that a stable DOA may be achieved. This implies that the classical method of anaesthetic drug delivery, by bolus doses or using the constant infusion rate scheme is not adequate. The use of computer-assisted continuous infusion schemes is discussed as a solution.

Patients Demography

The patients studied in this research work were undergoing surgery under general anaesthesia at the Royal Hallamshire Hospital in Sheffield and all the cases were performed by a single anaesthetist who had previous knowledge in the measurement of auditory evoked potentials. Informed consent was obtained from all the patients prior to the procedure. All the patients studied were of the ASA standard I, II or III, as determined by the anaesthetist.

In this study, we were also particularly interested in relating the model-predicted concentration of the anaesthetic agent in the blood to the DOA, and this meant that the patients had to fulfil certain criteria. They had to be suitable for anaesthesia using a particular set of drugs, only minor blood loss would be acceptable so that the measure of the drug concentration would be more accurate, and also major surgical procedures were not studied for convenience. These factors, among others, greatly narrowed the number of patients that could be studied.

Anaesthetic Drugs

A particular anaesthetic regimen was adhered to as much as possible in all the cases carried out unless further medication or a change in medication was required due to a change in the patient or surgical condition. In most cases, the Target Controlled Infusion (TCI) scheme was used; in some cases, we had to use a constant rate infusion procedure and in another, anaesthesia was maintained using an inhalational anaesthetic agent.

The anaesthetic drug used should ideally be able to induce anaesthesia quickly and have a rapid clearance. This rapid clearance means that recovery from anaesthesia is rapid although large doses may have to be used. Also, the drug may be used for induction as well as maintenance of anaesthesia. Propofol is such an anaesthetic drug. It has been in common clinical use since 1986. It produces rapid and smooth induction of anaesthesia and causes no pain on injection. It causes a depression of the cardiovascular system and respiratory system, thus making such clinical measurements appropriate as measurements of DOA with propofol.

Since propofol has negligible analgesic properties, an analgesic drug is also administered to the patient as part of the balanced anaesthesia technique. Fentanyl, which is a highly potent analgesic drug with an analgesic potency of approximately 100 times that of morphine, was used. It was administered in bolus doses as and when required and its rapid onset (1-2 min) and fast distribution make it suitable for general use. The combination of propofol and fentanyl is in common use in the operating theatre and is also widely reported in the literature. In some cases, muscle relaxation was also required, and when this was so, vecuronium was used.

Drug Administration using Controlled Infusion

The controlled drug infusion system is based on a well-known three-compartment open-loop model (Shafer et al, 1988) which is used to predict the propofol concentration in the central compartment of the patient, which is subsequently used to calculate the infusion rate. The drug concentration in this central compartment is believed to be the most highly correlated with the DOA since the brain is highly blood-profused. The pharmacodynamic effect of drug is closely related to the concentration in the central compartment (after equilibration); this is why it is desirable to maintain a stable concentration of the anaesthetic drug in the blood plasma as this would relate to maintaining a stable DOA. Also, as explained in the next section, there are many anaesthetists (those familiar as well as those unfamiliar with computer assisted controlled infusion (CACI)) who have shown a strong preference for the CACI systems.

The TCI system used in the operating theatre for this research was connected to a Graseby 3400 Anaesthetic Pump to automatically titrate the anaesthetic drug to the patient. The program runs on a Palmtop computer and is connected to the pump via a serial cable. Before start of induction, the anaesthetist enters the patient weight in the system as well as the desired concentration of the drug in the plasma. This initial value of the concentration is based on the anaesthetist's experience as to the probable patient requirement. This was usually between 3000 and 5000 ng ml^{-1} and could be changed according to patient requirement at the start of surgery based on the first skin incision. The anaesthetist could enter new desired concentrations using the palmtop computer depending on whether the patient responded to that first incision.

The Three-Compartment Model

The TCI system used in this study is based on a three-compartment patient model and uses the pharmacokinetics (PK) parameters reported by Glass et al (1989). The three compartment PK model of the patient as well as the PK parameters (in min^{-1}) describing the flow rate of the drug between the various compartments are shown in Figure 3.

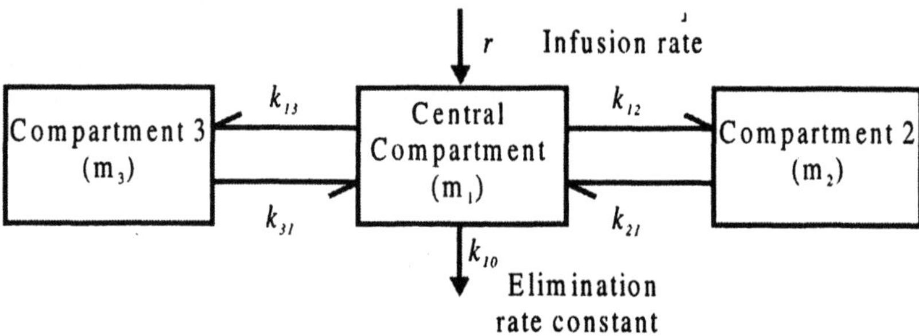

Figure 3: This figure describes the three-compartment PK model of the patient for the anaesthetic drug propofol. Also shown are the PK parameters describing the flow rate of the drug between the various compartments. k_{10} is the elimination rate from the central compartment only. m_1, m_2 and m_3 are the masses of the anaesthetic drug in compartments 1, 2 and 3 respectively.

The values of the PK parameters describing the patient model are shown in Table 1. V_1 is used to derive V_c, the volume of the central compartment (also sometimes referred to as compartment 1) from the mass of the patient using the equation V_c = mass * 0.159. These values were used in (Glass et al, 1989).

Table 1: PK parameters reported by Glass et al (1989) describing a three compartment patient model. V_1 is used to calculate the volume of the central compartment and hence the volumes of the other two compartments.

V_1 (litres Kg^{-1})	k_{10} (min^{-1})	k_{12} (min^{-1})	k_{13} (min^{-1})	k_{21} (min^{-1})	k_{31} (min^{-1})
0.159	0.152	0.207	0.040	0.092	0.0048

The three-compartment model described here is a linear model since the pharmacokinetic parameters describing the model are constant over time. The rate of transfer of the drug from one compartment to another is proportional to the amount of drug present in the first compartment. The equations below describe the rate of change of masses in the three compartments when the infusion rate is *r*:

$$\frac{dm_1(t)}{dt} = r(t) + k_{21} * m_2(t) + k_{31} * m_3(t) - m_1(t) * (k_{10} + k_{12} + k_{13})$$

$$\frac{dm_2(t)}{dt} = k_{12} * m_1(t) - k_{21} * m_2(t)$$

$$\frac{dm_3(t)}{dt} = k_{13} * m_1(t) - k_{31} * m_3(t)$$

The above equations describe the rate of change of the mass of propofol in each of the three compartments. m_1(t), m_2(t) and m_3(t) are the masses at time *t* in the central compartment and compartments 2 and 3 respectively and *r*(t) is the infusion rate at time *t*. The problem is to solve these equations to calculate the infusion rate *r*(t) required to achieve a target mass in the central compartment of the model. Solutions also have to be derived for cases when the target is changed (increased or reduced) so that the target concentration may be achieved and maintained as quickly as possible.

Assessment of Depth of Anaesthesia

Fourteen patients were studied after obtaining their informed consent. They were all premedicated with 10-20 mg temazepam. All the patients were also given fentanyl as part of the balanced anaesthetic procedure. After loss of consciousness in the anaesthetic room, they were intubated. In some cases, if apnoea occurred, the patients were manually ventilated. The patient was then transferred to the operating theatre. In this set of experiments the TCI system was used for ten of the patients, three were anaesthetised using a manually controlled infusion pump, and the last patient was anaesthetised using enflurane.

During the surgical procedure, the DOA as determined by the anaesthetist was noted at relevant stages and these were used to label the data collected. Four DOA levels (Awake/Light (AWAKE), OK Light (OKL), OK and OK Deep (OKD)) were used as they were considered to be the most clinically significant.

Features Extraction

The advantages of using a MRWA of event-related potentials (of which the AEP is one) was demonstrated by Samar (1995). An analysis in the time domain is usually carried out by selecting the few peaks of interest, measuring their amplitudes and/or latencies, and discarding the rest of the waveform information. Also, this time-series analysis can easily be corrupted by noise, even when the signal has been band-pass filtered. This method loses all the information coded within the peaks, intermittent peaks, time-relations between peaks, slopes and other higher derivatives. In contrast, the wavelet transform is able to retain this information.

The MRWA using Daubechies Wavelets (Daubechies, 1988) was used to decompose the signal into approximations at different scales of resolution. The Daubechies 6 Wavelet with 12 wavelet coefficients was found to give very satisfactory results, and was used to carry out a decomposition of the original MLAEP signal into its Detail components and the Residual component. Before the AEP is analysed using the MRA, it is padded with zeroes to make the sequence length 128 samples instead of 121; the MRA requires the length be a power of 2 number. Since each decomposition level is also accompanied by decimation by 2, the complete decomposition process produces six detail sequences and a residual sequence, giving a total of 128 wavelet coefficients (due to the orthogonality of the transform). The six detail components are called D1, D2, D3, D4, D5 and D6 and the numbers of coefficients in each sequence are 64, 32, 16, 8, 4, and 2 respectively. Thus, each wavelet coefficient of D1 spans a time of 2 ms, that of D2 spans a time of 4 ms, and similarly for the others. Also, D1 contains the highest frequency components and D6 the low-frequency components of the AEP signal.

Selected Detail components were used to create the features used, and the selection was based on the results obtained from a student *t-test* ($p<0.05$) on the Detail components. The components D6 and the Residual were not used since they contain mostly the residual EEG. The early and late components of Details D1-D4, not part of the MLAEP, were removed, and the energy contained in the remaining samples of each detail was computed. For D5 (the core of the MLAEP signal) each of the four samples (D5_1, D5_2, D5_3 and D5_4) was analysed individually. The first and last samples of D5, as expected, did not produce consistently significant difference when the data were obtained at different DOA levels, and were thus discarded. Thus, the feature vector used consisted of the six values D1-D4, D5_2 and D5_3.

The features from the first nine patients were used to construct a training/validation set, and the data from the remaining five patients were used for testing. The student *t-test* was again used to test for significant difference between the data, for all the patients, between the different DOA levels, as shown in Table

2. There is no significant difference between AWAKE and OKL for D5_2 and D5_3, since the AEPs still have high frequencies at these DOA levels. A set of 1000 features, with 250 patterns from each of the classes was created for training the classifier.

Table 2: Results of carrying out a student *t-test* test of significance between different DOA levels.

	D5_2	D5_3	D4	D3	D2	D1
AWAKE-OKL	0.248	0.129	0.000	0.000	0.000	0.000
OKL-OK.	0.000	0.000	0.000	0.000	0.000	0.000
OK-OKD	0.000	0.000	0.000	0.000	0.002	0.000

Adaptive Fuzzy Classifier

The primary bottleneck of knowledge-based systems is the tedious nature of rule-base acquisition. It is the determination of these fuzzy rules from the data that plays an important role in the performance of the fuzzy system. While for some systems, the knowledge obtained from the expert is sufficient to create a fuzzy system for classification, this is not true for all. Still, for many systems where the expert knowledge is available, this is usually dependent on one or very few experts' opinions. In cases where enough data are available, it may prove to be better to directly implement these fuzzy rules from the data through a learning process. The membership functions determined from the experts are also rarely optimal in terms of carrying out the classification process as required: they differ from person to person as well as from time to time.

Neural networks, where the network weights can be used to represent knowledge, can be substituted for fuzzy systems in the event that the rule base acquisition proves to be difficult. The adaptivity of the neural network's weights means that knowledge may be imparted to the system from input/output data. However, this learning in neural networks would produce a black box model which is not transparent, unlike fuzzy systems. Furthermore, *a priori* knowledge cannot be used to improve the neural network's performance. In the last decade, researchers have been showing much interest in the combination of both techniques and the term neuro-fuzzy system has often been coined in the literature (Isermann, 1977).
When input/output data are available, it might prove sufficient or indeed beneficial to implement the fuzzy rules from these data. In our case, the data obtained during surgery was labelled and could thus be used to train the neuro-fuzzy system. The expert knowledge is acquired during data collection through interaction with the anaesthetist. This expert knowledge is then implemented in

the fuzzy classifier by using the labelled data set to optimise the rules that were obtained. The neuro-fuzzy system used in this study is the one reported in Bersini and Bontempi (Bersini and Bontempi, 1997). This trainable Fuzzy Inference System (FIS) is based on the Takagi and Sugeno approach (Takagi and Sugeno, 1985) and uses Gaussian membership functions. The centres of the rules are initialised using a fuzzy clustering algorithm (Bezdek and Adderson, 1985). The centres and widths of the membership functions are optimised using the gradient-based Levenberg-Marquardt algorithm (Bishop, 1995) and the outputs are found using the pseudo-inverse method. The system uses the 10-fold cross-validation method: train on 9 subsets and test on the remaining subset. The FIS architecture is shown in Figure 4.

An FIS network of 16 rules was found to give the best compromise between network complexity and performance. Although performance could be increased using a more complex network, this was not significantly so, and thus the less complex network of 16 rules was used.

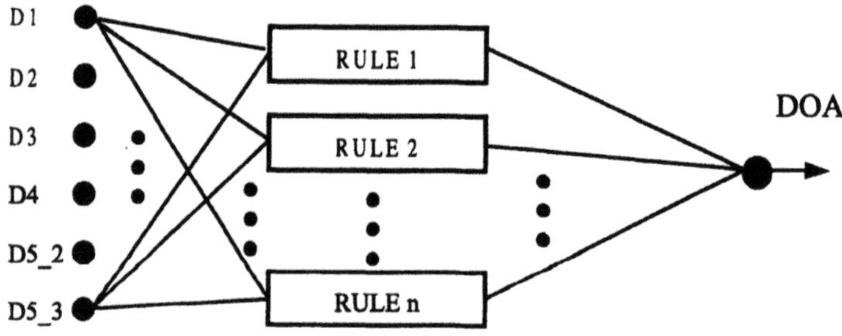

Figure 4: The neuro-fuzzy inference system with the six inputs, n rules and one output

Pharmacodynamics Patient Models

Fuzzy Logic Modelling

Modelling and identification are essential stages in the design of a control system (Babuška and Verbruggen, 1996). However, because of the complexity of many systems, modelling becomes a very complicated procedure. It would certainly be difficult to use conventional linear methods to describe the effects of the drug dosages on the patient and his response to surgery. Furthermore, with the data gathered from actual experimental procedures and the accurate expert knowledge available, it would become more advantageous to use a technique whereby both could be used in a more effective manner to construct a model of the system. Fuzzy models (Chen et al., 1995; Takagi and Sugeno, 1985; Yager, 1995; Zadeh,

1994) can be used to describe processes where the underlying physical mechanisms are not completely known and where the understanding of the process behaviour is mostly qualitative.

The use of fuzzy logic as a tool for modelling biological system has been suggested from as far back as 1969 by Zadeh (1969). It is indeed this high complexity of the human organisms that forces us to accept a level of fuzziness in the description of the behaviour of biological systems.

The fact that anaesthetists are able to control successfully the anaesthetic depth of patients in a very complex environment suggests that they have an understanding of the mechanisms controlling the DOA, and thus, also, a conceptual model of the patient's response to anaesthetics and surgical stimulation. This model of the patient used by the anaesthetist would be in the form of *if...then...* rules yielding a purely qualitative description. It is this knowledge, held by the expert, that is formalised into an assemblage amenable to computer implementation using fuzzy logic.

Analgesic Effect Model

Since propofol (the anaesthetic agent used) does not have a very strong analgesic action, it is often titrated in conjunction with an analgesic drug, usually administered in bolus doses according to patient requirement and depending on the anaesthetist's opinion. In this study, the analgesic drug fentanyl was used. If propofol alone was to be used for surgical anaesthesia, a much higher concentration of it would have been required and this would have increased the recovery time of the patient.

Fentanyl has also been used on its own to produce surgical anaesthesia (high dose opioid anaesthesia) (Schwender et al, 1993); the authors report that it has a minimal effect on the MLAEP. It was observed that the pattern changes seemed similar to those recorded during sleep. There is no dose dependent effect of fentanyl on MLAEPs. This correlates with the higher incidence of intra-operative awareness observed with high-dose opioid anaesthesia. The high synergism between fentanyl and propofol means considerably less of each can be used to achieve surgical anaesthesia when they are both administered together.

The high synergism between propofol and fentanyl and the continuously varying concentration of each drug in the patient throughout the surgical procedure makes it imperative that the effects of both be accounted for in the complete patient model. The assumption of fentanyl concentration being constant would not be able to indicate the considerably higher concentration of propofol required in the case when little or no fentanyl is present.

Shieh (1994) described the pharmacodynamics of fentanyl, used in conjunction with propofol to achieve general anaesthesia, in terms of the parameters he used to determine DOA, namely heart rate (HR) and systolic arterial pressure (SAP). The fuzzy patient models he proposed described the effects of fentanyl bolus doses and propofol constant infusion rates on HR and SAP, ultimately describing the effects of both on the DOA.

The analgesic model should describe the increasingly reduced level of pain perceived in the presence of an increasing level of fentanyl. However, level of pain cannot be readily measured from the patient and there is no way of quantifying the level of pain perceived in the presence of surgical stimuli. As a result, other possible means of describing the analgesic actions have to be pursued. Three possible implementations are explained below and are discussed in greater detail in the next section. The proposed implementations of the pharmacodynamics of fentanyl are:

1) Fentanyl increases the potency of propofol
    - The effects of fentanyl concentration in the body could be modelled as the equivalent dose of propofol that would have achieved the same pharmacodynamic effect (Figure 5).
2) Fentanyl increases the sensitivity of the patient
    - The fentanyl concentration could be used to describe the patient's sensitivity to the anaesthetic drug. A high concentration of fentanyl in the blood would increase the sensitivity of the patient to the drug thereby decreasing the amount of propofol required for anaesthesia.
3) Fentanyl reduces the intensity of surgical stimulus
    - The fentanyl concentration in the blood plasma could be used to calculate the level of analgesia it produces and hence the patient's resistance to pain caused by surgical stimuli.

Any one of the three ways described above could be used to describe the effect of fentanyl on the patient model. They would be made more accurate if the actual concentration of fentanyl in the blood plasma at any time could be known. Since this is impossible using current technology, in this current work a pharmacokinetic model for fentanyl was used to obtain a model-predicted concentration of the drug from the bolus injections (Glass et al, 1990).

Anaesthetic Effect Model

In the pharmacodynamic modelling of the anaesthetic drug propofol, when the observed effect is the level of sedation induced in the patient, the input variables are the anaesthetic drug concentration in the plasma (since this is most closely related to the depressant effects on the brain, the latter being a highly perfused organ), and the second important factor is the level of surgical stimuli (since the latter is well-known to reverse the depressant actions of the anaesthetic drugs). In fact, the DOA can be described as the balance between the depression of the central nervous system by general anaesthesia and its stimulation by surgery. The aim in designing a pharmacodynamic patient model is therefore to produce a model that responds in the same way, according to the drug dosage, as would the individual patient. Inter-patient variability based on age, sex, obesity and height among others, and especially the complexity of the human organism makes such an aim unattainable.

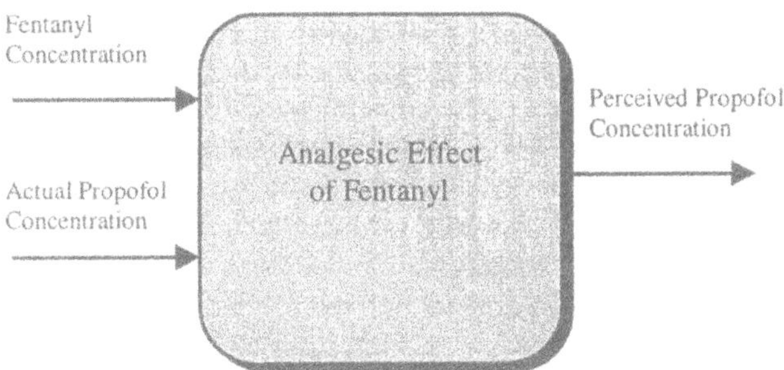

Figure 5: Pharmacodynamic modelling of the analgesic effect of fentanyl on the perceived effect of propofol concentration by the patient.

The very difficult nature of describing the effects of drugs in the body especially due to the high inter-patient variability. Therefore, much of the drug dosage is based, not on the individual patient requirements, but rather on the pharmacodynamic results obtained from a population study. A feedback mechanism would have allowed one to provide the exact drug dosage that would have achieved the required therapeutic effect, DOA in our case.

In the case of inhalational anaesthetic gases which are now delivered to a partial plasma pressure, which is a measure of the concentration of the anaesthetic drug in the blood plasma, the problem is easily solved as the desired concentration may be achieved and maintained, thereby maintaining a relatively constant anaesthetic depth. In the case of the intravenous drug, there is no direct feedback. At present, the intravenous drug concentration in the body cannot be measured on-line; blood samples obtained during the period of infusion (usually from the contra-lateral arm) have to be stored and the drug concentration measured at a later time through a long and complicated process of assaying. Thus, the pharmacokinetics, as well as the pharmacodynamics (based on the pharmacokinetic model output) of the anaesthetic drug can only be estimated through using open-loop models.

It is well accepted that there exists a high correlation between the concentration of anaesthetic drug in the blood and the DOA, though the different concentration levels required to achieve the same effect in different patients will be different.

Nevertheless, it would be extremely useful to obtain an accurate measurement of the drug concentration as in anaesthesia it is desirable to maintain the patient as much as possible at a constant DOA that is adequate for a particular surgical procedure. If the particular concentration producing the required level of sedation was known, then maintenance of the drug concentration in the blood at that level would produce a good quality of anaesthesia.

During surgery under general anaesthesia, however, due to the irregular occurrences of different surgical stimuli of varying intensities, a constant concentration of the drug in the body would not achieve the desired effect of a constant DOA. The drug concentration has to be constantly altered to achieve the desired anaesthetic depth under the current surgical conditions. Increasing surgical stimuli levels would require that a higher concentration of the anaesthetic drug be present in the plasma, and this can only be done if the pharmacokinetics of the drug for that particular patient are known so that the exact rate of drug may be titrated and if the pharmacodynamics of the drug on the central nervous system (the site of action) may be effectively measured. It has been shown that the MLAEPs (Schwender et al., 1994a; Schwender et al., 1994b; Thornton and Newton, 1989) effectively measure the level of sedation produced by intravenous as well as inhalational anaesthetic agents. They are also able to measure the reversal of the depressant effects of the anaesthetic drug on the central nervous system under surgical stimulation. In this study, features are extracted from the AEPs by using a multiresolution wavelet analysis method (Daubechies, 1988; Williams and Amaratunga, 1994). This effectively reduces the dimension of the MLAEP vector from 121 samples to a feature vector of only six values without much loss in information. Statistical analysis of the features has demonstrated that these wavelet features are able to distinguish between different DOAs as required for a monitoring system.

As previously mentioned, there has not been much reported work on the design of a pharmacodynamic patient model for intravenous anaesthetics. Shieh (1994) described a pharmacodynamic patient model that described the changes in the SAP and HR in terms of the change in the propofol rate and the amount of fentanyl bolus during maintenance. For the induction stage, he used the fentanyl bolus and the initial rate of propofol (300, 600 or 1200 mls/hr) to describe the changes in SAP and HR. Only the drug rates and boluses were used to describe the pharmacodynamics of the patient. The surgical stimuli were not entered as fuzzy inputs but rather as set increases/decreases in SAP and HR for intubation and incision (short period stimulation) and Gaussian Random Noise Sequence (GRNS) or Pseudo Random Binary Sequence (PRBS) were added to the SAP and HR for long surgical periods.

Elkfafi (1995) developed a patient model during the maintenance stage based on the current propofol rate and the change in the propofol rate. Rules were learnt from the change in DOA from data from 10 patients and the patient model's output was the change in DOA (anaesthetic depth was defined on a scale of 0-500, with 0 indicating awake and 500, deep anaesthesia).

Veng-Pedersen and Modi (1992) used a dynamically grown neural network (NN), in which sub-units are added every time a new infusion rate is encountered, to predict the heart rate of rabbits upon infusion of alfentanil. Only two different non-zero drug rates were used. They report that the ability of the NN to emulate the system was excellent and that it had good predictive extrapolation capabilities. The pharmacodynamic model system is one step towards being able to administer drug to the required effect as opposed to the drug level.

Closed-Loop Control and Simulation

In the community of researchers on the control of DOA, the ultimate system would probably be a closed-loop (CL) control of DOA whereby the minimum amount of anaesthetic drug was titrated according to the patient's requirements under the surgical conditions at that time. In other words, the minimum amount of drug to achieve the required therapeutic effect could be efficiently calculated and the correct dosage could be accurately determined and used.

This is however an enormous task made even more difficult because of the critical safety aspects involved. At present there is still ongoing work on the measurement of DOA. Over the years several physiological measurements have been proposed as indicators of anaesthetic depth. Most of them, though promising at the start, have eventually been superseded by other more accurate and reflective measurements. The search for other indicators of DOA apart from the usual clinical signs (e.g. heart rate, arterial pressure, patient movement, pupil response) has gained even more significance with the introduction of balanced anaesthesia whereby a plethora of drugs are used to achieve the triad of hypnosis, muscle relaxation and analgesia in the patient; these clinical signs are now no more reliable and some are even abolished.

With advances made in the production of a reliable index for DOA, more and more work has started on the closed-loop (CL) control of anaesthesia. Most of them have been carried out in a simulation stage (Elkfafi, 1995; Shieh, 1994; Webb et al., 1996) and there have also been CL control of anaesthetic depth carried out on animals (Nayak and Roy, 1998; Sharma *et al.*, 1993), and real patients (White *et al*, 1999; Dio *et al*, 1997; 1999; Gajraj *et al*, 1998; Mortier *et al*, 1998). The production of a reliable index for anaesthetic depth is only one of the major stages towards creating a CL anaesthesia system.

In the CL simulation studies, a pharmacodynamic model of the patient is required to describe the patient's response to changes in the drug concentration in the blood and to changes in the surgical stimuli.

Predictive Closed-Loop Control

The implementation of this proposed simulated CL system follows from the implementations of several other modules described in the preceding sections: the TCI system for delivering the anaesthetic drug to a TC, the extraction of significant features from the MLAEPs, the successful interpretation of these features to obtain an accurate indication of the DOA level, and finally the development of patient models to describe the effects of the analgesic and anaesthetic drugs on the patient. It is the latter that permit the simulation studies. If the CL system was to be used during a surgical case, then the anaesthetic patient model would be replaced by the actual patient.

The initial design of the controller subsystem of the CL system was modified so that a more intelligent TC of propofol could be chosen that would maintain adequate anaesthesia using an appropriate TCI profile, similar to the approach used by the anaesthetist. This removed the oscillatory TCI profile that was generated (in preliminary simulations) due to the system being overly sensitive to changes in the DOA levels (that were often due to noise) and the stimuli levels, and also because the time for any effects of a change in TCI to take place was not accounted for.

The basic controller comprised a look-up table as shown in Table 3. The table indicates, for each combination of DOA level and C1, the change in TCI level that should be made. PR (problem) is used to indicate those situations that are unlikely to occur. F indicates that as well as increasing the TCI level by 1000 to a maximum of 8000, the use of more fentanyl can be recommended.

The increase in concentration of propofol when the TCI level is low is relatively higher than when the concentration is high. However, as will become clear later when the prediction system is used, this does not limit the system to these set increases; it is known that in many instances, during the course of anaesthesia, the TCI level may be increased by values higher than those described in the table. The values in this table are intentionally set to low values so that the minimum concentration of propofol required to achieve the desired effect is used. Figure 6 shows a more detailed schematic of the CL infusion system. The user inputs to the system are made distinct from the inputs and outputs within the system.

Figure 7 shows how the basic controller system built around the look-up table was modified to one incorporating prediction. The CL control simulator is a replication of the CL system of Figure 6 and is the block that performs the prediction. It is called the predictor.

In this figure, t refers to a particular time during anaesthesia using the CL system, $DOA_{CL}(t)$ is the DOA level obtained from the classifier based on the patient's current MLAEP features, $C1(t)$, $C2(t)$ and $C2(t)$ are the propofol concentrations in the three respective compartments, D(*t*) is the wavelet feature from the patient model, $TC_{LUT}(t)$ is the TC obtained from the look-up table, $TC_{SIM}(t+M)$ is the TC from the predictor, $DOA_{SIM}(t+M)$ is the DOA from predictor, and $TC_{CON}(t)$ is the final controller output from the controller logic block. *M* is called the prediction time and defines the time for which the simulator prediction is run to produce the required outputs.

Table 3: This table shows the controller lookup table. The cells describe the amount by which C1 should be raised for each combination of DOA level and C1. PR indicates a problem and is used for those combinations that are not likely to occur and F indicates that more fentanyl is recommended and the concentration should be increased by 1000 to a maximum of 8000.

C1	**DOA Level**			
	AWAKE	OKL	OK	OKD
0	3000	PR	PR	PR
500	2500	2500	PR	PR
1000	2500	2000	PR	PR
1500	2000	1500	PR	PR
2000	2000	1000	0	PR
2500	2000	1000	0	-500
3000	2000	1000	0	-500
3500	1500	1000	0	-500
4000	1500	1000	0	-500
4500	1500	1000	0	-500
5000	1000	1000	0	-500
5500	1000	1000	0	-1000
6000	F	1000	0	-1000
6500	F	500	0	-1000
7000	F	500	0	-1000
7500	F	F	0	-1000
8000	F	F	0	-1000

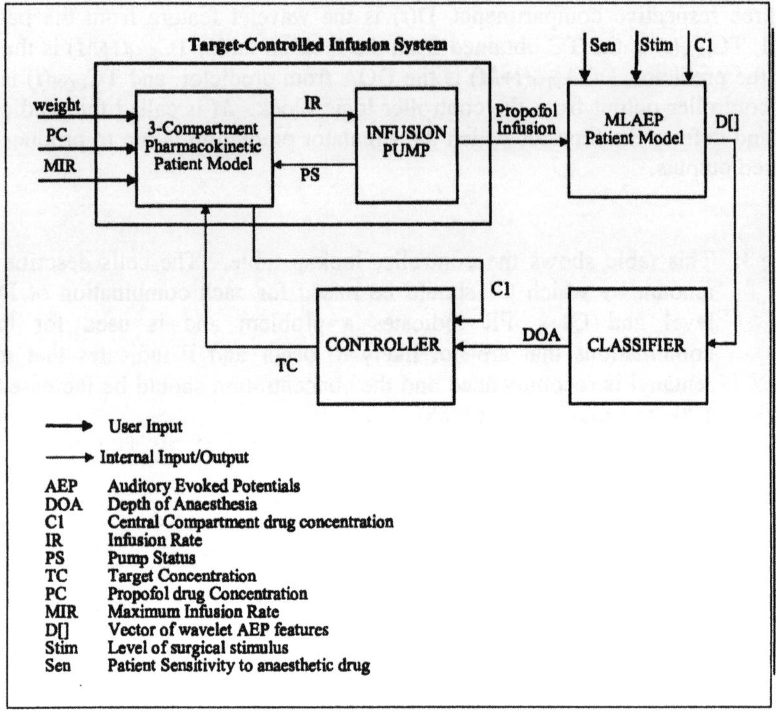

Figure 6: Schematic overview of the CL simulator system for the control of DOA.

The predictor is a copy of the CL system of Figure 6. During simulation, the simulator is initialised with the values from the actual CL system: state of the patient model, states of the pharmacokinetic systems for propofol and fentanyl (i.e. the concentrations in the compartments), the DOA level, the stage of anaesthesia (induction, maintenance or recovery) and the time into it, and the anaesthetist's estimate of the predicted stimulation level. These states would all be available during the course of the actual anaesthetic period if the CL system was to be used on-line: the state of the patient model would be the actual features from the MLAEP, and the concentrations could be obtained from the TCI systems. However, the stimulus level cannot be thus obtained, since it cannot be measured from the patient. In the simulator, an estimate for the current stimulus level was obtained by using the fuzzy logic pharmacodynamic patient model. The stimulus level (ranging from 0 to 1, in steps of 0.05) that produced the output (from the fuzzy-logic patient model) closest to the actual wavelet feature D(t) was selected as the best estimate of the stimulus level. A further modification to the simulator was the incorporation of the predicted stimulus level discussed earlier. The stimulus level input used in the predictor was the maximum of the stimulus estimate and the predicted stimulus level so that the worst-case scenario could be simulated.

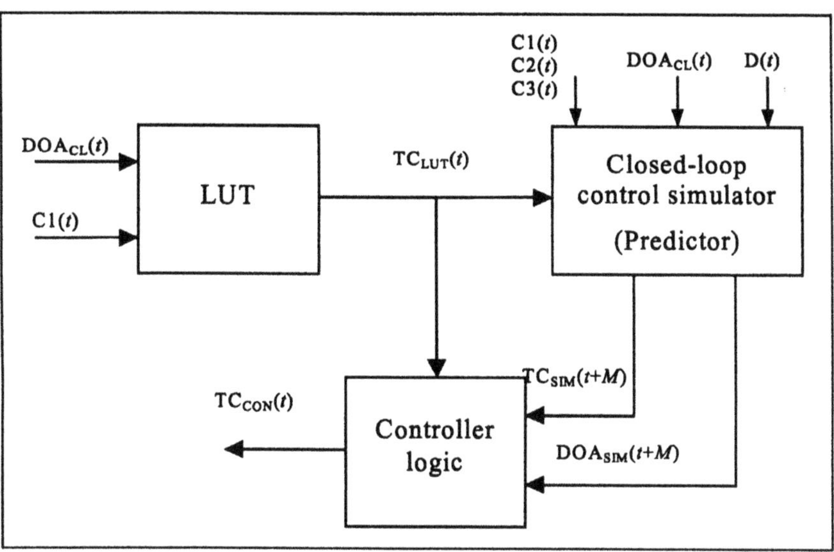

Figure 7: This figure shows the schematic of the controller subsystem incorporating prediction using the predictor

The predictor was run for *M* seconds (2 minutes used in the simulations) using a copy of the actual states of the CL system to produce $TC_{SIM}(t+M)$ and $DOA_{SIM}(t+M)$, the predicted TC and DOA levels after *M* minutes. These values predict the state of the patient and the concentration required to achieve it if the surgical conditions were to remain similar. By running the predictor, the adequacy of the TC from the LUT may be determined. The following scenario gives an example of how the simulator output would be used.

If during a TC of 3000 the DOA level goes to OKL due to larger stimuli, the LUT table would increase the TC level to 4000. If the simulator was then run with that new value of 4000 and a copy of the current surgical and anaesthetic conditions, the effects of that new TC level of 4000 could then be evaluated. If it was sufficient, then the simulator output would still produce an output of 4000, but if however that TC level was inadequate the simulator TC level would be higher, indicating an insufficient increase.

Results

The graphs shown in this section show the results obtained when the drug infusion was automatically controlled by the CL control system. They show the DOA level of the patient, the TC and the actual concentration of propofol, the advised TC (from the predictor), the concentration of fentanyl, and the actual and perceived stimuli levels. Results from the five patients whose data were not used to construct the patient model or train the neuro-fuzzy classifier are shown.

The CL control system program was run in two different modes. In the first one, the program was run in its normal mode and the TCI system was automatically controlled by the controller logic and the TC adjusted without any interference from the user. In the second mode, the controller logic's output was overridden by the TC that was used by the anaesthetist during the actual surgical procedure. Such results are shown for the four cases when the TCI was used to maintain anaesthesia in the patient by the anaesthetist. The first mode results are presented. By comparing the DOA levels achieved in both cases, it would be possible to compare both when the stimuli levels are similar (the stimuli levels used as input to the CL system is only an approximation of the actual stimuli levels).

It must however be appreciated that because only an estimate of the stimulus level is used, the DOA profile produced when the anaesthetist's TCI profile is used to control the drug infusion will not be similar to the one during the actual surgical period. However, if both the CL control TCI profile and the anaesthetist's TCI profile are compared under the same simulated surgical conditions, then a comparison of the TCI profiles based on the DOA profile achieved would be informational.

Patient Case 1

Figure 8 shows the performance obtained when the surgical profile of patient Case 1 was used as input to the system. The effects of the concentration of fentanyl on the actual surgical stimulus is seen as a decrease in the perceived intensity. C1, the concentration of propofol in the plasma closely follows the TC during the maintenance phase as expected.

Patient Case 2

Figure 9 shows the results when the CL control system was used to control the DOA using the simulated environment based on patient Case 2

Patient Case 3

Figure 10 shows the results when the CL control system was used to control the DOA using the simulated environment based on patient Case 3.

Patient Case 4

Figure 11 shows the results when the CL control system was used to control the DOA using the simulated environment based on patient Case 4.

Patient Case 5

Figure 12 shows the results when the CL control system was used to control the DOA using the simulated environment based on patient Case 5.

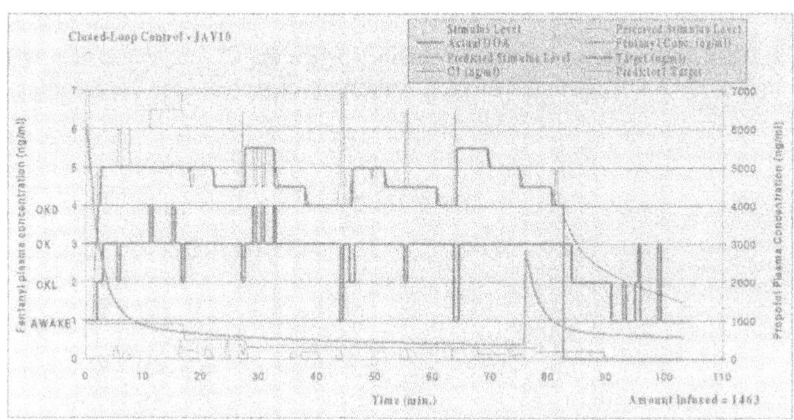

Figure 8: This figure shows the results obtained when the CL control system was used to control the DOA when the surgical conditions of patient case 1 were used

Validation of Closed-Loop System

There are difficulties inherent in the validation processes, the most obvious one being probably the use of other drugs that would also affect the DOA. While some of these drugs, such as fentanyl for analgesia and bupivacaine (often used as a local block at the site of surgery) can be accounted for, others such as vecuronium (for muscle relaxation), nitrous oxide (with both analgesic and anaesthetic effects), have not. Thus, administration of such drugs can be expected to cause a difference in the amount of propofol infused, as well as on the profile of the drug.

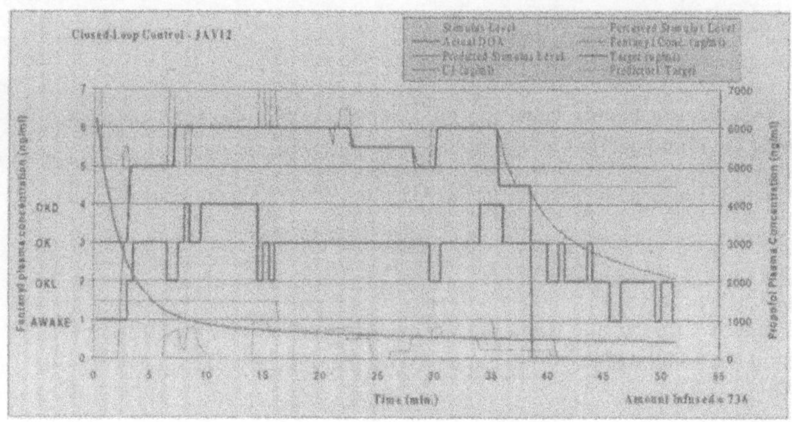

Figure 9: This figure shows the results obtained when the CL control system was used to control the DOA when the surgical conditions of patient case 2 were used.

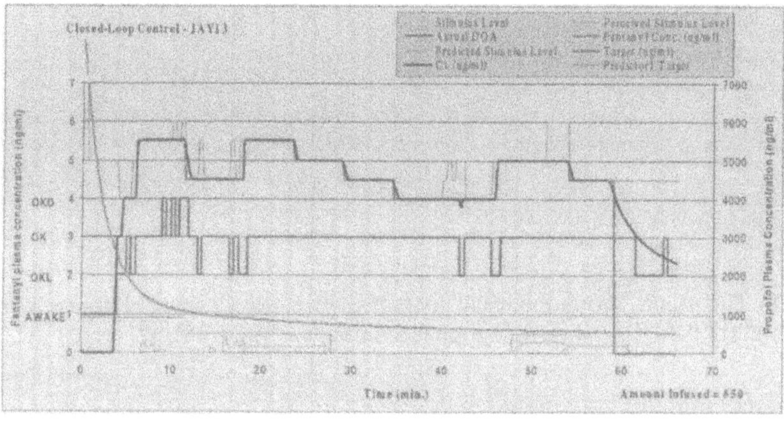

Figure 10: This figure shows the results obtained when the CL control system was used to control the DOA when the surgical conditions of patient case 3 were used.

One of the methods used to validate the CL control system was to compare, for each of the four cases, the total amount of propofol infused during the whole of the surgical procedure by the anaesthetist and the CL system. The TCI profiles may vary over the anaesthetic period, while both producing acceptable DOA levels. While one may use a higher TC which is then reduced, the converse might be true for the other, so that over time, the DOA is maintained at an adequate level, and the total amount of drug infused then becomes an appropriate method to validate the CL system.

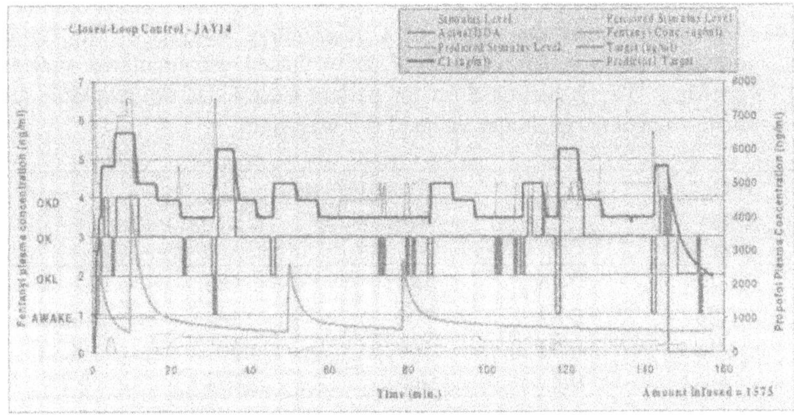

Figure 11: This figure shows the results obtained when the CL control system is used to control the DOA when the surgical conditions of patient case 4 are used as the model.

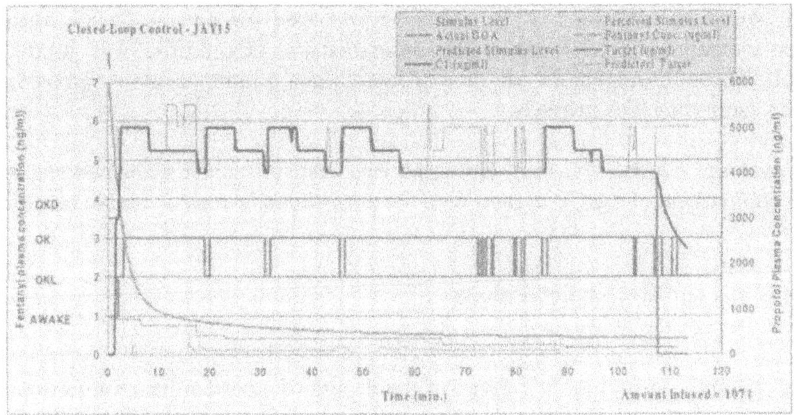

Figure 12: This figure shows the results obtained when the CL control system was used to control the DOA when the surgical conditions of patient case 5 were used.

Table 4 shows the results obtained when the total amount of propofol infused by the anaesthetist and the CL system are compared. The last column of the graph shows the % difference in the amount infused. A positive difference indicates that the CL control system infused more drug than that infused by the anaesthetist.

Table 4: This table shows the results of a quantitative analysis on the results obtained from a CL control of DOA based on simulated surgical profiles. The induction dose for patient Case5 was not available and hence a patient sensitivity value of 0.5 was used.

Patient	Induction Dose (mg/Kg)	Patient Sensitivity	Total Infused		% error
			Anaesthetist	CL Control	
Case1	1.12	0.48	1481	1463	-1.22
Case2	1.34	0.63	790	736	-6.84
Case3	1.185	0.52	709	650	-8.32
Case5	—	0.5	985	1071	8.73

The total amount infused by the CL system for patient Case1 is similar to that infused by the anaesthetist, with only a difference of 1.22 %. There are, however, significant differences in the total amount infused for patients Case2 and Case3. For patient Case2 and Case3, the greater amount infused by the anaesthetist correlated with the more frequent incidences of OKD levels achieved under similar surgical conditions. The converse was true for patient Case5, with a greater incidence of OKL when the anaesthetist's TCI profile was used for control. These discrepancies can be explained when a more accurate comparison is made using the DOA profile.

For Case4 the inhalational drug enflurane was used to maintain anaesthesia, and thus a comparison of the CL system with the anaesthetist's control cannot be done.

Conclusions and Recommendations

In this chapter, a description is given of the design of a system for monitoring the anaesthetic state of patients during surgical interventions under general anaesthesia. Mid-Latency Auditory Evoked Potentials obtained during general anaesthesia are used to design a neuro-fuzzy system for the determination of the level of unconsciousness after feature extraction using MRWA. The MLAEP has been shown to produce graded changes with increasing concentration of anaesthetic drugs and they have also been shown to indicate the balance between the depression of the nervous system caused by the anaesthetic drugs and arousal caused by surgical stimuli.

The neuro-fuzzy system proved to be a useful tool in eliciting knowledge for the fuzzy system: the anaesthetist's expertise is indirectly coded in the knowledge rule-base through the learning process with the training data. The anaesthetic depth of the patient, as deduced by the anaesthetist from the clinical signs and other haemodynamic variables, noted down during surgery, was subsequently used to label the MLAEP data accordingly. This anaesthetist-labelled data, used to train the neuro-fuzzy system, was able to produce a classifier that successfully interprets unseen data recorded from other patients. This system is not limited, however, to the combination of drugs used here. Indeed, the similar effects of inhalational and analgesic anaesthetic drugs on the MLAEPs demonstrate that the system could potentially be used for any anaesthetic and analgesic drug combination.

A closed-loop architecture has been developed that would automatically provide the drug profile necessary to maintain the patient at a safe level of sedation. The Measured DOA is combined with other cardiovascular signals to provide a reliable measure for the purpose feedback control. Based on the classified DOA, a target concentration is decided by a rule-based fuzzy logic controller which feeds the target to a Target Controller Infusion (TCI) algorithm.

The system has been validated using a simulated model of the patient based on a combination of qualitative and mathematical models. The system forms a closed-loop controller for monitoring the DOA for patients undergoing surgical operation. Finally, the system is being used on-line in the operating theatre for clinical trials in the Royal Hallamshire Hospital, Sheffield. This procedure required connecting the system (including the MLAEP monitor) to a DATEX AS/3 device for recording heart rate and blood pressure, as well as a Graseby 3400 syringe pump via the RS232 serial ports.

References

1. Babuška, R., and Verbruggen, H.B. (1996). "An overview of fuzzy modelling for control," Control Engineering Practice, 4(11), 1593-606.
2. Bersini, H., and Bontempi, G. (1997). "Now comes the time to defuzzify neuro-fuzzy models", Fuzzy Sets and Syst., 90, 161-169.
3. Bezdek, J.C., and Adderson, I.M. (1985). "An application of the c-varieties clustering algorithms to polygonal curve fitting," *IEEE Transactions on Systems man and Cybernetics*, **15**(5), 637-41.
4. Bishop, C.M. (1995). *Neural Networks for Pattern Recognition*, Oxford University Press, New York
5. Chen, G., Pham, T.T., and Weiss, J.J. (1995). "Fuzzy modelling of control systems," IEEE Transactions on Aerospace and Electronic Systems, 31(1), 414-428.

6. Daubechies, I. (1988). "Orthonormal bases of compactly supported wavelets," Communications on Pure and Applied Mathematics, 41, 909-96.
7. Dio, M., Gajarj, R.J., Mantzaridis, H., and Kenny, G.N. (1997). "Relationship between calculated blood concentration of propofol and electrophysiological varialbs during emergence from anaesthesia: comparison of bispectral index, spectral edge frequency, median frequency and auditory evoked potential index," British Journal of Anaesthesia, 78(2), 180-184.
8. Dio, M., Gajarj, R.J., Mantzaridis, H., and Kenny, G.N. (1999). "Prediction of movement at laryngeal mask airway insertion: comparison of auditory evoked potential index, bispectral index, spectral edge frequency and median frequency," British Journal of Anaesthesia, 82(2), 203-207.
9. Elkfafi, M. (1995). "Intelligent signal processing in anaesthesia," PhD Thesis, University of Sheffield, Sheffield.
10. Gajarj, R.J., Dio, M., Mantzaridis, H., and Kenny, G.N. (1998). "Analysis of the EEG bispectrm, auditory evoked potentials and the EEG power spectrum during repeated transitions from consciousness to unconsciousness," British Journal of Anaesthesia, 80(1), 46-52.
11. Glass, P.S., Goodman, D.K., Ginsberg, B., Reeves, J.G., and Jacobs, J.R. (1989). "Accuracy of pharmacokinetic model-driven infusion of propofol," Anesthesiology, 71(3A), A277.
12. Glass, P.S.A., Jacobs, J.R., Smith, L.R., Ginsberg, B., Quill, T.J., Bai, S.A., and Reves, J.G. (1990). "Pharmacokinetic model-driven infusion of fentanyl: assessment of accuracy," Anesthesiology, 73, 1082-1090.
13. Isermann, R. (1997). "Special Issue: Application of neuro-fuzzy systems - Preface," Fuzzy Sets and Systems, 89(3), 275.
14. Linkens, D.A., Shieh, J.S., and Peacock, J.E. (1994). "Machine-learning rule-based fuzzy logic control for depth of anaesthesia," Proc. of the IEE Int. Conf. on Control '94, Coventry, 31-36
15. Linkens, D.A., Abbod, M.F., and Backory, J. (1996a). "Fuzzy logic control of depth of anaesthesia using auditory evoked responses", IEE Colloquium, Fuzzy Logic Controllers in Practice, London, 4/1-4/6
16. Linkens, D.A., Elkfafi, M., and Peacock, J.E. (1996b). "Intelligent processing of evoked potentials for monitoring depth of anaesthesia," 16th International Symposium on Computing in Anaesthesia and Intensive Care, Rotterdam, The Netherlands.
17. Mortier, E., Struys, M., De-Smet, T., Versichelen, L., and Rolly, G. (1998). "Closed-loop controlled administration of propofol using bispectral analysis," Anaesthesia, 53(8), 749-754.
18. Nayak, A., and Roy, R.J. (1998). "Anaesthesia control using midlatency auditory evoked potentials," IEEE Transactions on Biomedical Engineering, 45(4), 409-21.
19. Samar, V.J., Swartz K.P., and Raghuveer, M.R. (1995). "Multiresolution analysis of event-related potentials by wavelet decomposition", Brain and Cognition, 27, 398-438.
20. Schwender, D., Rimkus, T., Haessler, R., Klasing, S., Pöppel, E., and Peter, K. (1993). "Effects of increasing doses of alfentanil, fentanyl and morphine

on mid-latency auditory evoked potentials," British Journal of Anaesthesia, 71(5), 622-628.

21. Schwender, D., Golling, W., Klasing, S., Faber-Züllig, E., Pöppel, E., and Peter, K. (1994a). "Effects of surgical stimulation on midlatency auditory evoked potentials during general anaesthesia with propofol/fentanyl, isoflurane/fentanyl and flunitrazepam/fentanyl", Anaesthesia, 49, 572-578.
22. Schwender, D., Faber-Züllig, E., Klasing, S., Pöppel, E., and Peter, K. (1994b). "Motor signs of wakefulness during general anaesthesia with propofol, isoflurane and flunitrazepam/fentanyl and midlatency auditory evoked potentials," Anaesthesia, 49(6), 476-84.
23. Shafer, S.L., Siegel, L.C., Cooke, J.E., and Scott, J.C. (1988b). "Testing computer-controlled infusion pumps by simulation," Anesthesiology, 68, 261-266.
24. Sharma, A., Griffith, R.L., and Roy, R.J. (1993). "An adaptive controller for the administration of closed-circuit anaesthesia during spontaneous and assisted ventilation," Journal of Clinical Monitoring, 9, 25-30.
25. Shieh, J.S. (1994). "Hierarchical fuzzy logic monitoring and control in anaesthesia," PhD Thesis, University of Sheffield, Sheffield.
26. Smith, W.D., Dutton, R.C., and Smith, N.T. (1996). "Measuring the performance of anaesthetic depth indicators," Anesthesiology, 84(1), 38-51.
27. Takagi, T., and Sugeno, M. (1985). "Fuzzy identification of systems and its applications to modelling and control," IEEE Transactions on Systems, Man and Cybernetics, 15(1), 116-132.
28. Thornton, C., Heneghan, C., Navaratnarajah, M., Bateman, P., and Jones, J. (1985). "Effect of Etomidate on the auditory evoked response in man," BJA, 57, 554-561.
29. Thornton, C., and Newton, D.E.F. (1989). "The auditory evoked response: a measure of depth of anaesthesia," Baillière's Clinical Anaesthesiology, 3(3), 559-585.
30. Thornton, C. (1991). "Evoked potentials in anaesthesia," *European Journal of Anaesthesiology*, **8**(2), 89-107
31. Tracy, J. (1993). "Awareness in the operating room: a patient's view", Memory and Awareness in Anesthesia, P.S. Sebel, B. B. Bonke, and E. Winograd, eds., Prentice Hall, New Jersey, 349-353.
32. Veng-Pedersen, P., and Modi, N.B. (1992). "Perspectives in Pharmacokinetics. Neural Network in pharmacodynamic modelling. Is current modelling practice of complex kinetic systems at a dead end?," Journal of Pharmacokinetics and Biopharmaceutics, 20(4), 397-412.
33. Webb, A., Allen, R., and Smith, D. (1996). "Closed-loop control of depth of anaesthesia," Measurement + Control, 29, 211-215.
34. White, M., Schenkels, M.J., Engbers, F.H., Vletter, A.,Burm, A.G., Bovill, J.G., and Kenny, G.N. (1999). "Effect sitemodelling of propofol using auditory evoked potentials," British Journal of Anaesthesia, 82(3), 333-339.
35. Williams, J.R., and Amaratunga, K. (1994). "Introduction to wavelets in engineering," International Journal for Numerical Methods in Engineering, 37, 2365-88.

36. Yager, R.R. (1995). "Fuzzy sets as a tool for modelling," Lecture Notes in Computer Science, 1000, 538-48.Thornton, C. (1991). "Evoked potentials in anaesthesia," European Journal of Anaesthesiology, 8(2), 89-107.
37. Zadeh, L.A. (1969), "Biological application of the theory of fuzzy sets and systems," Proceedings of the International Symposium on Biocybernetics of the Central Nervous system, 199-212.
38. Zadeh, L.A. (1994). "The role of fuzzy logic in modelling, identification and control," Modelling, Identification and Control, 15(3), 191-203.

Depth of Anesthesia Control with Fuzzy Logic

Xu-Sheng Zhang, Johnnie W. Huang and Rob J. Roy

Department of Biomedical Engineering
Rensselaer Polytechnic Institute
110 8th Street
Troy, NY 12180
U.S.A.
E-mail: royr@rpi.edu

Introduction

The anesthetic management of a surgical patient is a process that relies on the experience of an anesthesiologist, since currently there is no direct means of assessing a patient's level of consciousness during surgery. The decision for the initial anesthetic level is generally made by using the recommended drug dosages based on various patient characteristics, such as age and weight. The anesthesiologist determines any subsequent alteration in the anesthetic level by observing signs from the patient. These signs, the indirect indicators of the depth of anesthesia (DOA), may include changes in blood pressures or heart rate, lacrimation, facial grimacing, muscular movement, spontaneous breathing, diaphoresis, and other signs that may predicate awareness. However, they are not reliable indicators of changes in a patient's level of consciousness. Although an anesthesiologist can adjust recommended anesthetic dosages based on individual patient characteristics, these adjustments cannot always account for variability in patient responses to anesthesia or changes in anesthetic requirements during the course of surgery.

Anesthetic underdosing can cause intraoperative awareness [1], and explicit cognizance, resulting in postoperative psychological consequences. The lack of a reliable technique for controlling the anesthetic titration has prompted anesthesiologists to overdose in order to prevent possible intraoperative awareness. However, anesthetic overdosing prolongs the recovery period, which increases the healthcare costs and the utilization of post-recovery care. Furthermore, anesthetic overdosing in critically ill patients may cause severe hemodynamic depression. Central to this problem is our poor understanding of the complex levels of consciousness during anesthesia and our inability to assess the DOA. Reliable and noninvasive monitoring of the DOA would be highly desirable for infusing the right amount of drugs needed by the patient.

Design of an effective DOA automated control system therefore involves two essential challenges: reliable estimation of the DOA and proper controlling of anesthetic administration. Models of anesthesia are poorly understood (i.e. being a typical ill-defined system) and described only in natural language terms, and moreover, it is a complex and nonlinear system. The variables such as those traditional signs of DOA are not deterministic and there is not a direct (1:1) correlation between any of these variables and the DOA. Estimations of these variables are required due to the complex interactions in an unknown system with unpredictable physiological delays. Traditional control strategies are applicable only to well-structured problems, such as linear or piecewise linear dynamic systems. To control such an ill-defined system, anesthesiologists consequently make decisions heuristically based on knowledge and experience, as those deterministic rules are not available in determining the DOA. Fuzzy logic is therefore naturally applicable to anesthesia management, since it can quantify imprecise natural language, and convert an anesthesiologist's experiences to systematic and mathematical enumeration with fuzzy if-then rules for creating a control surface. The architecture of the fuzzy rule-base is conveniently flat and the knowledge is collaterally constructed to provide the relationships among all the fuzzified state variables. These convenient features facilitate the building of controllers even if the understanding of the underlying mathematical behavior of the system, such as the consciousness, is incomplete. Fuzzy logic therefore effectively enables the transference of an anesthesiologist's knowledge to the controller for anesthetic titration.

Recently, fuzzy logic has found applications in DOA control and some preliminary results have been obtained [2-7]. An automated closed-loop control system [7] has been constructed at Rensselaer based on their previous studies of fuzzy logic in multiple drug hemodynamic control [1-3] and DOA control [1]. The testing results using dog experiments [7] is promising: The system monitors multiple variables for meaningful changes, integrates this information with anesthesiologist's knowledge and experience, and continually make decisions concerning present status, appropriate interventions, and expected results.

In this chapter, the use of fuzzy logic concepts in DOA control will first be illustrated through a simple fuzzy control system utilizing a fuzzy physician knowledge model. This simplified model emulates the thought processes of an anesthesiologist in managing anesthesia for patients under surgery. However, in order to make the control process feasible in operating rooms, a more sophisticated fuzzy controller based on a knowledge model derived from a reliable technique for grading DOA is then presented. The detailed results obtained by this model during animal experiments under propofol anesthesia [12] are shown for demonstrating the clinical feasibility for human. Further discussions on advanced topics relating to current research challenges in the area of anesthesia estimation and control are discussed at the end.

Fuzzy Knowledge Models

Currently, the two most commonly used fuzzy logic systems were originally introduced by Mamdani and Assilian [13], and Sugeno, Kang, and Takagi [14-15], respectively. Correspondingly, fuzzy control is classified into two categories: a) first generation (Mamdani type): rule-based feedback control with the rules being interpolated by fuzzy sets, and b) second generation (Takagi-Sugeno type): fuzzy augmentation of crisp control laws [16]. The Takagi-Sugeno type of fuzzy system is implemented in the derived knowledge model for estimation DOA. The Mamdani type of fuzzy control is introduced in the physician knowledge model and will be used again later for supervising anesthetic control in the derived knowledge model.

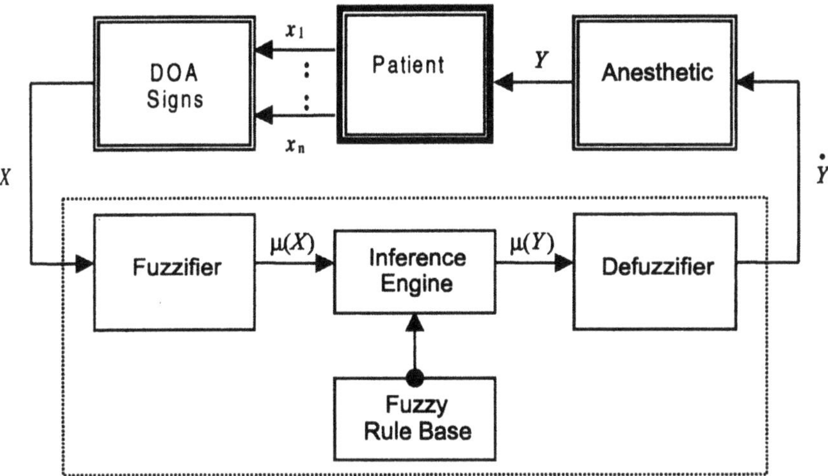

Figure 1 - Basic architecture of a fuzzy logic controller based on some physician knowledge model. The DOA signs may be any of the "traditional observable inputs" such as hemodynamics, body temperature, patterns of spontaneous breathing, and other indications of awareness. The fuzzy rule base stores the empirical knowledge of the anesthesiologists relating anesthetic titration requirements to changes in DOA signs.

Fuzzy Physician Knowledge Model

Model Concept

An anesthesiologist controls the level of anesthetic titration based on observable measurements of state variables such as hemodynamics, body temperature, spontaneous breathing, and other signs of DOA from the patient. The decision-making process that ultimately leads to changes in the anesthetic titration level is a complex process that very much relies on the experience and knowledge of the anesthesiologist in interpreting those state variables. A simple fuzzy logic controller can thus be substituted for the operation of anesthesia management where the anesthesiologist's knowledge is transcribed and modeled as fuzzy rules for the task of state variable transformation into controlled actions. The flow of this fuzzy control process is illustrated in Figure 1.

The *x's* are the signs of DOA measured or secondarily computed, obtained via the sensors placed on the patient. An input variable of the *x's* can be any of the current state (arterial blood pressure), state error (change in arterial blood pressure), state error derivative (rate of change in arterial blood pressure), and state error integral. The output of the fuzzy controller changes the current level of anesthetic titration as necessary based of the fuzzy inference process relating the *x's* to that of the anesthetic needs. This process emulates the thought processes of an anesthesiologist in determining the need for changing the titration level based on a collection of observable parameters.

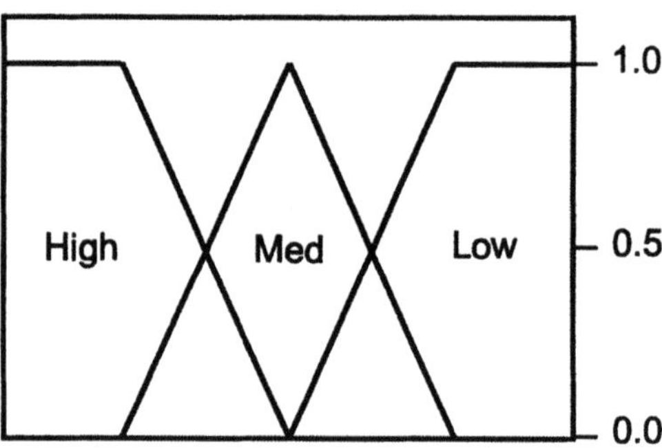

Figure 2 - A typical fuzzy membership term set with three membership functions: High, Medium, and Low, can be used semantically in the ruleset to represent knowledge. This term set is therefore applied for fuzzifying the input and output variables in the ruleset. A finer term set with more membership gradation can possibly provide a finer control, however, it also depends on the number of inputs and the size of the ruleset.

Fuzzy Inference Process

In the fuzzy physician knowledge model, the fuzzy interference process is based on the Mamdani system approach. The individual-rule based inference process is conducted by computing the degree of match between the fuzzified input value X and the fuzzy sets describing the meaning of the rule-antecedent as prescribed in the fuzzy ruleset. The fuzzy ruleset contains a series of if-then rules transcribed from an anesthesiologist (expert knowledge). The primary format for each rule is n numbers of "if" conditions as antecedents, which are the fuzzy linguistic DOA signs described earlier, and one or several "then" outcomes as the consequents. The fuzzy consequents are the fuzzy linguistic actions that an anesthesiologist will normally take for changing the anesthetic titration based on the conditions of the antecedents.

Each output is represented by one membership in the ruleset, but in order to reduce the number of rules, an input may have a range of fuzzy memberships. The output μ is produced by clipping the fuzzy member describing the rule-consequent to the degree to which the rule-antecedent has been matched by X. The possibility distribution function is then found by finding the minimal of all μ's:

$$\pi(x_1, \cdots, x_n) = \mu(x_1) \wedge \cdots \wedge \mu(x_n) \quad (1)$$

The minimized value of all μ's therefore determines the degree of applicability for each rule. As π's are aggregated on the fuzzy anesthetic depth term set, the value of the overall output $\dot{Y}$ can then be determined. The rule-consequent is then inferred on the fuzzy anesthetic depth term set. In this example, the defuzzification process utilizes the standard center of gravity method (COG):

$$DEFUZ_{COG}(X) = \frac{\int \mu(x) dx}{\int x dx} \quad (2)$$

The $DEFUZ_{COG}(X)$ determines the output $\dot{Y}$, which is the abscissa of the center of gravity of the area describing the output of the inference engine in the fuzzy anesthetic depth term set.

Feasibility

Although a fuzzy controller based on the fuzzy physician knowledge model emulates the actions of an anesthesiologist, there are still several challenges present making the controller feasible only in limited clinical settings:

Input Weighting Scheme - The fuzzy controller weights all the input parameters equally as prescribed by the ruleset, whereas an anesthesiologist considers all the observable parameters but weights each parameter differently according to its relevance as the condition of the patient changes. We can overcome this difficulty by developing a feedback mechanism for adaptively changing the rules or by passing inputs though a series of sophisticated adaptive filters. However, the convergence of the controlled parameters may be severely challenged.

Size of Input Dimension - Ideally, *n*, the number of inputs into the fuzzy controller as shown in Figure 1 should be maximized. In flat knowledge representation, the expansion of the number of the input parameters should not increase the level of complexity in transcribing anesthesiologist's knowledge into rules. However, this expansion of the number of the parameters will greatly increase the number of rules involved. Although fuzzy systems are generally considered robust even if the knowledge may not be complete, however any missing rules in the ruleset may potentially cause devastating consequences in the outcome, such as overdosing the patient because the control surface is not smooth.

Patient Sensitivity - There are both intra-patient and inter-patient sensitivity differences to anesthetics. The anesthetic effect in a given patient may alter depending upon the stimulus and the patients state. These differences have made the task of adjusting the universe of discourse laborious and the convergence of the controlled parameters uncertain.

Impartial DOA Knowledge - Elevated input parameters such as the blood pressure or heart rate may be caused by insufficient anesthesia, but they are only the *indirect* indicators of intraoperative awareness. This inability to rely on a measurable indicator of DOA is the fundamental challenge in maintaining anesthesia for an anesthesiologist. However, a fuzzy controller based on a fuzzy physician knowledge model faces even greater challenge since it does not monitor all the outputs nor tracks all the inputs into the plant. For example, the infusion of a vasoactive drug by the anesthesiologist or surgical stimulus will alter the hemodynamic state of the patient.

A robust method for estimating DOA can overcome some of these fundamental challenges in designing an effective automated anesthesia management system. In the following section, a closed-loop fuzzy system based on a derived fuzzy knowledge model is detailed.

Derived Fuzzy Knowledge Model

System Overview

In Figure 3, the schematic diagram of the closed-loop fuzzy system based on a derived fuzzy knowledge model for controlling DOA is shown. It mainly consists of three parts: 1) a derived fuzzy knowledge model for accurate DOA estimation, 2) a fuzzy supervisor for supervising the whole closed-loop operation and for determining drug concentrations based on the confidence level estimator for enhancing the performance of the DOA estimation, and 3) a drug infusion system for directly driving pumps or ventilators to administer drugs. The derived fuzzy knowledge model now plays the key role in estimating the DOA for the overall system instead of relying on secondary parameters such as blood pressures that are indirectly influenced by the anesthetics.

The system will initially use the age, gender, and the BSA (body surface area calculated from the weight and height of the subject) as inputs for determining a starting drug concentration setpoint. In this system, the initial setpoint is computed fuzzily with a multiple-input-single-output fuzzy integrator. Special considerations are made for deducing a lower setpoint for infants and elderly patients [7]. The electroencephalogram (EEG) collected via patient monitor is processed by novel signal processing techniques, and the extracted characteristics are fed into the adaptive network-based fuzzy inference system (ANFIS) for determining the depth of anesthesia. In order to minimize any erratic behaviors caused by external disturbances the confidence level of each ANFIS output is calculated by the confidence estimator for rejecting inconsistent ANFIS outputs.

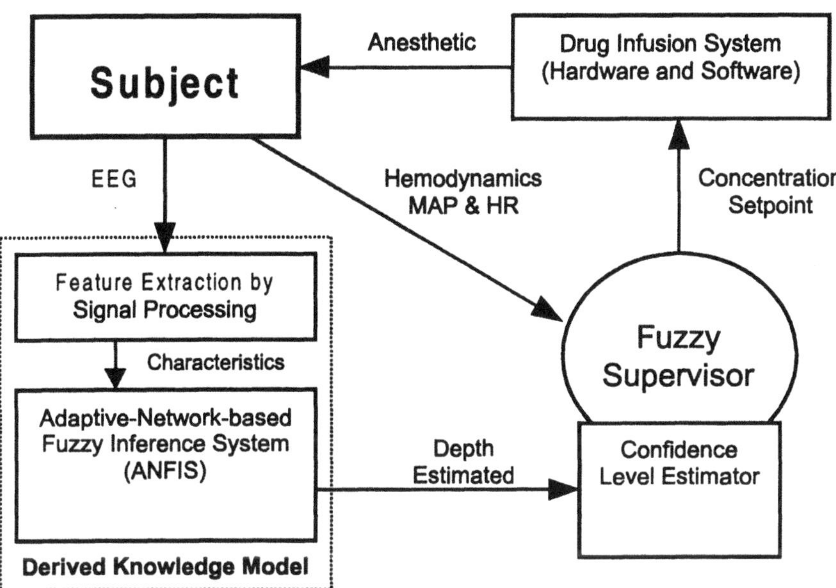

Figure 3 - Flowchart of the fuzzy control system for estimating and controlling depth of anesthesia. The derived fuzzy knowledge model is encircled by the dotted rectangle.

The fuzzy inference engine monitors the heart rate (HR) and mean arterial pressure (MAP) in response to the delivery of anesthetic medication for calculating the effectiveness of the current medication level based on these vital signs. The supervisor makes the last decision to raise or lower the anesthetic set-point concentrations as needed. Various safety mechanisms have been tested and built into the supervisor to safeguard the patient from anesthetic overdosing or underdosing caused by excessive disturbances. Depending on the type of anesthetic preferred, we can use syringe pumps for intravenous (IV) drugs (e.g. propofol or/and fentanyl) or anesthetic vaporizer for inhalational drugs (e.g. isoflurane, desflurane, or sevoflurane). In this example, we will use IV drugs. The syringe pump is driven by the drug's 3-compartment pharmocokinetic and pharmocodynamic (PK/PD) model.

Derived Knowledge Model Concept

Since a target site of action of general anesthetics is the brain, it is reasonable to monitor its activity by examining the brain waves (i.e. EEG and MLAEP), which can quantitatively measure anesthetic effects [17-21]. We prefer to use the EEG, since it is easier to collect under the clinical situation without too much trouble for the patient. In order to secure more DOA-related information by quantitative analyses for assessing the effects of anesthetic agents, we should combine different signal processing techniques. Moreover, the EEG signal is generated by a nonlinear mechanism, therefore, its non-linearity is an important factor to be taken into consideration during preprocessing of the signal. Nonlinear quantitative analysis in addition to spectral analysis of the EEG can improve the discrimination of sleep stages in human adults [22]. In our study, two new derived EEG nonlinear characteristics, complexity and regularity, along with spectral entropy will be used as input variables for the model.

The derived variables should be fuzzily weighted in order to weight each method differently as the EEG changes nonlinearly from light to deep anesthesia as well as with varying degrees of stimulation. The weighting scheme will optimize the strength of a particular signal processing method to correlate with the behavior of the EEG. Fortunately, this can be automatically accomplished by an adaptive-network-based fuzzy inference system (ANFIS), one kind of Takagi-Sugeno type fuzzy logic system, since it can automatically refine the coarse fuzzy if-then rules obtained from human's heuristics and experience, or derive the fuzzy if-then rules if human experts are not available (i.e., automatic elicitation of knowledge in the forms of fuzzy if-then rules). This capability is very important for designing the automated DOA control system, where there will be not enough expertise available to directly build the if-then rules, because anesthesiologists are not used to using the EEG derived parameters for monitoring DOA.

Moreover, complexity measure $C(n)$ and approximate entropy *ApEn* quantify complexity and regularity in a manner consistent with human intuition, and they are all model-independent statistics, which can be applied to any time series, deterministic or/and stochastic. The EEG is considered to contain both types of components. These measures help to understand and assess the complex levels of consciousness during anesthesia.

Methods

Feature Extraction and Data Set

Complexity Measure C(n): The complexity of the brain's activity under anesthesia can be measured from the 1-dimensional EEG signal by complexity analysis [23], initially proposed by Lempel and Ziv [24]. The EEG signal first is transformed into a finite symbol sequence S. For simplicity, we only consider a *0-1* string $s_1s_2\ldots s_n$, where $s_i \in \{0,1\}$, n is the length of data segment to be analyzed, i.e. the window length (*WL*). Thus, within the window the mean value of the data points $\{x_i \mid i=1,2,\ldots, n\}$ is estimated as $x_m = (1/n)\sum_{i=1}^{n} x_i$. Then x_i is compared with x_m for transforming the signal data into *0-1* string $s_1s_2\ldots s_n$: if $x_i < x_m$, $s_i=0$, otherwise $s_i=1$. According to [24], the computational algorithm of $c(n)$ can be described as below: Let S and Q denote, respectively, two strings, and SQ be the concatenation of S and Q, while string $SQ\pi$ is derived from SQ after its last character is deleted (π means the operation to delete the last character). Let $v(SQ\pi)$ denote the vocabulary of all different substrings of $SQ\pi$. At the beginning, $c(n)=1$, $S=s_1$, $Q=s_2$, therefore, $SQ\pi=s_1$. For generalization, now suppose $S=s_1s_2\ldots s_r$, $Q=s_{r+1}$; if $Q \in v(SQ\pi)$, then s_{r+1} is a substring of $s_1s_2\ldots s_r$, therefore S doesn't change, and renew Q to be $s_{r+1}s_{r+2}$, then judge if Q belongs to $v(SQ\pi)$ or not; and doing so this way until $Q \notin v(SQ\pi)$, now $Q=s_{r+1}s_{r+2}\ldots s_{r+i}$, which is not a substring of $s_1s_2\ldots s_rs_{r+1}\ldots s_{r+i+1}$, thus increase $c(n)$ by one. Thereafter combine S with Q, and S is renewed to be $S= s_1s_2\ldots s_rs_{r+1}\ldots s_{r+i}$, at the same time take Q as $Q=s_{r+i+1}$. Repeat above procedures until Q is the last character. At this time the number of different substrings of $s_1s_2\ldots s_n$ is $c(n)$, i.e. the measure of complexity.

In our study, we use the normalized complexity measure $C(n)$, since in practical application only relative values of $c(n)$ are meaningful and in particular it is the comparison with the $c(n)$ for a random string that is meaningful. The definition is as follow:

$$C(n) = \frac{c(n) \cdot \log_2{}^{n}}{hn} \qquad (3)$$

$0 \le C(n) \le 1$. where n is the length of the string, and h denotes the normalized source entropy. $C(n)$ reflects the rate of new patterns arising with the increase in string length. When n=3000, the time needed to estimate $C(n)$ is about 94 ms with an Intel 266 MHz Pentium II processor.

Compared with other complexity measure, such as correlation dimension, $C(n)$ is very easy to implement and does not require a large amount of data.

Approximate Entropy (ApEn): The degree of regularity in EEGs can be measured by *ApEn* without any *a priori* hypothesis about the system structure generating them. *ApEn* is a nonnegative number that will distinguish among data sets, with larger numbers indicating more irregularity and randomness.

Let the raw data be $\{x(1), x(2), \ldots, x(N)\}$, where N is the total number of data points. Two parameters must be fixed before *ApEn* can be computed: embedding dimension m of the vector to be formed, tolerance r functioning as a noise filter.

(1) Construct m-vectors $X(1)$~$X(N-m+1)$ defined by: $X(i)=[x(i), x(i+1), \ldots, x(i+m-1)]$, $i=1$~$N-m+1$.

(2) Define the distance between $X(i)$ and $X(j)$, $d[X(i), X(j)]$, as the maximum absolute difference between their corresponding scalar elements, such as the following equation where $d[X(i), X(j)] = \max_{k=0\sim m-1} [|x(i+k) - x(j+k)|]$.

(3) For a given $X(i)$, count the number of j ($j=1$~$N-m+1$, $j \neq i$) such that $d[X(i),X(j)] \leq r$, denoted as $N^m(i)$. Then, for $i=1$~$N-m+1$, $C_r^m(i) = N^m(i)/(N-m+1)$.

(4) Take the natural logarithm of each $C_r^m(i)$, and average it over i,

$$\phi^m(r) = \frac{1}{N-m+1} \sum_{i=1}^{N-m+1} \ln C_r^m(i)$$

(5) Increase the dimension to $m+1$. Repeat steps (1)~(4) and find $C_r^{m+1}(i)$, $\phi^{m+1}(r)$.

(6) Theoretically, the approximate entropy is defined as

$$ApEn(m,r) = \lim_{N \to \infty} [\phi^m(r) - \phi^{m+1}(r)]$$

In actual practice, the number of data points N is finite and the result obtained through the above steps is the estimate of *ApEn* which can be denoted as $ApEn(m,r,N) = \phi^m(r) - \phi^{m+1}(r)$. Obviously, the value of the estimate depends on m and r. As suggested by Pincus *et al.* [25], m and r can be taken as 2 and $(0.1\sim0.25)SD_x$, respectively, where SD_x is the standard deviation of the original data sequence. In our study, m=2, r=$0.25SD_x$, N=1000.

The needed calculation time for *ApEn* is about 3911 ms, which exponentially increases with the window length. Obviously, it is far slower than the computation of $C(n)$. This further demonstrates the advantages of $C(n)$: simper and faster calculation.

Spectral Entropy Analysis : In addition to nonlinear quantitative measures, spectral entropy (*SE*) is selected as the third derived parameter in our study. This measure quantifies the spectral complexity of the EEG signal. The power spectral density (PSD) $\hat{P}(f)$ can be obtained from the EEG signal by a fast Fourier transform (FFT). $\hat{P}(f)$ is a density function, i.e., it represents the distribution of power as a function of frequency. The normalization of $\hat{P}(f)$, with respect to the total spectral power, will yield a probability density function (*pdf*). Application of Shannon's channel entropy gives an estimation of the spectral entropy (*SE*) of the underlying EEG process, where entropy is given as

$$H = \sum_f p_f \ln(1/p_f) \qquad (4)$$

p_f is the *pdf* value at frequency *f*. Heuristically, the entropy has been interpreted as a measure of uncertainty about the event at *f*. High uncertainty (entropy) is due to a large number of processes, whereas low entropy is due to a small number of dominating processes, which make up the EEG signal. The *SE* calculated by FFT with a window length of 1024 data points consumes about 7 ms.

Data Set: These three derived parameters and the corresponding dog's state (movement "0" and asleep "1") are constructed into a data set.

Adaptive Network Based Fuzzy Inference System (ANFIS)

Combining neural-nets and fuzzy logic, ANFIS [26], a five-layer adaptive network architecture, represents a Takagi-Sugeno type fuzzy system [14] using a continuous linear function as the output instead of a group of fuzzy membership functions used in Mamdani type fuzzy system. A neuro-fuzzy learning control system, such as ANFIS, has many advantages, including integrating the greater learning capability of neural networks with fuzzy logic systems to form the initial membership functions to manage the system efficiently and accurately.

Figure 4 shows a simple ANFIS that has two inputs *x* and *y*, one output *f*, and two fuzzy if-then rules:

Rule 1: If x is A_1 and y is B_1 then $f_1=p_1x+q_1y+r_1$
Rule 2: If x is A_2 and y is B_2 then $f_2=p_2x+q_2y+r_2$

where, A_i and B_i are linguistic labels of fuzzy sets, stipulated by membership functions. "x is A_i" means that x belongs to the fuzzy set labeled A_i with a membership degree $0<\mu_{Ai}\leq 1$.

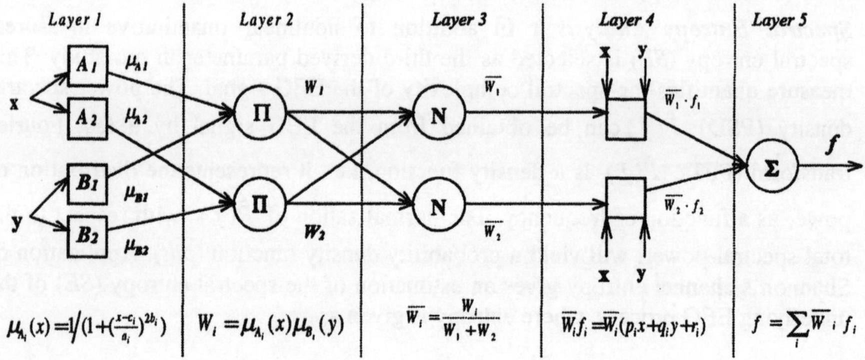

Figure 4 - A two inputs one output ANFIS based on Takagi-Sugeno model.

Layer 1: Each node in this layer generates bell-shaped membership grades of a linguistic label. Parameters $\{a_i, b_i, c_i\}$ are referred to as *the premise parameters*, which change the shape and position of the membership function.

Layer 2: Each node in this layer calculates the firing strength (W_i) of a rule.

Layer 3: Node i in this layer calculates the ratio ($\overline{W_i}$) of the i-th rule's firing strength to the total of all firing strengths.

Layer 4: Node i in this layer computes the contribution ($\overline{W_i} \cdot f_i$) of i-th rule toward the overall output. Parameters $\{p_i, q_i, r_i\}$ are referred to as the *consequent parameters*, which specify the output of each rule.

Layer 5: The single node in this layer computes the overall output (f) as the summation of contribution from each rule.

The ANFIS employs a hybrid learning scheme that combines a back-propagation-type gradient descent algorithm for adjusting the *premise parameters*, with a recursive least-squares estimation algorithm for adjusting the *consequent parameters* [26]. A step in the learning procedure has two parts. In the first part, the input patterns are propagated, and the optimal consequent parameters are estimated by a recursive least mean squares procedure, while the premise parameters are assumed to be fixed for the current cycle through the training set. In the second part the patterns are propagated again, and in this epoch back-propagation is used to modify the premise parameters by gradient descent, while the consequent parameters remain fixed. This procedure is then iterated. The structure of ANFIS ensures that each linguistic term is represented by only one fuzzy set. By learning, ANFIS can get the last member function and consequent parameters.

The proposed ANFIS architecture can identify the near-optimal membership functions and other parameters of a rule base for achieving a desired input-output mapping. Without resorting to human experts, using ANFIS we can construct a fuzzy controller to perform a prescribed control task. However, ANFIS does not exclude *a priori* knowledge, which can generally provide a better starting point to train the ANFIS, thus reducing the convergence time and improving the results.

In our study, the ANFIS used contains 8 rules, with 2 membership functions being assigned to each input variable (total 3 variables, *C(n)*, *ApEn*, and *SE*) and the total number of fitting parameters is 50, which are composed of 18 premise parameters and 32 consequent parameters. Such an ANFIS model has the potential to improve DOA estimation accuracy while retaining the structural knowledge, which is particularly useful for anesthesiologists to understand the process of the model.

After being trained, the ANFIS only need perform forward computing for estimating DOA. The time needed is about 1 ms.

The derived knowledge about DOA in the form of fuzzy if-then rules along with the three derived parameters is constructed as a "derived knowledge model" (in Figure 3). Such model has the potential to improve DOA estimation accuracy while retaining the structural knowledge, which is particularly useful for anesthesiologists to understand the process of the inference system, since it expresses the relationship between DOA and the EEG-derived parameters in the form of if-then rules.

The main concern about the derived knowledge model (see Figure 3) in real-time clinical application is the time needed to estimate the DOA. Adding the times needed to calculate *C*(*n*), *ApEn*, and *SE*, as well as the ANFIS forward computing time, we obtain the total time needed to estimate the DOA: 3911+94+7+1=4015 ms = 4.015 s. Therefore, our proposed scheme is computationally fast, feasible and suitable for real-time on-line application, where every 10 s one DOA estimation is enough. One example of the results in continuously estimating DOA during a dog experiment is shown in Figure 7.
The software for performing this system is developed using the Borland C++ language.

Fuzzy Supervisor

Patient safety is one of the most critical issues in designing any automated systems suitable for any clinical use. To this end, we have designed a rule-based supervisor to oversee the closed-loop operation and take necessary actions to safeguard the subject. The basic concept regarding the supervisor design is found in [27], according to which the supervisor has 3 levels. Because fuzzy systems are, in essence, expert systems dealing with uncertainty, perhaps the most appropriate application for them in DOA control is in the design of the supervisor.

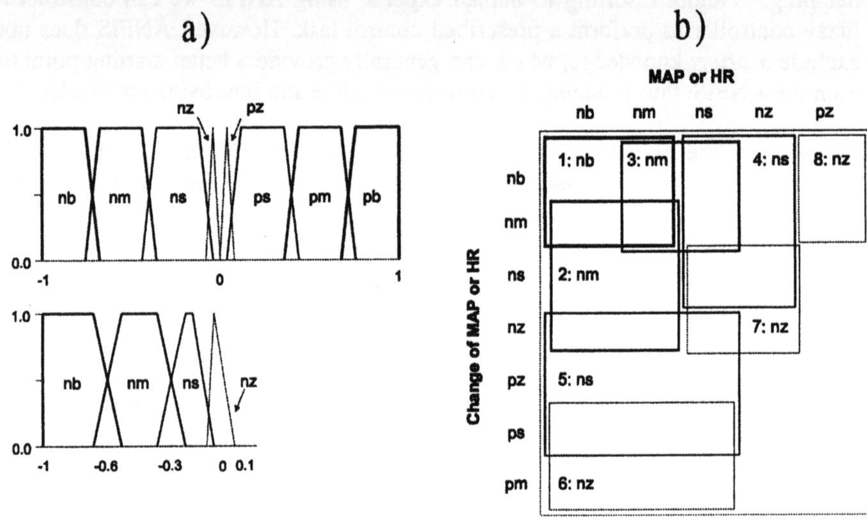

Figure 5 - Fuzzy Inference Engine for $[Prop]_{sp}$ Decrementation. **(a)** Fuzzy membership function set for the fuzzification of HR and MAP (up). Fuzzy membership function set for the fuzzification of Propofol reduction (bottom). The shapes of the memberships were designed for a exponential reduction. Notice the non-symmetrical membership function of 'nz' which allows Propofol reduction level to lower down to zero. **(b)** Two-input-one-output fuzzy rule table used by the inference engine when either HR or MAP is not present. The labels for "MAP or HR" and "Change of MAP or HR" include all possible antecedents. Each rule is represented by a block with a corresponding rule number and the fuzzified consequence. These rules are obtained from anesthesiologists. (The four-input-one-output fuzzy rule table contained 90 rules is available online. This four-dimensional rule table is used when both MAP and HR are present).

When the ANFIS has determined that the subject is not responsive, it is often necessary to ensure that it has not been a consequence of over-dosing, which may result in depression of the hemodynamics. A dual-ruleset fuzzy inference engine (Figure 5) based on the Mamdani type of fuzzy control [13] is incorporated as part of the supervisor for lowering the anesthetic by evaluating either or both MAP and HR. The defuzzification process utilizes the center of gravity approach (Equation 2) where the current levels of MAP and HR and the rates of their changes are used as inputs for determining the amount of anesthetic reduction required using a four-input-one-output rule set (90 rules). However, when either MAP or HR is not available or is corrupted, the inference engine will switch automatically to using a two-input-one-output ruleset (8 rules) as shown in Figure 5 (b).

The supervisor continuously monitors the controller's output (i.e. the concentration set-point), if there is a conflict between the set-point and the DOA, it will take some actions to avoid the conflict or to override erratic controller actions caused by external disturbances. The supervisor is equipped with rules intended for basic patient safety. For example, the maximum input concentration will be limited to 12 ug/ml and minimum 2 ug/ml for propofol. The limit will prevent the possibility of patient overdose and also awareness due to light anesthesia, given the chance that there could be an equipment malfunction. If the systolic blood pressure drops below a critical lower limit the anesthetic will be shut off. In this event, the user is directed to increase the rate of fluid infusion to support the MAP, and if necessary, infuse vasoactive drugs [28].

Drug Infusion System (Hardware and Software)

Since direct means of sampling the concentrations of intravenous anesthetics is not available on a continuous basis, the Propofol concentrations are estimated by a 3-compartment mathematical model,

$$Concentration = Ae^{-\alpha t} + Be^{-\beta t} + Ce^{-\gamma t} + D \qquad (5)$$

The Tackley *et al.* parameter set [29] is used which has been found to have a lesser bias and a greater accuracy as compared to most existing parameter sets [30, 31]. The three compartmental analysis is performed by estimating the three rate constants α, γ, and β (rapid and slow distribution, and elimination). A, B, C, and D are constant when describing a constant rate infusion and are complex functions of time when characterizing an exponentially decreasing infusion.

The program STANPUMP [45] uses this model to control the rate of propofol infusion, via syringe pump, to obtain the desired plasma concentration of the drug.

Experiments and Results

Dog Experiments and EEG Data

The dog experiments (approved by the Institute Animal Care Committee) were conducted using mongrel dogs weighing 15-20 kg under propofol anesthesia. A rapid, ultrashort-acting intravenous anesthetic, Brevital (2mg/kg), was used for initial induction of anesthesia. This was followed by a short-acting muscle relaxant Succinylcholine Chloride (1mg/kg) for facilitating orotracheal intubation. The dog's lungs were ventilated mechanically with 100% oxygen using a Ohmeda 7000 ventilator, and body temperature was maintained 35.5 to 37 °C during the experiment. A peripheral vein catheter was used to infuse propofol and to replace fluids (6-8 ml/kg/h lactated Ringer's solution), and a radial artery catheter was used for continuous measurement of arterial blood pressure. Anesthesia was maintained with propofol titrated by one computer-controlled Harvard Apparatus Syringe Infusion Pump (Model 2400-003). STANPUMP software was used to simultaneously control the pump and to estimate the internal propofol concentrations using the 3-compartment PK/PD model. End-tidal CO_2 ($EtCO_2$) and arterial oxygen saturation were monitored using a Criticare Systems POET Capnograph and a Nellcor Oximeter. The ECG leads were placed by needle electrodes or Red dot™ Ag/AgCl electrodes. The EEG platinum subdermal needle electrodes, type E2 (Grass Instrument Company, Quincy, MA), were placed to collect two channels of EEG (right frontal-right occipital and left frontal-left occipital) simultaneously. Arterial pressure and ECG were monitored using a Mennen Horizon monitor, and EEG signals were monitored by an Axon Systems Sentine-4 EEG/EP monitor. Thus, total monitoring included heart rate (HR), ECG, systolic and diastolic blood pressure, respiration, two EEG channels, and movement (by visualization). All analog signals were collected by a DELL Optiplex (Intel 266 MHz) computer equipped with a Data Translation™ analog to digital input board. The digital data (heart rate and blood pressure) were directly collected into the computer via serial ports.

The training and the testing data were gathered during the experiment by changing propofol concentration set-points between 2 and 12 ug/ml in steps of 1.0ug/ml. At each new set-point, a minimum of a 10-min stabilization period was allowed for the equilibration between the plasma and effect site concentrations. Towards the end of each interval, a 30-s tail clamping, considered as a supramaximal stimulus in dogs [32], was applied to assess response. During each tail clamping, the determination for grading a positive response (awake)(depth 0) and a negative response (asleep)(depth 1) were estimated by observing (1) any animal head or extremities movements, (2) spontaneous changes in $EtCO_2$ respiration pattern, (3) changes in HR or blood pressure.

Throughout the study, the dog was observed for inadequate ventilation. Inadequate ventilation was defined as an end-tidal carbon dioxide partial pressure exceeding 46 mmHg, and/or an oxygen saturation of less than 90%. If necessary, ventilation was assisted with a mask and bag to maintain the end-tidal carbon dioxide partial pressure below 46 mmHg, and the oxygen saturation greater than 90%.

Results

Fuzzy if-then Rules of the Derived Knowledge Model and Test Results

Before training, the consequent parameters of the ANFIS are all set (initialized) to zero. As a conventional way of setting parameters in a fuzzy system, the premise parameters are set (initialized) in a way that the membership function (MF) can cover the domain interval (or the universe of discourse) completely, with sufficient overlapping (see Figure 2).

After training by only propofol EEG data sets, the 8 fuzzy rules are obtained for the ANFIS as follows, where $\vec{X}^T$=[*C(n)*, *ApEn*, *SE*, 1] and $\vec{c}_i$ is the *i*th row of the following *consequent parameter* matrix ***C***:

if *C(n)* is $SMALL_1$ and *ApEn* is $SMALL_2$ and *SE* is $SMALL_3$, then
OUTPUT=$\vec{c}_1 \cdot \vec{X}$
if *C(n)* is $SMALL_1$ and *ApEn* is $SMALL_2$ and *SE* is $LARGE_3$, then
OUTPUT=$\vec{c}_2 \cdot \vec{X}$
if *C(n)* is $SMALL_1$ and *ApEn* is $LARGE_2$ and *SE* is $SMALL_3$, then
OUTPUT=$\vec{c}_3 \cdot \vec{X}$
if *C(n)* is $SMALL_1$ and *ApEn* is $LARGE_2$ and *SE* is $LARGE_3$, then
OUTPUT=$\vec{c}_4 \cdot \vec{X}$
if *C(n)* is $LARGE_1$ and *ApEn* is $SMALL_2$ and *SE* is $SMALL_3$, then
OUTPUT=$\vec{c}_5 \cdot \vec{X}$
if *C(n)* is $LARGE_1$ and *ApEn* is $SMALL_2$ and *SE* is $LARGE_3$, then
OUTPUT=$\vec{c}_6 \cdot \vec{X}$
if *C(n)* is $LARGE_1$ and *ApEn* is $LARGE_2$ and *SE* is $SMALL_3$, then
OUTPUT=$\vec{c}_7 \cdot \vec{X}$
if *C(n)* is $LARGE_1$ and *ApEn* is $LARGE_2$ and *SE* is $LARGE_3$, then
OUTPUT=$\vec{c}_8 \cdot \vec{X}$

$$C = \begin{bmatrix} \vec{c}_1 \\ \vec{c}_2 \\ \vec{c}_3 \\ \vec{c}_4 \\ \vec{c}_5 \\ \vec{c}_6 \\ \vec{c}_7 \\ \vec{c}_8 \end{bmatrix} = \begin{bmatrix} 0.26 & -0.95 & 1.14 & -2.38 \\ -1.51 & 0.47 & 2.88 & -9.46 \\ -7.32 & 7.48 & -0.75 & -0.77 \\ -0.73 & 0.06 & 0.03 & 0.46 \\ -158.52 & 206.01 & -68.93 & 171.67 \\ 105.13 & -52.98 & 3.07 & -33.00 \\ 58.49 & 1.22 & 4.72 & -58.15 \\ -1.75 & -4.08 & 0.30 & 5.26 \end{bmatrix}$$

The linguistic labels *SMALL$_i$* and *LARGE$_i$* (i=1 to 3) are defined by the bell membership function (with different *premise parameters a, b,* and *c*):

$$\mu_A(x) = 1 \Big/ \left(1 + \left[\left(\frac{x-c}{a}\right)^2\right]^b\right) \quad (6)$$

The membership functions are shown in Figure 6. Table 1 lists the linguistic labels and the corresponding parameters in Equation 6.

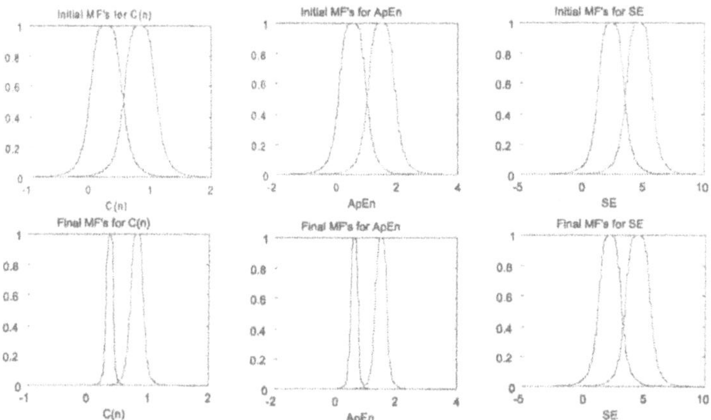

Figure 6 - The initial and final membership functions for the ANFIS trained by Propofol EEG.

Table 1 - The final premise parameter obtained by training the ANFIS using Propofol EEG.

Parameters	Linguistic Labels	Final MF's Parameters		
		a	*b*	*C*
$C(n)$	SMALL_1	0.0634	2.0993	0.3669
	LARGE_1	0.1181	2.0214	0.8165
ApEn	SMALL_2	0.1269	2.0702	0.6208
	LARGE_2	0.2060	2.0576	1.4990
SE	SMALL_3	0.9843	1.9516	2.1717
	LARGE_3	1.0848	2.1092	4.4549

By learning, ANFIS can automatically elicit knowledge in the form of fuzzy if-then rules. Therefore, in a sense its ability of knowledge acquisition can help the anesthesiologist use these new EEG derived-parameters for assessing DOA.

There are 134 EEG recordings, each approximately 10 minutes in length. To determine the estimation ability of the obtained derived knowledge model, a cross-validation method using the "*leave-one-out*" procedure is used. In short, a model is constructed from the data obtained from n-1 dogs by leaving one dog out and the data from this dog is used for testing. This is repeated for all n dogs. Because the excluded dog's data are not used to develop the model, the difference between the model output and the true anesthesia states is nearly unbiased estimate of the estimation ability of the model. The performance of the obtained final model is quantified by the results of the n cross-validations. Test results are tabulated in Table 2.

Table 2 - Test results by the derived knowledge model using the "leave-one-out" procedure for the Propofol experiments.

State	**Sensitivity** (%)	**Specificity** (%)	**Accuracy** (%)
Awake	92.3	88.4	90.3
Asleep	88.4	92.3	90.3

Sensitivity = TP/(TP+FN),
Specificity = TN/(TN+FP),
Accuracy =(TP+TN)/(TP+FN+TN+FP),

where: TP =true positive, FN =false negative, TN =true negative, FP =false positive.

By just using 95% spectral edge frequency to discriminate the awake and asleep states, the accuracy is 70.2% over the same EEG database. Also by dog experiments under propofol anesthesia, MLAEPs achieved a 89.2% accuracy for classifying the awake and asleep states [7]. Therefore, our results in Table II are comparable with these results and demonstrate a little better.

Simulation on the On-line Operation of the Model

Using the derived if-then rules, we obtain a derived knowledge model (see Figure 3). We have applied this model to analyze part of the raw EEG data collected during one dog experiment under Propofol anesthesia (see Figure 7). The windows for calculating the three characteristics ($C(n)$, *ApEn*, and *SE*) move forward 500 data points (5 sec.) every time for the next DOA estimation. Thus, for the calculation of $C(n)$ there is an overlap (2500 data points) in EEG data segments between two consecutive DOA estimations, for *ApEn* the overlap is 500 data points, for *SE* 524 data points.

During the experiment, the anesthesia state is being changed by adjusting the Propofol concentration setpoint (Cs). The estimated DOA continuously demonstrates different values to track anesthesia states and state transitions in real time, and the value of DOA is consistent with the dog's true anesthesia states assessed by the clinician at observation points. The deeper the depth of anesthesia, the higher the value of the output of the model. The value decreases while decreasing the depth of anesthesia (from asleep to awake). Moreover, the output of the model is sensitive enough to the changes in the EEG caused by the anesthetic agent, which correlates well with the depth of anesthesia (see the test result for all Propofol EEG data sets in Table II).

In Figure 7 we can see that an intuitive idea for discriminating asleep and awake states is to compare the output of the model with one pre-selected threshold (e.g. 0.5), above which is asleep and below which is awake. Figure 7 a, c, and d show that the estimated DOA has decreased to a lower value for a period of time before the dog starts moving or responds from an asleep state. This means, by use of a "lower threshold" (e.g. 0.3) the output of the model has the ability to predict movement during anesthesia. This is of important clinical significance since avoiding awareness during surgery is a major concern. Furthermore, monitoring the trend of the estimated DOA also allows the clinician to anticipate when the subject will recover. In the same way, by the use of a "higher threshold" (e.g. 0.8) we can avoid having the subject too deeply anesthetized.

Although we only grade the depth of anesthesia to awake (0.0) and asleep (1.0), just two levels, Figure 7 shows that after training the model can automatically estimate the intermediate states (between asleep and awake) and give a value between 1.0 and 0.0 to track the gradual transitions. This shows that the model has strong ability to implement non-linear decision boundaries and can handle the transition between awake and asleep states.

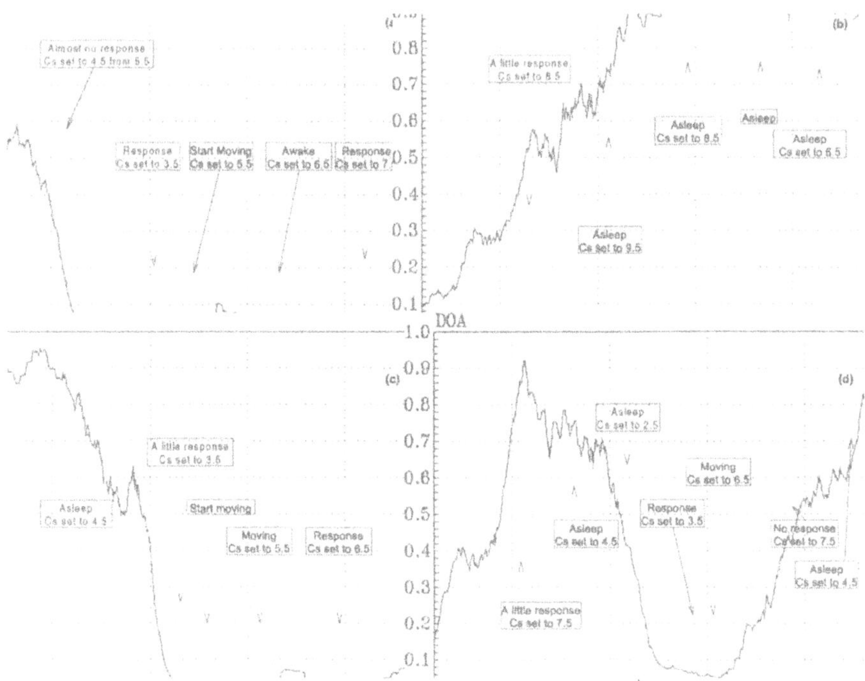

Figure 7 - The continuously estimated DOA by the derived knowledge model versus time under different anesthesia situations during part of one dog experiment using Propofol. Cs denotes the Propofol concentration (*u*g/ml) setpoint at the site of drug effect. The annotation on the figure indicates the state and the concentration set at that observation point.

Discussion and Future Progress

Regarding the Test Results

Based on ANFIS modeling, we construct a derived knowledge model for quantitatively estimating the depth of anesthesia. By effectively eliciting the fuzzy if-then rules, the model provides a semantically transparent way for anesthesiologist to address the DOA estimation problem by using the EEG-derived parameters. It demonstrates good performance for the Propofol anesthetic regimen (Table 2) and real-time feasibility (see the previous section). All these make it a promising candidate as an effective tool for continuous assessment of the depth of anesthesia under clinical situations. However, more experiments and studies are needed to test its effectiveness on other types of anesthetics (inhalational and intravenous).

Simultaneous Administration of Two IV Drugs

Although the use of inhalational agents in surgical anesthesia remains popular, anesthesiologists are increasing the use of intravenous (IV) anesthesia techniques, often relying totally on IV methods. The advantages are shorter induction and recovery time, reduced major side effects and complications, and firmer control of pharmacodynamic effects. Moreover, the following factors also make it easy to effectively use intravenous techniques in clinical practice: pharmacokinetic/ pharmadynamic (PK/PD) studies on the drugs; the availability of small, reliable, easy-to-use, computer-controllable syringe pumps; and the availability of PK/PD model-driven drug delivery software. In this chapter we have used the IV drug, propofol, as an example to design our DOA fuzzy control system.

There is not an IV anesthetic which can alone provide all the necessary components of general anesthesia, so in clinical practice a sedative-hypnotic (e.g. propofol) and an opioid analgesic (e.g. fentanyl) are usually used in combination to produce total intravenous anesthesia (TIVA). TIVA can reduce the dose requirements of the individual agents, supplement one another and provide satisfactory anesthetic conditions to various noxious stimuli [33-35], and increase the speed and quality of emergence, thereby prevent excessive intraoperative dosing and subsequent delayed post-anesthetic recovery [33, 36]. Therefore, to make our system feasible for TIVA clinical practice, we have extended the system to control two or more IV drugs.

When a hypnotic and an analgesic are used in combination, the anesthesiologist is confronted with the dilemma of whether to vary the hypnotic or the opioid. The latest studies of the quantitative interaction of hypnotic and opioids [33, 37-42] can help overcome this dilemma. We built a Propofol and Fentanyl interaction model (see the simulation results shown in Figure 8) according to the population-based interaction relationship between Propofol and opioid [41, 42], and incorporated it into our Automated Anesthesia Management System [7, 43] for realizing the simultaneous administration of two drugs for TIVA. According to the interaction model, the system can optimally determine the infusion rate of one drug while another one is being infused.

Once the two-drug interaction model is obtained, the DOA fuzzy control system can be easily extended to simultaneously control two drugs. The Drug Infusion System in Figure 3 is replaced by Figure 9. The Modified STANPUMP software [44] is used by one computer to simultaneously drive two pumps for delivering two different IV drugs, such as Propofol and Fentanyl. It is modified from the STANPUMP software [45] initially developed by Professor S. Shafer for one IV drug delivery.

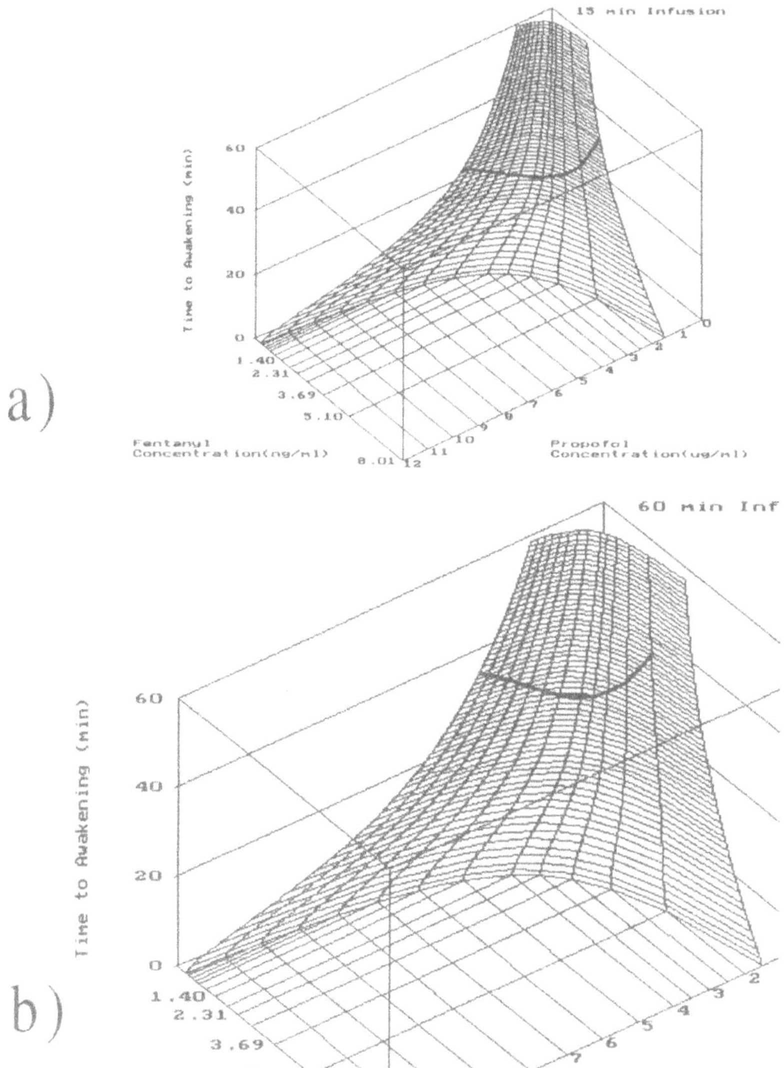

Figure 8 - Computer simulation of the effect site Propofol and Fentanyl concentrations *vs.* time during the first 60 min after termination of target-controlled infusions of Propofol and Fentanyl that had been maintained for 15 and 60, respectively, at constant target concentration combinations associated with a 95% probability of no response to surgical stimuli. These concentration combinations are represented by the curved line on the bottom of the figure in the x-y plane. The decrease in the concentrations after various intraoperative Propofol-Fentanyl combinations is represented by the curves running upward from the x-y plane. The curved lines in parallel to the x-y plane represent consecutive 1-min intervals. The bold line represents the Propofol-Fentanyl-time relationship at which return of consciousness occurs in 50% of the patients. The optimal concentration combination is represented by the lowest point on the bold awakening line. The estimated time to awakening is represented by the distance between this point and the nearest point on the curve in the x-y plane.

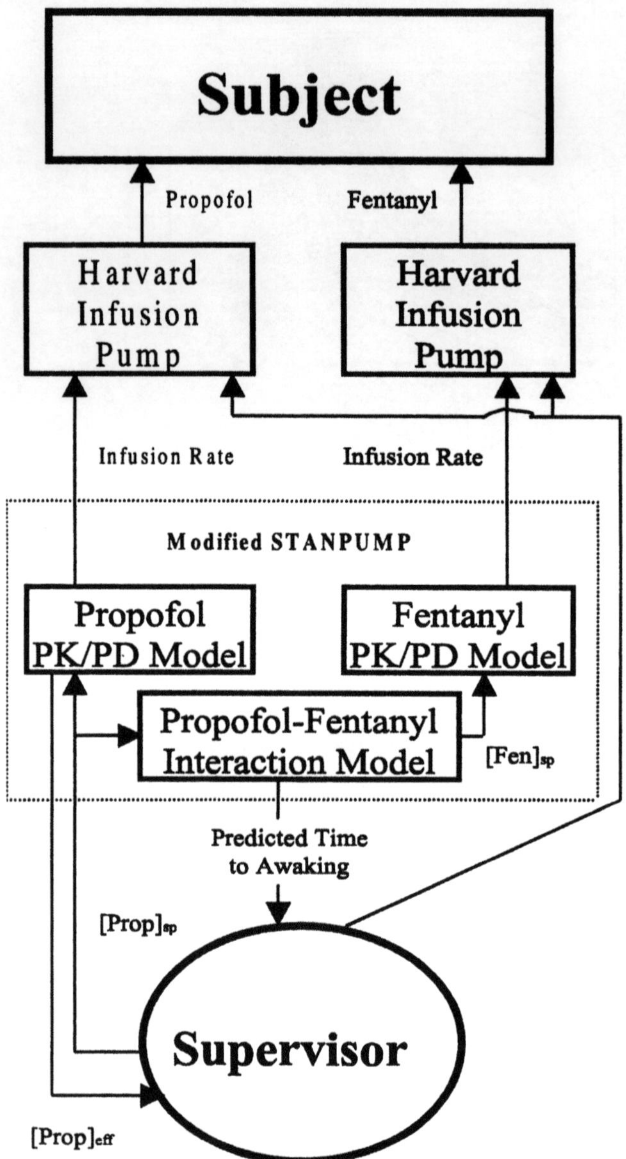

Figure 9 - System diagram of the closed-loop TIVA administration (just showing the Drug Infusion System part in Figure 3, other parts being the same as Figure 3). $[Prop]_{sp}$, $[Fent]_{sp}$, and $[Prop]_{eff}$ denotes Propofol set-point concentration, Fentanyl set-point concentration, and Propofol effect-site concentration, respectively.

Adaptivity of Fuzzy Logic System in Anesthesia Control

Regardless of the adaptation method used, there are several interconnected means of allowing a fuzzy system to adapt. These methods [46, 47] include the management of the weights attached to the rules, the dynamic hedging of the fuzzy regions, the structural modification of the fuzzy sets, the redefinition of truth in the fuzzy model, the selection of alternative methods of defuzzification, and the refining of fuzzy ruleset. Some of the concepts that are applicable to fuzzy control of anesthesia delivery are as follows:

Fuzzy Rule-Weight Management

The *Fuzzy Rule-Weight Management* is different from the *Input Weight Scheme*, one of the major challenges stated earlier in the design of a fuzzy controller based on a physician-knowledge model. The *Input Weight Scheme* places weight on each of the input variables, which are dynamically adjusted to emulate an anesthesiologist's emphasis on some observable input parameters over the others. In *Fuzzy Rule-Weight Management*, weights are placed on each of the fuzzy rules to reflect the adjustments made by an anesthesiologist in compensating the intra-patient differences in drug sensitivity on the observable parameters.

Its implementation is similar to that of neural networks and the training can be done with back propagation, where the error is determined by some arbitrary transfer function for the anesthetic infused and the state variables. The outcome of active rule-weight management are the amplification of those rules that consistently contributed more to the output and dampening of those rules that have contributed less. Effectively, the central control region is shifted in response to the changes in the localization of the inputs as the weight for each rule is adjusted. The results are faster convergence and multi-dimensional adaptation permitting dynamic handling of a wider patient population.

Fuzzy Regions Dynamic Hedging

The shape broadening and narrowing of the fuzzy terms has always been an active area of research in adaptive fuzzy systems. Essentially, if the controller output is lower/higher than the desired output, then all the fuzzy terms accessed during that iteration would be broadened/narrowed, respectively. The shape alteration of the fuzzy terms is therefore proportional to the error feedback from the previous output cycle. Although this adaptation is analogous to adjustments made by the anesthesiologist for a particular patient, mathematically, the control actions are refined and smoothed while providing localization effects on the inputs during the inference process. Therefore, the rate of convergence is often enhanced, and at the same time, less erratic system responses are observed.

In addition, dynamic hedging can be applied to the output fuzzy terms when not all the inputs are available. For example, when one of the multiple inputs is not available, the output of a particular rule that considers the missing input is therefore less certain. Hedging therefore increases its ambiguity.

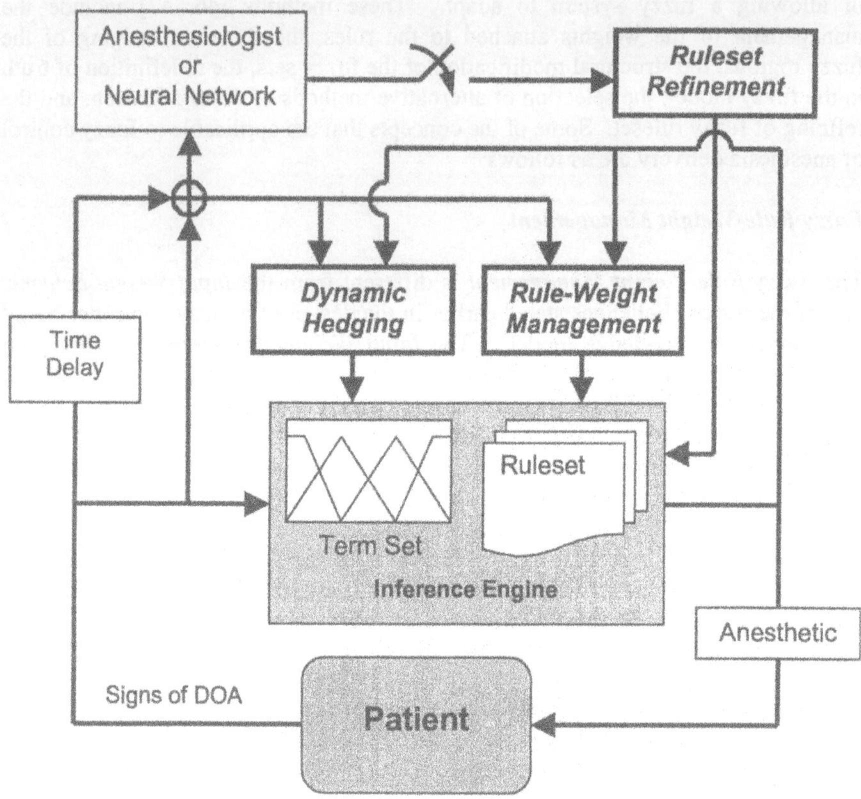

Figure 10 - Three of the fuzzy controller adaptation methods applicable in anesthesia delivery control are shown. Dynamic hedging modifies the fuzzy term set while rule-weight management manipulates the contributions of each rule in the ruleset. Activated only during the learning phase, ruleset refinement enhances the fuzzy ruleset and sharpens the fuzzy term set on the original basic fuzzy rule and fuzzy term "factory-sets".

Fuzzy Ruleset Refinement

Refining the fuzzy ruleset opens up the possibility of handling different anesthetics or physician's preferences by a control system using a rule table that can be adaptively refined as the system is being used online. There are several approaches to refining the ruleset online. For example, in the case of having a new anesthetic used (or added), a default system can start with only three fuzzy members and a limited fundamental basic ruleset written by the developer. The control system starts as an open loop system during initialization period. The original ruleset is refined with the creation of more members and with new rules written by the physician added during the learning mode. After a while, the control system closes the loop when some error function is minimized. Alternatively, this process can be assisted with a neural network similar to the ANFIS system discussed previously to minimize the involvement of an operator.

Task-Oriented Control

Many of the applications of fuzzy control are task control systems rather than "set point" control systems. Currently, the field is moving toward task-oriented control [16]. The DOA control can be treated as a problem of task-oriented control from the prospective of an anesthesiologist. When this task is viewed from this prospective, we need to get away from the thinking of "set point control" and embrace the concept of "task control" for replacing human functions. The success of such a DOA control system would benefit from the comprehensive application of signal processing and intelligent technology, such as rule-based algorithms, artificial neural networks, expert systems, and fuzzy logic.

Nomenclature

ANFIS	Adaptive Network-based Fuzzy Inference System
ApEn	Approximate Entropy
BSA	Body Surface Area
$C(n)$	Complexity Measure
COG	Center of Gravity
DOA	Depth of Anesthesia
ECG	Electrocardiogram
EEG	Electroencephalogram
$EtCO_2$	End-tidal CO_2
HR	Heart Rate
IV	Intravenous
MAP	Mean Arterial Pressure
MF	Membership Function
MLAEP	Mid-Latency Auditory Evoked Potentials
pdf	probability density fucntion
PK/PD	Pharmocokinetic / Pharmocodynamic
$[Prop]_{sp}$	Propofol set-point concentration
PSD	Power Spectral Density
SE	Spectral Entropy
TIVA	Total Intravenous Anesthesia
WL	Window Length

References

1. Ranta SOV, Laurila R, Saario J, Ali-Melkkila T, and Hynynen M, "Awareness with recall during general anesthesia: incidence and risk factors." *Anesth Analg*, 86:1084-9, 1998.
2. Guignard B, Menigaux C, Dupont X, and Chauvin M. "Fuzzy logic closed loop system for propofol administration using bispectral index and hemodynamics", *Anesthesiology*, 89(3A):A1218, 1998.
3. Zhang X.-S. and Roy RJ, "Depth of anesthesia estimation by adaptive-network-based fuzzy inference system", *Proceedings of The First Joint BMES/EMBS Conference*, Atlanta, Georgia, p.391, Oct. 1999
4. Asbury AJ and Tzabar Y, "Fuzzy logic: new ways of thinking for anaesthesia", *British Journal of Anaesthesia*, vol.75, no.1, pp.1-10, 1995.
5. Abbod MF and Linkens DA, "Anaesthesia monitoring and control using fuzzy logic fusion", *Biomedical Engineering Application, Basis Communications*, vol. 10, no.4, pp.225-235, 1998.
6. Elkfafi M, Shieh JS, Linkens DA, and Peacock JE, "Fuzzy logic for auditory evoked response monitoring and control of depth of anaesthesia", *Fuzzy Sets and Systems*, vol. 100, no.1, pp.29-43, 1998.
7. Huang JW, Lu Y-Y, Nayak A, and Roy RJ, "Depth of anesthesia estimation and control", *IEEE Transaction on Biomedical Engineering*, 46(1): 71-81, 1999.
8. Huang JW, and Roy RJ, "Multiple-drug hemodynamic control using fuzzy decision theory", *IEEE Transaction on Biomedical Engineering*, 45(2):213-228, 1998.
9. Held CM, and Roy RJ, "Multiple drug hemodynamic control by means of a supervisory-fuzzy rule-based adaptive control system: validation on a model", *IEEE Transaction on Biomedical Engineering*, 42(4): 371-385, 1995.
10. Huang JW, Held CM, and Roy RJ, "Hemodynamic management with multiple drugs using fuzzy logic", in (Teodorescu H-N, Kandel A, and Jain LC, eds): *Fuzzy and neuro-fuzzy systems in medicine*, CRC Press (Boca Raton, London, New York, and Washington DC), chapter 11(pp.319-340), 1999.
11. Nayak A, and Roy RJ, "Anesthesia control using midlatency auditory evoked potentials", *IEEE Trans. on Biomedical Engineering*, 45(4):409-421, 1998.
12. Sebel PS and Lowdon JD, "Propofol: A new intravenous anesthetic", *Anesthesiology*, vol.71, pp. 260-277, 1989.
13. Mamdani EH, and Assilian S, "An experiment in linguistic synthesis with a fuzzy logic controller", *Int. J. Man-Machine Studies*, 7(1):1-13, 1975.
14. Takagi T, and Sugeno M, "Fuzzy identification of systems and its applications to modeling and control", *IEEE Trans. on Systems, Man, and Cybernetics*, 15:116-132, 1985.
15. Sugeno M, and Kang GT, "Structure identification of fuzzy model", *Fuzzy Sets and Systems*, 28:15-33, 1988.
16. Abramovitch DY and Bushnell LG, "Report on the fuzzy versus conventional control debate", *IEEE Control Systems*, pp.88-91, June, 1999.

17. Schwender D, Daunderer M, Mulzer S, Klasing S, Finsterer U, and Peter K, "Midlatency auditory evoked potentials predict movements during anesthesia with isoflurane or porpofol", *Anesth Analg*, 85:164-173, 1997.
18. Zhang X-S, Roy RJ, Schwender D, and Daunderer M, "Discrimination of anesthetic states using midlatency auditory evoked potentials and artificial neural networks", *Anesth. Analg.* (under review).
19. Scott JC, Cooke JE, and Stanski DR, "Electroencephalographic quantitation of opioid effect: comparative pharmacodynamics of fentanyl and sufentanil", *Anesthesiology*, 74: 34-42, 1991.
20. Stanski DR, "Pharmacodynamic modeling of anesthetic EEG drug effects", *Annu. Rev. Pharmacol. Toxicol.*, 32: 423-447, 1992.
21. M.M. Todd, "EEGs, EEG Processing, and the Bispectral Index", *Anesthesiology*, 89:815-7, 1998.
22. Fell J, Roeschke J, Mann K, and Schaffner C, "Discrimination of sleep stages: a comparison between spectral and nonlinear measures", *Electroencephal Clin. Neurophysiol*, 98(5):401-410,1996.
23. Zhang, X-S, and Roy RJ, "Predicting movement during anesthesia by complexity analysis of the EEG", *Medical & Biological Engineering & Computing*, 37(3):327-334, 1999
24. Lempel A, and Ziv J, "On the complexity of finite sequences", *IEEE Trans. on Information Theory*, IT-22:75-81, 1976.
25. Pincus SM, Gladstone, IM, and Ehrenkranz RA, "A regularity statistic for medical data analysis", *J Clin Monit*, 7:335-345, 1991.
26. Jang J-SR, "ANFIS: Adaptive-network-based fuzzy inference system", *IEEE Trans. on Systems, man, and cybernetics*, 23(3):665-684, 1993.
27. Martin JF, Schneider AM, Quinn ML, and Smith NT, "Improved safety and efficacy in adaptive control of arterial blood pressure through the use of a supervisor", *IEEE Trans. on Biomedical Engineering*, 39(4):381-388, 1992.
28. Rao R, Bequette WB, Huang JW, Roy RJ, Kaufman H, "Modeling and Control of Anesthetic and Hemodynamic Drug Infusion", AIChE 1997 Fall Meeting, LA - Session 08b12.
29. Tackley RM, Lewis GTR, Prys-Roberts C, Boaden RW, Dixon J, and Harvey JT, "Computer Controlled Infusion of Propofol," *British Journal of Anaesthesia*, vol. 62, pp. 46-53, 1989.
30. Coetzee JF, Glen JB, Wium CA, and Boshoff L, "Pharmacokinetic Model Selection for Target Controlled Infusions of Propofol - Assessment of Three Parameter Sets", *Anesthesiology*, vol. 82, pp. 1328-1345, 1995.
31. Vuyk J, Engbers FHM, Burm AGL, Vletter AA, and Bovill JG, "Performance of Computer-Controlled Infusion of Propofol: An Evaluation of Five Pharmacokinetic Parameter Sets", *Anesth. Analg.*, vol. 81, pp. 1275-1282, 1995.
32. Eger EI, Saidman LJ, and Brandstater B, "Minimum alveolar anesthetic concentration: a standard of anesthetic potency", *Anesthesiology*, vol.26:756-763, 1965.
33. Smith C, EcEwan AI, Jhaveri R, Wilkinson M, Goodman D, Smith LR, Canada AT, Glass PSA, "The interaction of fentanyl on the Cp50 of propofol

for loss of consciousness and skin incision", *Anesthesiology*, 81:820-828, 1994.
34. Vuyk J, Mertens MJ, Olofsen E, Burm AGL, and Bovill JG, "Propofol anesthesia and rational opioid selection," *Anesthesiology*, 87:1549-1562, 1997.
35. Kazama T, Ikeda K, and Morita K, "The pharmacodynamic interaction between propofol and fentanyl with respect to the suppression of somatic or hemodynamic responses to skin incision, peritoneum incision, and abdominal wall retraction", *Anesthesiology*, 89:894-906, 1998.
36. Kazama T, Ikeda K, and Morita K, "Reduction by fentanyl of the Cp50 values of propofol and hemodynamic response to various noxious stimuli", *Anesthesiology*, 87:213-227, 1997.
37. Katoh T and Ikeda K, "The effects of fentanyl on sevoflurane requirements for loss of consciousness and skin incision", *Anesthesiology*, 88:18-24, 1988.
38. Kazama T, Ikeda K, Morita K, Kàtoh T, and Kikura M, "Propofol concentration required for endotracheal intubation with a laryngoscope or fiberscope and its interaction with fentanyl", *Anesth Analg* 86:872-879, 1998.
39. Vuyk J, Lim T, Engbers FHM, Burm AGL, Vletter AA, and Bovill JG, "Pharmacodynamics of alfentanil as a supplement to propofol or nitrous oxide for lower abdominal surgery in female patients", *Anesthesiology*, 78:1036-1045, 1993.
40. Kazama T, Ikeda K, Morita K, and Sanjo Y, "Awakening propofol concentration with and without blood-effect site equilibration after short-term and lόg-term administration of propofol and fentanyl anesthesia", *Anesthesiology*, 88:928-934, 1998.
41. Vuyk J, Lim T, Engbers FHM, Burm AGL, Vletter AA, and Bovill JG, "The pharmacodynamic interaction of propofol and alfentanil during lower abdominal surgery in women", *Anesthesiology*, 83:8-22, 1995.
42. Vuyk J, Engbers FHM, Burm AGL, Vletter AA, Griever GER, Olofsen E, and Bovill JG, "Pharmacodynamic interaction between propofol and alfentanil when given for induction of anesthesia", *Anesthesiology*, 84:288-299, 1996.
43. Roy RJ, and Huang JW, "Closed loop intravenous anesthetic administration," *Anesthesiology*, 87(3A): A461, Sep. 1997.
44. Zhang, X-S, Roy RJ, and Huang JW, "Closed-loop system for total intravenous anesthesia by simultaneously administering two anesthetic drugs", *Proc. of 20th Annual Int. Conf. of the IEEE Engineering in Medicine and Biology Society*, Hong Kong, 20:3052-3055, 1998.
45. Shafer S, STANPUMP software, Stanford University Medical Center, http://pkpd.icon.palo- alto.med.va.gov.
46. Cox E, "Adaptive fuzzy systems", *IEEE Spectrum*, pp. 27-31, Feb. 1993.
47. Kang H and Vachtsevanos G, "Adaptive fuzzy logic control", *Proc. of the IEEE Int. Conf. on Fuzzy Systems 1992*, San Diego, Mar. 1992; 407-14.

Intelligent Alarms for Anaesthesia Monitoring Based on a Fuzzy Logic Approach

A. Jungk[1], B. Thull[2] and G. Rau[1]

[1] Ergonomics in Medicine
Helmholtz-Institute for Biomedical Engineering
Aachen University of Technology (RWTH)

D-52074 Aachen, Germany
[2] Department of Information and Design
University of Applied Science
Darmstadt, Germany

E-mails: {jungk, thull, rau}@hia.rwth-aachen.de

Introduction

One of the most important tasks of the anaesthetist is to monitor the patient's vital signs in order to evaluate the patient's state, and to control it according to the needs of the surgical procedure. To support the anaesthetists' decision making process sensor techniques have been continuously developed by the medical industry. Hence, an increasing large number of vital parameters (e.g.: blood pressures, EEG, ECG, inspired and expired gas fractions etc.) are nowadays displayed by modern monitoring devices especially during highly invasive surgery [1-3]. As a result of this development, over 95% of anaesthesia based critical incidents could be *theoretically* detected only with the help of a monitor (over 65% without any organ damage) [4]. Obviously, these new measurement techniques have improved the patient's safety during the surgical procedure significantly.

However, several studies analysing the workflow and human errors in the anaesthesia workplace have shown that the alarming and visualisation techniques of the monitoring devices have not yet been appropriately adapted to this development [5-17]. Usually, directly measured vital parameters are still separately presented as trends along a timeline and the alarm management is still based on simple threshold alarms for each vital parameter. Both, the confusing presentation of many physiologic parameters as well as the large amount of the pre-set threshold alarms lead to a limitation of the anaesthetists' perception of the patient's state and to an increase of the anaesthetists' cognitive load during critical incidents. This section is about intelligent alarms, hence we now focus on the alarm problems.

Typically, a significant change of a monitored vital parameter is reported by a sound alarm if its value lies outside a predefined range. Upper and lower alarm thresholds are chosen by the monitors' default values, or by the physicians' selection. The choice of the alarm limits is rather difficult. Wide limits result in fewer false alarms but increase the risk of missing a true alarm and hence, increase the risk of the patients' safety. On the other hand, tight limits result in too many unnecessary alarms, in a high cognitive load, and in the long term in a lack of vigilance towards true alarms. In any case false, unnecessary, and incorrect alarms are so frequent that, in practice, alarms often fail to have their desired function (e.g. [5, 16, 17]). As a result Block et. al [16] reported that more than 70% of their surveyed anaesthetists stated they sometimes turn alarms off.

What are the reasons? Alarm problems are mainly of twofold nature: (1) frequent false-alarms, e.g. due to uncritical artefacts caused by the surgical procedure [5, 15-17], and (2) alarm cascades which may occur in critical situations due to the complex physiologic interrelations of all parameters and which reasons can then be difficult to trace back [18].

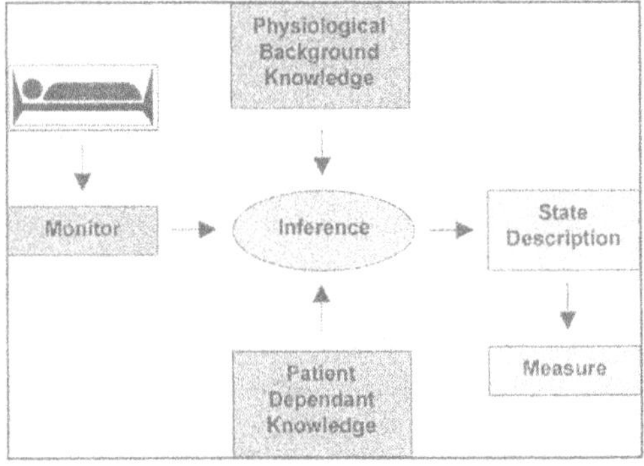

Figure 1. The anaesthetist's decision making model.

Consequently, most of the parameters contain different kinds of uncertainty and vague information has to be assessed in combination with temporal reasoning. Fuzzy logic offers a possibility to describe this kind of information in a decision making model. Hence, we designed our concept of intelligent alarms for the anaesthesia workplace based on a fuzzy logic approach.

Our first fuzzy logic approaches were based on so-called hemodynamic state variables [19, 20]. We now enlarged this concept by including trends and defining additional state variables for the respiration mechanics, gas management, and the oxygen supply. The intelligent alarm concept was integrated in a new display type which served as an explanation facility for the alarms. It was based on the principle of ecological interface design [21]. The idea of ecological interface design is to map the anaesthetists' mental model of a patient (e.g.: parameter relationships, functionality, context dependence) on the display.

Table 1. Intelligent systems in patient monitoring: fuzzy logic approaches

Researcher	Description
Guez et al. (Philadelphia, USA)	**ARTAA:** Real-time intelligent anaesthetist associate system for reduction of false alarms; neuro-fuzzy approach, classification of incoming measured vital parameters with a multi-layer neural network; system under development [25]
de Graaf et al. (Delft, NL)	**DSS:** Intelligent alarms for anaesthesia monitoring using an anaesthetists' decision-driven model; neuro-fuzzy approach, classification of incoming data with neural networks, fuzzification of these classes, using fuzzy rules for intelligent alarms; proof-of-concept, system under development [26]
Lowe et al. (Auckland, NZ)	**Diagnostic monitoring:** Diagnosis system for the anaesthesia workplace; formal framework for 'fuzzy trend templates': combined fuzzification of vital parameter values, their trends (fuzzy courses) and their temporal segmentation; first evaluations using recorded data [27, 28]
Shieh et al. (Sheffield, UK)	**Control of depth of anaesthesia:** Design of a hierarchical fuzzy control system for an intelligent adviser for drug selection; fuzzification of vital parameters and drug doses, definition of context dependent complex fuzzy rules; system under development and in proof-of-concept stage [29]
Oberli et al. (Santiago, Chile)	**Intelligent alarm system** for cardiac surgical patients; fuzzification of vital parameters, definition of fuzzy rules to infer the patient state, no trend analysis of vital parameters; first evaluations, system under development [30]
Vila et al. (Santiago, Spain)	**SUTIL:** Monitoring of patients in the coronary care unit, detection of ischemic episodes in the ECG; fuzzification of ECG parameters such as the amplitude of the T wave to infer the patient state; first evaluations, system under development [31]
Steimann et al. (Vienna, Austria)	**DiaMon-1:** On-line monitoring of ICU patients; event- and trend-based abstract description of a patient's cardiovascular and oxygenation status by using a combined fuzzification of measured vital parameters and their trends (fuzzy courses); system off-line, retrospectively evaluated [32]
Hayes-Roth et al. (Stanford, USA)	**GUARDIAN:** Diagnosis and intelligent monitoring system for post-cardiac surgery patients; a complex blackbox architecture using temporal fuzzy pattern recognition and qualitative temporal reasoning models; system evaluated with simulated scenarios [33, 34]

State-of-the-art

Since the 1970s various approaches towards expert systems for patient monitoring e.g. in the intensive care unit (ICU) or the operation room (OR) as well as especially towards intelligent alarms for anaesthesia monitoring have been suggested and discussed in several surveys (e.g. [22-24]).

As mentioned above intelligent alarms for anaesthesia monitoring require models for temporal and abstract reasoning. Hence, we mainly surveyed intelligent systems in patient monitoring designed in the last decade focussing this kind of purpose. All projects, their approaches and their evaluation status are shown in Table 1 and Table 2 and classified using Uckun's taxonomy [22].

Following this taxonomy, expert systems can be classified in three main tasks of interest with different levels of abstraction:

- diagnosis: interpretation of a pathophysiological state,
- prediction: assessment of future pathophysiological state trajectories, and
- control: treatment of a pathophysiological state.

In *diagnosis systems* the methods for the reasoning process have two orthogonal dimensions: level of data interpretation (single parameters, physiological state, or disorders) and temporal abstraction (single data points or data trends). Consequently, at one edge of the interpretation spectrum only simple parameters were classified whereas at the other edge complex reasoning models for pathophysiological disease trajectories over time have to be defined.

Structural, behavioural, or functional *prediction systems* use qualitative or quantitative model-based reasoning techniques and they are used mainly for therapy planning and management.

Open- or closed-loop *control systems* are mainly used for therapy planning and management, too. Whereas open-loop systems only give recommendations to the clinician who is still responsible for any treatment, closed-loop systems execute treatments directly (e.g.: administration of drugs).

These expert systems are designed following four major development concepts which can be combined [22]. This comprises real-time performance and resource management, handling of noisy data, context sensitivity, and intelligent alarms. The latter two are based on similar ideas but serve to a different purpose:

Context sensitivity bases an interpretation of the patient's state on a highly developed knowledge-base and all facts relevant to the current situation. An example is the interpretation of a measured vital parameter due to the administration of drugs (e.g.: a bolus of atropine should appropriately increase the heart rate).

Table 2. Intelligent systems in patient monitoring: non-fuzzy approaches

Researcher	Description
Larizza et al. (Pavia, Italy)	**M-HTP:** Assist monitoring and therapy planning for heart transplanted patients; using linear regression methods for trend analysis, combining qualitative and temporal abstractions for a measured vital parameter, reasoning models for therapy planning; prototype under development [35]
Sittig et al. (New Haven, USA)	**ICM:** Intelligent cardiovascular monitoring; based on the process trellis parallel computing architecture, trend detection using multi-state Kalman filtering algorithms, applying Bayesian statistical techniques to chose appropriately data models; prototype monitor under development [36]
Miksch et al. (Vienna, Austria)	**VIE-VENT:** Intelligent alarm and real-time system for monitoring and therapy planning for artificial ventilation of new-born infants; linear regression methods for trend detection, assessment and classification of ventilation parameters and their trends with respect to their temporal predictions and constraints; evaluation with recorded data [37-39]
Westenskow et al. (Salt Lake City, USA)	**Intelligent alarm system:** Intelligent alarms for ventilation problems; using a multi-layer neural network, classification of pulmonary resistance and compliance for spontaneous and controlled breathing; first evaluations with recorded and simulated data [40, 41]
Sukuvaara et al. (Kuopio, Finland)	**InCare:** Intelligent alarm system for monitoring cardiac operated patients; using linear regression and prediction methods, assessment of measured parameters with respect to their predicted parameter, definition and assessment of abstract cardiovascular state variables; system validated [42-44]
Haimowitz et al. (Cambridge, USA)	**TrendDX:** Diagnosis of paediatric growth; using regression-based trend templates in combination with event-based temporal reasoning methods; under development and tested for other domains [45]
Shahar et al. (Stanford, USA)	**RÉSUMÉ:** Monitoring insulin-dependent diabetes and therapy planning; general framework for the creation of abstract, interval-based concepts from time-stamped clinical data; system tested for other domains, in final stages of the development [46]
Dawant et al. (Vanderbilt, USA)	**SIMON:** Architecture for patient monitoring in an ICU; using a qualitative/quantitative reasoning ontology for a model-based reasoning to reduce false alarms; in development [47]

Context sensitivity reasoning must be performed in order to manage *intelligent alarms*. The purpose of intelligent alarms is to interpret the situational context to increase the number of correct alarms. Regarding the above mentioned simple example this means to set an alarm if the heart rate does not increase.

Materials and Methods

Figure 2 shows the architecture of the intelligent alarm system. Vital parameters of a patient undergoing surgery are measured and afterwards pre-processed by calculating their trends and mean values. In a next step all quantitative input parameters are transformed to a qualitative linguistic level with respect to the situational context (fuzzification). For each input variable of the inference procedure (fuzzy rules) which is determined by the knowledge base, the term set of a linguistic variable and its specific membership functions have to be identified. The output of the inference procedure are linguistic state variables which are relevant for decision making and which are defuzzified in a next step. They are displayed as a colour-coded alarm visualisation on the user interface which serves as the explanation facility together with the pre-processed vital parameter values and the situational context (normal values). Due to the patient's state the anaesthetist decides to initiate necessary measures.

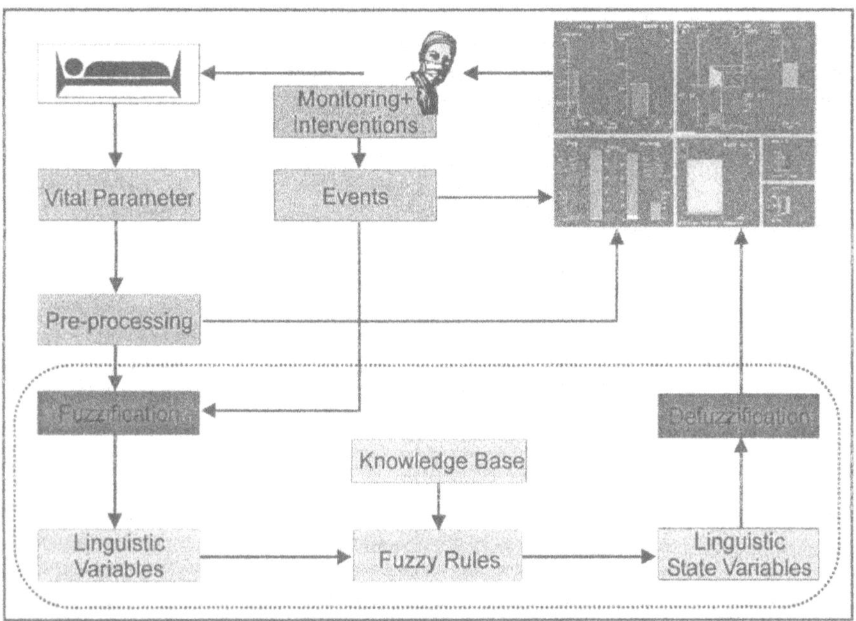

Figure 2. Architecture of the intelligent alarm system. The fuzzy sub-system is surrounded by the dotted line.

The pre-processing unit as well as the user interface are only shortly described in the following parts. All data necessary for the verification of our approach were generated by a commercially available anaesthesia software simulator (BODY Simulation™, Advanced Simulation Corporation, San Clemente, CA).

Pre-Processing of Vital Parameters

This module handles the task of data storage and low-level signal processing in terms of filtering the incoming vital parameters which are transmitted from the anaesthesia simulator every 600ms and trend detection.

Many different filter techniques are described in the literature. Beside complex filter systems (e.g.: Kalman-filter [36], neuronal networks [48]), Salman and Hunter [49] investigated different simple methods such as lowpass, median, or bandpass filter. In their investigations the median filter showed best results. In our approach we implemented the median as well as a filter based on the harmonic mean (HM) [50] (Eq. 1). We calculated the quadratic deviation of the two means from the original data to investigate which of the two methods better fits the trend of the data. The results have shown that the HM is a better approach (cf. Fig. 3).

$$HM = n \Big/ \sum_{i=1}^{n} 1/v_i \quad with:\ v_i = Value(i),\ n = number\ of\ values \qquad (1)$$

For each vital parameter, every 5 seconds, the last 10-seconds-HM of the 600ms-data is calculated to smooth data oscillation. Also, every 5 seconds the harmonic means' last 90-seconds-trend was calculated by using linear and polynomial regression methods which is a common technique to quantitatively describe trends (e.g. [45]). Following the results of Haimowitz et al. [45] we used the linear regression methods for in general more or less constant vital parameters (e.g.: airway pressure and tidal volume). Whereas polynomial regression better fits the data course for continuously slightly oscillating vital parameters (e.g.: heart rate, blood pressure).

Fuzzification of incoming vital parameter values and trends

For the fuzzy inference approach, all input parameters (harmonic means and trends) have to be transformed to a linguistic level. This procedure is called fuzzification and is done every 5 seconds.

A linguistic variable consists of a set of linguistic descriptions (terms) as values which are based on the anaesthetists' mental model for the qualitative description of the input parameters. The mental model was derived in co-operation with anaesthetists in interviews and by using questionnaires [51] as well as with the help of corresponding literature (e.g. [52, 53]) and the analysis of simulated scenarios. Also verbal protocols of the anaesthetists' critical incident management during simulated scenarios [54] were included in the knowledge acquisition process.

As result, each term is a semantic description of a specific range of the base variable in the universe of discourse X, x are the current quantitative values of the base variable. Regarding trends x is the value of the gradient of the regression curve, or regarding the means x is the difference (D) between the harmonic mean (HM) of a parameter and its normal value with respect to the current situational context. The linguistic variables for the input parameters commonly consist of five linguistic terms (D: 'very low', 'low'. 'good', 'high', and 'very high'; trend: 'decreasing', 'little decreasing', 'constant', 'little increasing', and 'increasing'). The terms of a linguistic variable are defined as fuzzy sets (Eq. 2). $\mu_{term}(x)$ yields the membership value to a term for a specific base variable measurement x.

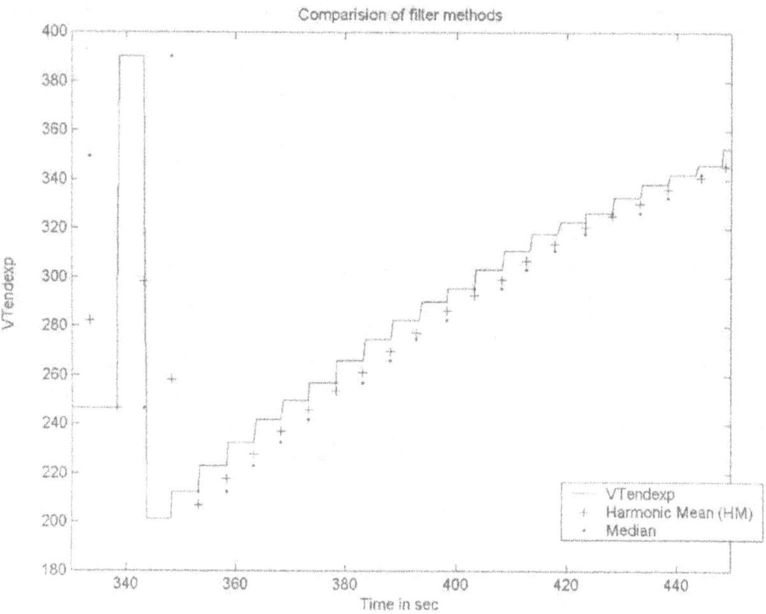

Figure 3. Comparison of the filter methods for the endexpiratory tidal volume using the median filter and the harmonic mean filter to fit the data.

$$\tilde{F}_{var}(term): \tilde{F}_{var}(term) = \{(x, \mu_{term}(x))\ x \in X\} \quad (2)$$

Example: The linguistic input variable 'Differenence of Pulmonal arterial diastolic pressure to its normal value' $\tilde{F}_{PAPdiasD}$ is defined in the universe of discourse $x \in$

[-6 mmHg, 6 mmHg] and consists of the above mentioned five terms. Its corresponding trend variable $\tilde{F}_{PAPdiasTrend}$ is defined in the universe of discourse $x \in$ [-0.3 mmHg/s, 0.3 mmHg/s]. The definition of their membership functions $\mu_{\text{term}}(x)$ are shown in Fig. 4.

Example: An on principle healthy patient undergoing surgery may have a decreasing PAPdias of 11.6 mmHg with an decreasing rate of -0.22 mmHg/s. The normal value of PAPdias for such a patient is said to be 10 mmHg. Hence, PAPdias_D is 11.6 mmHg - 10 mmHg = 1.6 mmHg. The precise crisp values of these parameters yield the following term memberships:

$\mu_{\text{PAPdiasD good}}(1.6 \text{ mmHg}) = 0.33$
$\mu_{\text{PAPdiasD high}}(1.6 \text{ mmHg}) = 0.67$
$\mu_{\text{PAPdiasTrend little\_decreasing}}(-0.22 \text{ mmHg/s}) = 0.6$
$\mu_{\text{PAPdiasTrend decreasing}}(-0.22 \text{ mmHg/s}) = 0.4$

All other term memberships are equal to zero.

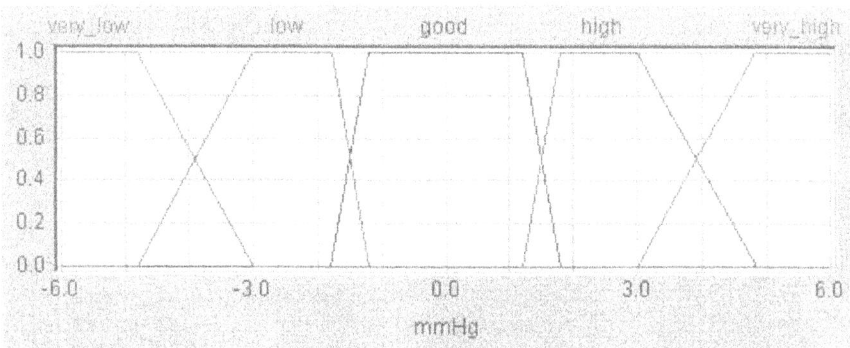

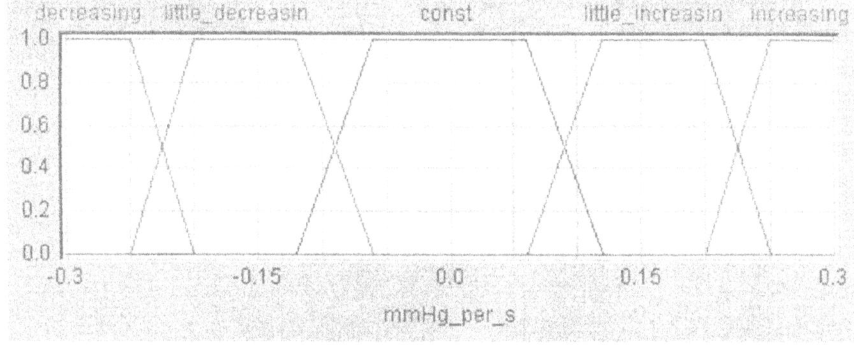

Figure 4. Topdown: Membership functions $\mu_{\text{term}}(x)$ of PAPdias_D and $\text{PAPdias}_{\text{Trend}}$.

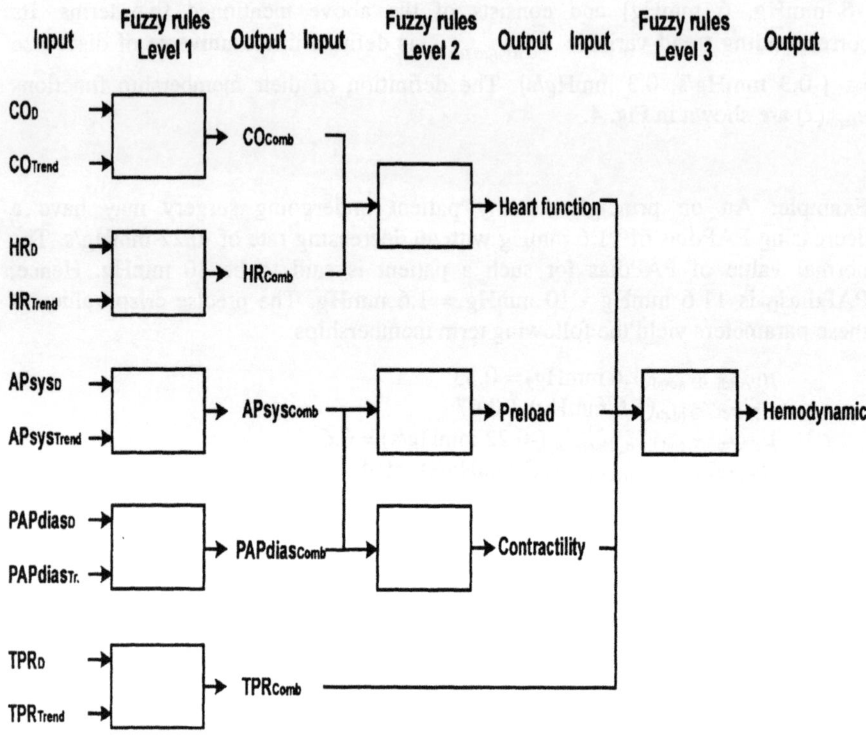

Figure 5. The three-levels structure of the fuzzy logic system which defines the abstract state variable 'Hemodynamic' including rule blocks, inputs and outputs. The connecting lines symbolise the data flow. Abr.: CO: cardiac output, HR: heart rate, APsys: arterial systolic pressure, PAPdias: pulmonal arterial diastolic pressure, TPR: total periphery resistance.

Definition of Abstract State Variables and Evaluation of Fuzzy Rules

In this module the linguistic statements on the input parameters are combined on different levels by using fuzzy rules. According to the complexity of the four main subsystems we defined two or three levels of abstraction: i.e., 'Hemodynamic' (three levels, s. Fig. 5) , 'Respiration mechanics' (two levels), 'Respiration gases' (two levels), and 'Oxygen supply' (two levels). The fuzzy rules are expressed in natural language and therefore easy to understand and to generate for domain experts.

Level 1: The fuzzified outputs of a vital parameter P (i.e., P_D and P_{Trend}), are combined to the abstract state variable P_{Comb}, which has similar linguistic terms like P_D (cf. Fig. 6).

Level 2: The combination of two abstract state variables $P_{Comb,1}$ and $P_{Comb,2}$ was especially defined for the most complex subsystem of the intelligent alarm system: the patient's hemodynamic (cf. Fig. 5). The linguistic output variables represent qualitative ratings on certain for the anaesthetist relevant state variables, i.e. 'preload', 'contractility', and 'heart function'. These linguistic state variables consist of the terms 'good', 'little bad', and 'bad'.

Level 3: All linguistic outputs generated in level 1 and/or level 2 are used as inputs for one of the four above introduced main abstract state variables which are most important for the anaesthetists' decision making. The linguistic outputs of these have four terms: 'good', 'little bad', 'bad', and 'very bad'.

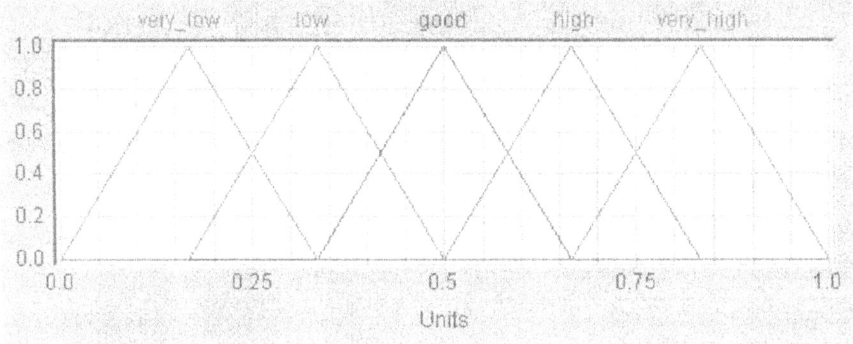

Figure 6. Membership functions $\mu_{term}(x)$ of $PAPdias_{Comb}$.

Table 3. Example for fuzzy rules of the first level to infer the state variable $PAPdias_{Comb}$

If $PAPdias_D$	and $PAPdias_{Trend}$	then $PAPdias_{Comb}$	DoS
High	Little deacreasing	High	0.9
High	Decreasing	High	0.8
High	Little decreasing	Good	0.1
High	Decreasing	Good	0.2
Good	Little decreasing	Good	0.8
Good	Decreasing	Good	0.5
Good	Little decreasing	Low	0.2
Good	Decreasing	Low	0.5

After the definition of all abstract state variables and their inputs the fuzzy rules for the inference process have to be defined. Fuzzy rules are production rules. They are of the form: 'If a set of conditions are satisfied, then a set of consequences can be produced'. To make them more flexible, the fuzzy associative memory approach (FAM) was used [55]. A degree of support (DoS) is attached to each rule which stands for the plausibility of this rule in the knowledge base. The plausibility factor has a value between 0 (implausible) and 1 (full plausibility). Altogether we defined 569 rules.

Table 4. Example for fuzzy rules of the second level to infer the state variables 'preload' and 'contractility'.

If $PAPdias_{Comb}$	and $APsys_{Comb}$	Then contractility	then preload	DoS
High	Low	Little bad		0.5
Low	Good	Good		1.0
High	Low		Little bad	0.3
Good	Very low		Little bad	0.1
Low	Good		Good	1.0

Table 5. Example for fuzzy rules of the third level to infer the state variable 'hemodynamic'.

If TPR_{Comb}	and contractility	and preload	and heart function	then hemodynamic	DoS
Good	Good	Little bad	Good	Little bad	1.0
Good	Little bad	Little bad	Good	Little bad	1.0
Good	Bad	Little bad	Good	Bad	1.0
Good	Bad	Little bad	Bad	Very bad	1.0

Using the above introduced example with the parameters $PAPdias_D$ and $PAPdias_{Trend}$ the corresponding fuzzy rules for the state variable $PAPdias_{Comb}$ of the first level are shown in Table 3.

In the next step e.g. $PAPdias_{Comb}$ and the abstract state variable for the arterial systolic pressure $APsys_{Comb}$ are combined to infer the higher level abstract state variables 'contractility' and 'preload' (exemplary rules are shown in Table 4).

In the last level all abstract state variables necessary for assessing the abstract state variable 'Hemodynamic' are combined as e.g. in Table 5.

After the definition of all linguistic variables and fuzzy rules the next step is the aggregation of the linguistic statements. During the last two decades, several empirical investigations on the properties of different families of operators have been performed. For the representation of a compensatory aggregation, the linguistic 'and', the γ-operator class showed good results [56]:

$$\mu_{\tilde{A}\Gamma\tilde{B}}(x,y,) = (\mu_{\tilde{A}}(x)\cdot\mu_{\tilde{B}}(y))^{1-\gamma}\cdot(\mu_{\tilde{A}}(x)+\mu_{\tilde{B}}(y)-\mu_{\tilde{A}}(x)\cdot\mu_{\tilde{B}}(y))^{\gamma}$$
$$\forall\ x\in X, y\in Y,\ \mu,\gamma\in [0,1] \qquad (3)$$

Our previous results have shown that a medium compensation ($\gamma = 0.5$) is the best choice for the evaluation of our kind of linguistic rules which are used for the knowledge base of the intelligent patient monitoring and alarm system [19, 51].

Example: Using the above introduced example ($PAPdias_D$ = 1.6 mmHg, $PAPdias_{Trend}$ = -0.22 mmHg/s) the corresponding rules for '$PAPdias_{Comb}$ is high' in Table 3.1 are aggregated as follows:

R1 If $PAPdias_D$ is **high** and $PAPdias_{Trend}$ is **little decreasing** then $PAPdias_{Comb}$ is **high** (DoS: 0.9).

$\mu_{PAPdiasComb\ is\ high}(1.6\ mmHg, -0.22\ mmHg/s)$
$= (0.67\cdot 0.6)^{0.5}\cdot(0.67+0.6-(0.67\cdot 0.6))^{0.5}\cdot(0.9)\approx 0.53$

R2 If $PAPdias_D$ is **high** and $PAPdias_{Trend}$ is **decreasing** then $PAPdias_{Comb}$ is **high** (DoS: 0.8).

$\mu_{PAPdiasComb\ is\ high}(1.6\ mmHg, -0.22\ mmHg/s)\approx 0.37$

In the next step all rules that fire to the same conclusion have to be aggregated. This is done by using the MAX ('or')-operator [56].

Example: With the above calculated membership values for the two fired rules the corresponding membership degrees $\mu_{term}(x)$ after rule aggregation are:

$$\mu_{PAPComb\ is\ high}(1.6\ mmHg, -0.22\ mmHg/s)\approx MAX(0.53; 0.37)\approx 0.53$$

These statements are used as the input parameters for the next step of the fuzzy inference to assess higher level state variables. For the four main abstract state variables (e.g.: the state variable 'Hemodynamic') also a quantitative result is needed which can be achieved by using defuzzification methods.

Defuzzification

If a real number is needed as mentioned above, the fuzzy outputs have to be transformed into a crisp value. Hence, a defuzzification method is necessary.

The results of the inference process are visualised as colour-coded alarm visualisation according to the membership of an abstract state variable to its linguistic description (i.e., 'good', 'little bad', 'bad', 'very bad'). In our case the well-known 'Center-of-Area' method (CoA) was used [57].

Visualisation - the ecological interface approach

An important aspect in the design of an intelligent patient monitoring and alarm system is the visual presentation of the results of the fuzzy inference procedure. User interfaces are an integral part of system design for anaesthesia monitoring (e.g.: [7, 17]). In order to support the physician to access the complex information about the patient state during the decision making behaviour we developed an user interface according to guidelines of ecological interface design [21]. Our preliminary studies [54, 58] have shown that this new approach may better support the anaesthetists' concept of decision making than traditional trend displays.

The idea of an ecological interface is to visualise all task- and goal-relevant information necessary for decision making in its different levels of abstraction (from the micro to the macro) in the interface to enhance knowledge-based behaviour [21]. According to Rasmussen et al. [59] the visual form of an ecological interface "has to serve as a symbolic representation - an external mental model" of the workplace. To meet these requirements it is necessary to "show relationships between the actual functional state, the target states, and the boundaries to be respected" [59]. That is for an interface designed for anaesthesia monitoring to combine and visually represent all relevant information necessary for decision making in one single display: i.e. measured vital parameters, physiological background knowledge, and patient dependant context (cf. Fig. 1).

We developed an ecological interface which visualises 35 measured and for a decision making process relevant parameters during anaesthesia monitoring (cf. Fig. 7). The variables are organised according to their function. For the most important values trend indicators close to the displayed number show their last 90-seconds trend. On the upper left side the functionality of the respiratory mechanics is visualised in terms of the endexpiratory tidal volume (Vt_{ex}) and expired minute volume (ExMV) as rectangles together with their dependencies (maximal and minimal airway pressure (Paw), airway compliance (Compl) and respiration rate (AF)). Normal values are visualised with green rectangles. On the lower left side, the respiration gases in terms of the inspired and expired tidal volumes and their various fractions (CO_2, O_2, N_2O, N_2, narcotic gas) are shown as bars. On the middle lower right side, the oxygen supply is visualised by a square which is determined by the two fractions of oxygen concentration in the blood on the y-axis and cardiac output on the x-axis. The normal value is shown as a green rectangle. The important number for the oxygen saturation (SaO_2) is displayed separately. On the upper right side, the functionality of the hemodynamic is visualised with the help of a schematic work diagram of the heart (Frank-Starling diagram) and the total periphery resistance (TPR) (for a detailed description s. [58]). On the lower right side the effect of the administered drugs in terms of the clinical relevant parameters "train of four" (TOF) for the neuromuscular relaxation, and "minimum alveolar concentration" (MAC) for the anaesthesia depth are visualised as bars and explicitly displayed as number. Normal values are shown as a green bar for the TOF and a grey bar for the MAC on the corresponding axes.

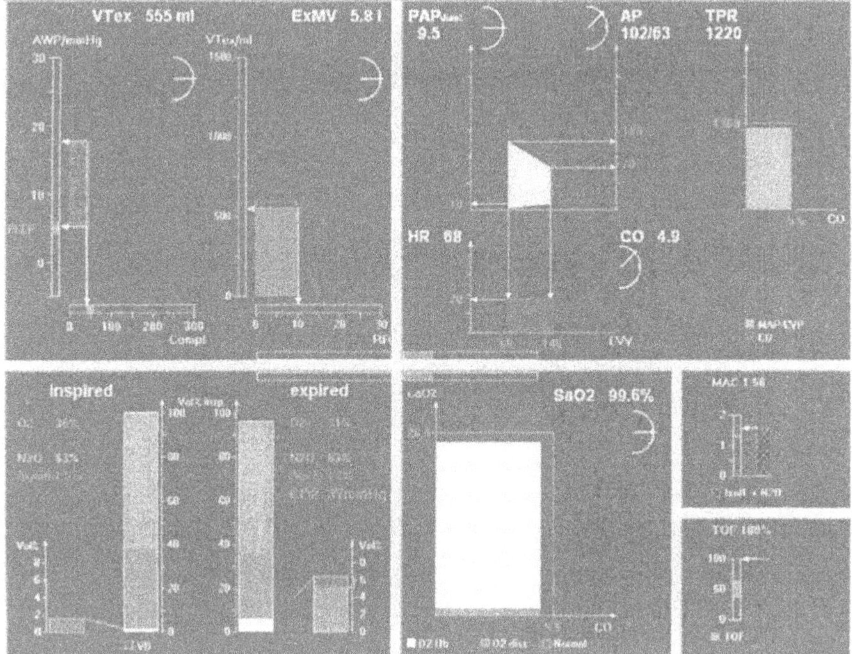

Figure 7. User interface of the intelligent patient monitoring and alarm system.

The result of the fuzzy inference procedure and the CoA-defuzzification for the abstract state variables 'Respiration mechanics,' 'Respiration gases', 'Oxygen supply' and 'Hemodynamic' is displayed as a continuously, in its size and colour changing profilogram for each variable in the middle of the display. For the full membership values the colours are defined as:

$\mu_{\text{good}}(x) = 1 \Rightarrow$ 'green'
$\mu_{\text{little bad}}(x) = 1 \Rightarrow$ 'yellow'
$\mu_{\text{bad}}(x) = 1 \Rightarrow$ 'orange'
$\mu_{\text{very bad}}(x) = 1 \Rightarrow$ 'red'

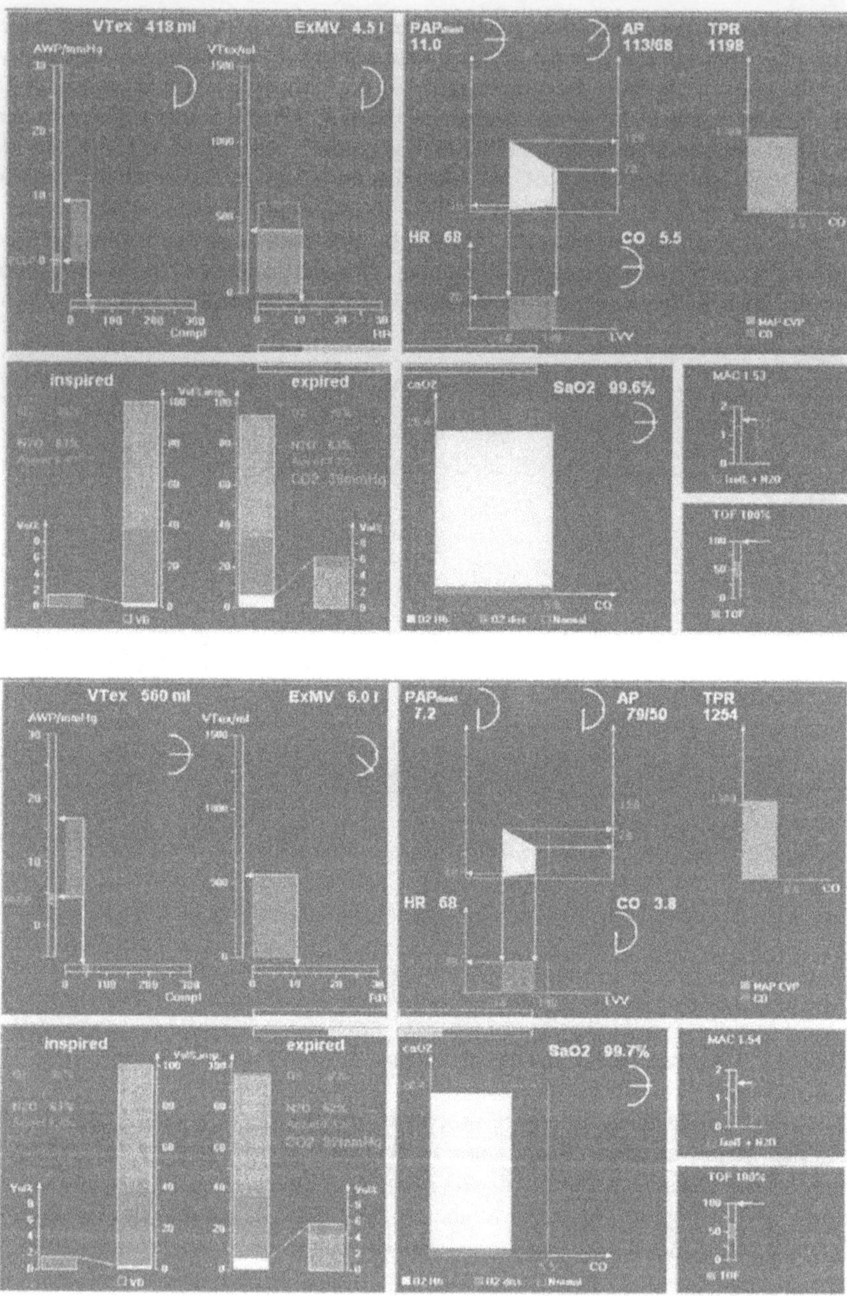

Figures 8a and 8b. Topdown examples for the visualisation of the incidents 'cuff-leakage' and 'blood loss'.

Evaluation

Experimental set-up

All necessary parameters, which are displayed on the ecological interface were transmitted from the anaesthesia simulator. The simulator offers various possibilities to simulate the anaesthetic procedure (e.g.: intubation, ventilation, administering drugs, and communication with the staff in the operation theatre). It includes a pulsoxymetre, two monitors for ventilation and hemodynamic parameters, and gives the possibility to simulate critical incidents.

In an experimental set-up, subjects had to anaesthetise a simulated 'patient'. During a trial one of two critical incidents, i.e., a blood loss (4 min after beginning of surgery, duration: 4 min, amount: 170 ml/min), and a cuff-leakage (5 min after end of surgery, leakage: 50%) were simulated.

Eight anaesthetists (working experience: 0.5-13yrs.) participated in the experiments. About 45 min time was allowed to make themselves familiar with the new display and the experimental set-up. They had no experience with our new display or with intelligent alarms. Each subject conducted at least two trials working with the simulator monitors in combination with the ecological interface. A 'blood loss' was simulated for a 'healthy' and a hypovolemic patient and a 'cuff-leakage' was simulated for a 'healthy' patient and a patient with severe respiration problems (COPD). Examples for the visualisation and the assessment of the two incidents are shown in Fig. 8a and Fig 8b.

The anaesthetists' task was to identify the incident and to assess the patient's state during the experiment. A trial was stopped as soon as a subject identified the incident or it was aborted by the test supervisor if there were no signs that an incident could be successfully identified.

Analysis methods

As described above, the intelligent patient monitoring and alarm system generates a continuous alarm visualisation for each abstract state variable in the direction 'good' to 'very bad'. In order to make the evaluation results transparent, the continuous scale was divided into three sections similarly to Becker et al. in [19] (cf. Fig. 9).

In our investigations the anaesthetists served as the reference for a correct evaluation. They had to assess the patient's state at least every minute. The intelligent patient monitoring and alarm system had to state its correctness compared to this reference. By this comparison the alarms generated by the system were classified according to Fig. 9.

After the determination of the described alarms we quantified the categories by calculating the sensitivity, specificity, and predictability [60] (Eq. 4-6).

$$sensitivity = \frac{\sum true\ positive\ alarms}{\sum true\ positive\ alarms + \sum false\ negative\ alarms} \tag{4}$$

$$specificity = \frac{\sum true\ negative\ alarms}{\sum true\ negative\ alarms + \sum false\ positive\ alarms} \tag{5}$$

$$predictability = \frac{\sum true\ positive\ alarms}{\sum true\ positive\ alarms + \sum false\ positive\ alarms} \tag{6}$$

To analyse the anaesthetists' performance, the time to identify an incident was measured. Moreover, to analyse the effect of our new alarm system display the times for the 'healthy' patient were compared with our previous results in [54]. In that study 8 anaesthetists had the same task and worked only with the conventional simulator monitors.

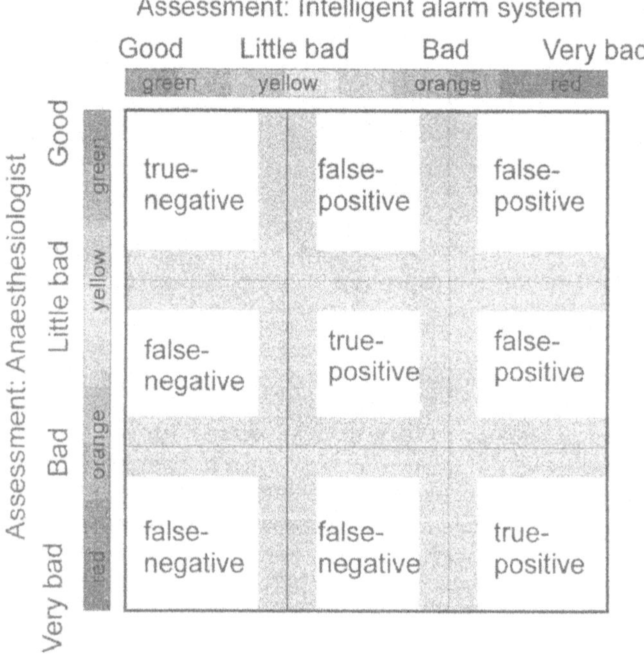

Figure 9. Alarm type definition matrix. The patient's state evaluation serves as the reference and the evaluation of the intelligent patient monitoring and alarm system is compared to this reference.

Results

Table 6 shows the results of the performance analysis. The anaesthetists improved their performance especially for the time to identify an incident when the new alarm system and display was available as source of information. Regarding the second parameter 'Number of identified incidents' we had similar results as in our previous experiments. Rather all incidents (26 of 28) could be identified.

Table 6. Comparison of the results of the anaesthetists' performance when working with the new display and only with conventional monitors.

Incident	'Blood loss'		'Cuff-Leakage'	
	No. of identified incidents	Time/s	No. of identified incidents	Time/s
Only simulator monitors [54]	100% (8 of 8)	217 ± 72	75% (6 of 8)	222 ± 187
Simulator monitors and new display	100% (15 of 15)	136 ± 67	85% (11 of 13)	62 ± 87

Table 7 shows the results of the validation. Altogether 1532 state variable evaluations were performed by the eight test persons during the simulated surgical procedures. The system's assessment was too sensitive especially for the state variables 'Hemodynamic' and 'Respiration mechanics' in the red warning zone. In total, the sensitivity of alarm recognition is 95.7%, the specificity is 95.3%, and the predictability is 87.4%.

Discussion and Conclusion

We designed an intelligent alarm system for the anaesthesia workplace on a fuzzy logic approach which is based on our previous systems described in [19, 20, 51] and which based on a concept of so-called abstract state variables. The idea of this concept is to combine directly measured vital parameters to more abstract ones such as 'Contractility of the heart' according to the anaesthetists' mental model of a patient. As a result we no longer have error-prone threshold alarms for every single measured parameter which are common in nowadays' alarm technology but a more qualitative description of the patient's state which is near to the clinical decision making process (e.g.: 'Contractility is good').

Table 7. Results of the validation of the intelligent alarm system during 12 simulated surgical procedures. Comparison between the system's (S) assessment and the anaesthetists' (A) validations and the alarm classification with its quantifying values.

Alarm type	Respiration mechanics	Respiration gases	Hemodynamic	Oxygen supply	Total
S green - A green	236	284	225	340	1085
S green - A yellow	5	0	6	1	12
S green - A red	0	0	0	0	0
S yellow - A green	7	3	6	2	18
S yellow - A yellow	53	36	84	40	213
S yellow - A red	2	1	2	0	5
S red – A green	3	0	0	0	3
S red – A yellow	14	1	18	0	33
S red – A red	63	58	42	0	163
True-negative	236	284	225	340	1085
True-positive	116	94	126	40	376
False-positive	24	4	24	2	54
False-negative	7	1	8	1	17
Total	383	383	383	383	1532
Sensitivity	94.3%	99.0%	94.0%	97.6%	95.7%
Specificity	90.8%	98.6%	90.4%	99.4%	95.3%
Predictability	82.9%	95.9%	84.0%	95.2%	87.4%

Our new approach as well as the above mentioned previous systems have in common that they offer a problem oriented modelling technique for medical domains where inter-individual differences of the patient have to be considered. Because of the high complexity of the biological system, accurate mathematical models fail. Hence, the fuzzy approach offers a well-defined solution to model the anaesthetists' qualitative assessment of uncertain and vague information about the patient's state on a higher level of abstraction.

We enlarged our previous approaches by additional abstract state variables not only for the patient's cardiovascular system but also for the patient's respiration and oxygen supply system. Altogether four main subsystems were defined: i.e., 'Hemodynamic', 'Respiration mechanics', 'Respiration gases', and 'Oxygen supply'. Each of them are subdivided in several levels which each has their own abstract state variables. Quantitative values of these variables are transferred to a qualitative linguistic level with the help of fuzzy sets. Relations between higher level and lower level abstract state variables are defined by fuzzy rules. Fuzzy rules have the advantage that they are easy to understand and to generate by the medical domain experts.

Including trend gradients of directly measured parameters in the intelligent alarm system was also an important issue since the temporal behaviour of a parameter is relevant for the anaesthetists' decision making process especially during critical incident management. Many approaches for intelligent systems exist using fuzzy logic, neural networks, or other non-fuzzy modelling techniques to qualitatively describe parameter values and their trends (cf. the second section). In contrast to e.g. Steimann et al. [32] and Lowe et al. [27, 28] who defined fuzzy sets (so-called fuzzy-courses) to combine a parameter's value and its trend gradient we transferred both variables apart on an linguistic level with the help of fuzzy sets and combined them to an abstract state variable with the help of fuzzy rules.

The intelligent alarm system was integrated in a new visualisation approach for anaesthesia monitoring which served as an explanation facility for the intelligent alarms. The design concept was based on Rasmussens' theory of ecological interface design (EID) [21, 59]. The principle of EID is to make the users' mental model of a system transparent on an interface. Hence, according to Rasmussen especially an expert user should better understand and faster identify system changes when using an ecological interface. To transfer this hypothesis to the anaesthesia work domain an anaesthetist should better understand the system 'patient' and the situational awareness as well as clinical decision making process should be improved with the help of an appropriately visualisation of the patient's state. Our previous results [54, 58] as well as e.g. Michels et al. [61] have shown that in fact an ecological interface approach might support the anaesthetists critical incident management.

To prove our new alarm and visualisation approach we evaluated the system by using an commercially available anaesthesia simulator and simulated critical incidents. The same incidents were simulated in our previous experiments when only conventional monitors were available [54]. As our results have shown, the anaesthetists identified an incident faster when the new display and intelligent alarm system was available. Hence, these result again support the hypothesis that an ecological interface designed for the anaesthesia workplace may enhance clinical decision making.

The validation of the knowledge base of the intelligent alarm system showed very good results since we achieved overall a sensitivity of 95.7%, a specificity of 95.3%, and a predictability of 87.4%. Only in 1.1% percent of cases the intelligent alarm system underestimated the situation (alarm level too low). The situation was overestimated by the system in 3.5% of cases (alarm level too high). To survey the overestimated alarms, it must be taken into account that only in 38.9% of these cases (1.4% of all alarm cases) there was no alarm necessary at all. Comparing our results with our previous approach [19, 51] or with other intelligent alarm systems for anaesthesia monitoring (e.g. [30]) seems to be difficult since the classification of the alarms were slightly different. Moreover, compared especially to these two systems we designed an intelligent alarm system with extended functionality. Nevertheless, Becker et al. [19, 51] as well as Oberli et al. [30] reported of a sensitivity of their alarms of over 92% which we also achieved for all components of our approach

Compared to monitoring systems used in daily clinical routine with threshold alarms where high false alarm rates of 30-76% are reported [16] the concept of continuos intelligent alarms seems to be very promising. Normally, the anaesthetists had the same impression of the patient's state as the intelligent alarm system. In cases of different impressions our system overestimated the situation in most cases. However, since our intelligent alarm system must not make therapy decisions but is rather designed as a 'self-referential' system for the anaesthetist it can be seen as a kind of safety net. I.e., if the anaesthetist has a different impression of the patient's state, the anaesthetist will check the patient's state and might faster recognise upcoming dangerous conditions.

References

[1] List WF, Metzler H, Pasch T (1995) Monitoring in Anästhesie und Intensivmedizin. Springer, Berlin, Heidelberg

[2] Petry A (1995) On-line Aufzeichung von Monitordaten. Anaesthesist 44: 818-825

[3] Martin E (1997) Facharztlehrbuch Anästhesiologie. Blackwell Wissenschaftsverlag, Berlin, Wien

[4] Webb RK, van der Valt JH, Runciman WB, Williamson JA, Cockings J, Russell WJ, Helps S (1993) Which Monitor? An Analysis of 2000 Incident Reports. Anaesthesia Intensive Care 21: 529-542

[5] Gaba DM (1991) Human performance issues in anesthesia patient safety. Problems in Anesthesia 5: 329-350

[6] Waterson C, Calkins JM (1986) Development directions for monitoring in anesthesia. Seminars in Anesthesia V(3): 225-236

[7] Coiera E (1993) Intelligent monitoring and control of dynamic physiological systems. Artificial Intelligence in Medicine 5: 1-8

[8] Chopra V, Bovill JG, Spierdijk J, Koornneef F (1992) Reported significant observations during anesthesia: a prospective analysis over a 18-month period. British Journal of Anesthesia 68: 13-17

[9] Chopra V, Bovill JG, Spierdijk J (1990) Accidents, near accidents and complications during anesthesia: A retrospective analysis of a 10-year period in a teaching hospital. Anesthesia 45: 3-6

[10] Short TG, O'Regan A, Lew J, Oh TE (1992) Critical incident reporting in an anaesthetic department quality assurance programme. Anaesthesia 47: 3-7
[11] Cooper JB, Newbower RS, Kitz RJ (1984) An analysis of major errors and equipment failures in anaesthesia management: Considerations for prevention and detection. Anesthesiology 60: 34-42
[12] Webb RK, Currie M, Morgan CA, Williamson JA, Mackay P, Russell WJ, Runciman WB (1993) The australian incident monitoring study: An analysis of 2000 incident reports. Anaesthesia Intensive Care 21(5): 506-519
[13] Boquet G, Bushman JA, Davenport H (1980) The anaesthetic machine- a study of function and design. British Journal of Anaesthesia 52: 61-67
[14] Weinger MB, Herndon OW, Zornow MH, Paulus MP, Gaba DM, Dallen LT (1994) An objective methodology for task analysis and workload assessment in anesthesia providers. Anesthesiology 80: 77-92
[15] Runciman WB, Sellen A, Webb RK, Williamson JA, Currie M, Morgan C, Russell (1993) Errors, Incidents and Accidents in Anaesthetic Practice. Anaesthesia Intensive Care 21: 506-519
[16] Block E, Nuutinen L, Ballast B (1999) Optimization of alarms: a study on alarm limits, alarm sounds, and false alarms, intended to reduce annoyance. Journal of Clinical Monitoring and Computing 15: 75-83
[17] Weinger MB, Englund CE (1990) Ergonomic and Human Factors Affecting Anesthetic Vigilance and Monitoring Performance in the Operating Room Environment. Anesthesiology 73: 995-1021
[18] Cook RI, Block FE, McDonald JS (1988) Cascade of Monitor Detection of Anesthetic Disaster. Anesthesiology 59(3A): A277
[19] Becker K, Thull B, Käsmacher-Leidinger H, Stemmer J, Rau G, Kalff G, Zimmermann H-J (1997) Design and validation of an intelligent alarm system based on a fuzzy logic process model. Artificial Intelligence in Medicine 11: 33-53
[20] Schecke T, Rau G, Popp H-J, Käsmacher H, Kalff G, Zimmermann H-J (1991) A Knowledge-Based Approach to Intelligent Alarms in Anesthesia. IEEE Engineering in Medicine and Biology 10(4): 38-43
[21] Vicente K, Rasmussen J (1992) Ecological interface design: theoretical foundations. IEEE Trans. System, Man, and Cybernetics 22(4): 589-606
[22] Uckun S (1994) Intelligent systems in patient monitoring and therapy measurement: A survey of research projects. International Journal of Clinical Monitoring and Computing 11: 241-253
[23] Mora FA, Passariello G, Carrault G, Le Pichon J-P (1993) Intelligent patient monitoring and management systems. IEEE Engineering in Medicine and Biology December: 23-33
[24] Adlassnig K-P (1982). A survey on medical diagnosis and fuzzy subsets. In: Gupta MM, Sanchez E (eds.): Approximate Reasoning in Decision Analysis, North-Holland, New York, pp 203-217
[25] Guez A, Nevo I (1996) Neural networks and fuzzy logic in clinical laboratory computing with application to integrated monitoring. Clinica Chimica Acta 248: 73-90

[26] de Graaf PMA, van den Eijkel GC, Vullings HJLM, de Mol BAJM (1997) A decision-driven design of a decision support system in anesthesia. Artificial Intelligence in Medicine 11(2): 141-153
[27] Lowe A, Jones RW, Harrison MJ (1999) Temporal Pattern Matching Using Fuzzy Templates. Journal of Intelligent Information Systems 13: 27-45
[28] Lowe A, Harrison MJ, Jones RW (1999) Diagnostic monitoring in anaesthesia using fuzzy trend templates for matching temporal patterns. Artificial Intelligence in Medicine 16, 183-199
[29] Shieh JS, Linkens DA, Peacock JE (1999) Hierarchical Rule-Based and Self-Organizing Fuzzy Logic Control for Depth of Anaesthesia. IEEE Trans. on Systems, Man, and Cybernetics Part C 29(1): 98-109
[30] Oberli C, Urzua J, Saez C, Guarini M, Cipriano A, Garayar B, Lema G, Canessa R, Sacco C, Irirrazaval M (1999) An expert system for monitor alarm integration. Journal of Clinical Monitoring and Computing 15: 29-35
[31] Vila J, Presedo J, Delgado M, Barro S, Ruiz R, Palacios F (1997) SUTIL: Intelligent ischemia monitoring system. International Journal of Medical Informatics 47: 193-214
[32] Steimann, F (1996) The interpretation of time-varying data with DiaMon-1. Artificial intelligence in medicine 8: 343-357
[33] Larsson JE, Hayes-Roth B, Gaba DM, Smith BE (1997) Evaluation of a medical diagnosis system using simulator test scenarios. Artificial Intelligence in Medicine 11: 119-140
[34] Drakopoulos JA, Hayes-Roth B (1998) tFPR: A fuzzy and structural pattern recognition system of multi-variate time-dependent pattern classes based on sigmoidal functions. Fuzzy Sets and Systems 99: 57-72
[35] Larizza C, Bernuzzi G, Stefanelli M (1995). A General Framework for Building Patient Monitoring Systems. In: Barahona P, Stefanelli M, Wyatt J (eds.): Lecture Notes in Artificial Intelligence, Springer Verlag, Berlin, pp 91-102
[36] Sittig DF, Factor M (1990) Physiologic trend detection and artifact rejection: a parallel implementation of a multi-state Kalman filtering algorithm. Computer Methods and Programs in Biomedicine 31: 1-10
[37] Miksch S, Horn W, Popow C, Paky F (1993). VIE-VENT: Knowledge-Based Monitoring and Therapy Planning of the Artificial Ventilation of Newborn Infants. In: Andreassen et al. (eds.): Artificial Intelligence in Medicine, IOS Press, Amsterdam, pp 218-229
[38] Miksch S, Horn W, Popow C, Paky F (1995). Therapy Planning Using Qualitative Trend Descriptions. In: Barahona P, Stefanelli M, Wyatt J (eds.): Lecture Notes in Artificial Intelligence, Springer Verlag, Berlin, pp 197-208
[39] Horn W, Miksch S, Egghart G, Popow C, Paky F (1997) Effective data validation of high-frequency data: time-point-, time-interval-, and trend-based methods. Comput Biol Med 27(5): 389-409
[40] Westenskow DR, Orr JA, Simon FH, Bender H-J, Frankenberger H (1992) Intelligent Alarms Reduce Anesthesiologist's Response Time to Critical Faults. Anesthesiology 77: 1074-1079

[41] Narus SP, Kück K, Westenskow DR (1995). Intelligent Monitor for an Anesthesia Breathing Circuit. In: Proc Annu Symp Comput Appl Med Care, AMIA Inc., pp 96-100

[42] Sukuvaara T, Koski EMJ, Mäkivirta A, Kari A (1993) A knowledge-based alarm system for monitoring cardiac operated patients – technical construction and evaluation. International J. of Clin. Monitoring and Computing 10: 117-126

[43] Sukuvaara T, Sydänmaa M, Nieminen H, Heikelä A, Koski EMJ (1993) Object-Oriented Implementation of an Architecture for Patient Monitoring. IEEE Engineering in Medicine and Biology December: 69-81

[44] Koski EMJ, Sukuvaara T, Mäkivirta A, Kari A (1994) A knowledge-based system for monitoring cardiac operated patients – assessment of clinical performance. International J. of Clin. Monitoring and Computing 11: 79-83

[45] Haimowitz IJ, Le PP, Kohane IS (1995) Clinical monitoring using regression-based trend templates. Artificial Intelligence in Medicine 7: 473-496

[46] Shahar Y, Musen MA (1996) Knowledge-based temporal abstraction in clinical domains. Artificial Intelligence in Medicine 8: 267-298

[47] Dawant BM, Uckun S, Manders EJ, Lindstrom DP (1993) The SIMON Project: Model-Based Signal Acquisition, Analysis and Interpretation In Intelligent Patient Monitoring. IEEE Engineering in Medicine and Biology December: 82-91

[48] Coiera E (1994) Monitoring in Anaesthesia and Intensive Care. W.B. Sounders, London

[49] Salatin A, Hunter J (1999) Deriving trends in historical and real-time continously sampled medical data. Journal of Intelligent Information Systems 13: 47-71

[50] Bronstein IN, Semendjajew KA (1989) Taschenbuch der Mathematik. Teubner Verlag, Leipzig

[51] Becker K (1996) Der Einsatz quantitativer und qualitativer Methoden bei der Implementierung und Validierung eines intelligenten Entscheidungsunterstützungs- und Alarmsystems für die Kardioanästhesie. Dissertation, RWTH Aachen

[52] Larsen R (1985) Anästhesie. Urban&Schwarzenberg Verlag, München

[53] Nemes C, Niemer M, Noack G (1982) Datenbuch Anästhesiologie. Gustav Fischer Verlag, Stuttgart

[54] Jungk A, Thull B, Rau G (1999). Evaluation of an ecological interface for the anaesthesia workplace by eye-tracking. In: Bullinger H-J, Vossen PH (eds): Adjunct Proc. of the 8th HCI International '99, Fraunhofer IRB Verlag, Stuttgart, pp 31-32

[55] Kosko B (1992) Neural Networks and Fuzzy Systems. Prentice Hall International, Englewood-Cliffs

[56] Zimmermann H-J (1996) Fuzzy Set Theory and its Applications. 2nd ed., Kluwer, Dordrecht

[57] Zimmermann H-J (1993) Fuzzy-Technologien: Prinzipien, Werkzeuge, Potentiale. VDI Verlag, Düsseldorf

[58] Jungk A, Thull B, Hoeft A, Rau G (2000) Ergonomic Evaluation of an Ecological Interface and a Profilogram Display for Hemodynamic Monitoring. Journal of Clinical Monitoring and Computing (in press)
[59] Rasmussen J, Mark Pejtersen A, Goodstein LP (1994) Cognitive System Engineering. John Wiley, New York
[60] Gravenstein JS, Paulus DA (1985) Praxis der Patientenüberwachung. Fisher Verlag, Stuttgart
[61] Michels P, Gravenstein D, Westenskow DR (1997) An integrated graphic data display improves detection and identification of critical events during anesthesia. Journal of Clinical Monitoring 13(4): 249-259

Fuzzy Clustering in Medicine: Applications to Electrophysiological Signal Processing

Amir B. Geva and Dan H. Kerem

Electrical Engineering Department
Ben-Gurion University of the Negev
P.O.B. 653
Beer-Sheva 84105
Israel
E-mail: geva@ee.bgu.ac.il

Introduction

The essence of modern medicine is a continuous process of decision-making based on the intelligent evaluation of voluminous yet often inconclusive data gathered from patients. In many clinical setups such as intensive care units and epilepsy care units, monitored patients produce a vast amount of biomedical data from online continuous recordings of ECG, EEG, blood pressure, temperature, etc., as well as from X-ray, CT and MRI imaging. In the current state of affairs, there are objective difficulties in processing and interpreting all this data with the aim of extracting the relevant information.

By looking for temporal structure in a data set, clustering is particularly suitable for biomedical data mining that would aid the process of decision making. As the data will be based on uncertain information due to both the inherent complexity of the biological system and the shortcomings of the monitoring instrumentation, fuzzy clustering would be the tool of choice. As the number and nature of classes may not always be known and dictated beforehand, an unsupervised approach is often called for. This approach is also suitable for use on individual subjects without the need to enforce universal thresholds that define the crossing into the pathological state.

Review of Past and Current Uses

The first obvious use of fuzzy clustering in the medical arena was in the diagnostic field: the assigning of patients to one of several pathological categories, based on a group of features comprised of continuous measurements and/or binary data (presence or absence of symptom).

It was shown that for stomach disease, a lower classifying error rate was obtained by the use of a fuzzy nearest prototype (1-NP) classifier as compared to the widely-used Euclidean k-NN designs (Bezdek 1981). In a more recent example, this use was extended to the sub-classification of patients within a single pathological category by O'Malley et al. (1997). The authors succeeded in ascribing children with spastic diplegia (a form of cerebral palsy) degrees of membership in each of 5 fuzzy clusters representing 5 different gait strategies, based on stride length and cadence, adopted by afflicted children. Changes in membership partitioning then allowed the tracking of walking improvement following corrective surgery.

As an example of data fusion, this approach may be further extended to the task of risk-stratification of patients by supervised fuzzy cluster analysis (FCA) of several binary, graded and continuous-measure risk factors of their illness. Thus, both the prediction of future cardiac events and the correlation with coronary angiography findings were significantly higher in patients categorized by performing FCA on a combination of several stress-test variables and ST-segment changes than by the latter alone (Peters et al. 1998).

An important area where fuzzy clustering is proving useful is in medical image analysis, specifically but not exclusively brain MRI image segmentation. The expressed aims are automatic definition of the volume and exact edge detection of normal anatomical structures as well as abnormal tissue masses such as tumors. Uncertainty and fuzziness are still intrinsic in this field due to acquisition noise and low resolution of sensors. Work by Hall and coworkers utilized the fuzzy-c-means algorithm (Cannon et al. 1986) to classify brain slice images in a 3-D feature space comprised from different intensity measures. Classes included normal tissue such as gray matter, white matter and cerebro-spinal fluid as well as pathological tissues such as tumor (gliomas), edema fluid and necrotic tissue.

Attempts were made at reconstructing and labeling volume and contours of normal brain tissues by a hybrid approach, combining knowledge gained from the distribution of cluster centers in feature space and from anatomical-tissue-structure based expert systems (inter-subject variability required the setting of thresholds and the adoption of qualitative models). In the initial phase, the identification of abnormal tissue, either directly or indirectly, from distortion of normal structure (mismatch between normal model and its imaged instance) halted the procedure (Clark et al. 1994). Later on, by using membership partitioning in uncertain regions for re-clustering iterations, fuzzy clustering aids in a better definition of the boundaries of tumor tissue in preparation for radiation therapy and/or for following its efficacy (Clark et al. 1998).

Several other groups have joined this area in an attempt to refine the algorithms or to form new ones more suitable to other anatomical shapes such as the ring-shaped heart ventricle contour in a transverse MRI image of the thorax (Gath and Hoori, 1995). Their efforts divided into supervised and unsupervised as well as two and three dimensional data methods are described in a recent review by Bezdek et al. (1997). Examples of more recent contributions are Suckling et al. (1999) in brain MRI, Tolias and Panas (1998) in defining ocular fundus vessels in retinal images and Masulli and Schenone (1999) in general image analysis. Other important and relevant fuzzy clustering algorithms were suggested over the recent years, like the Possibilistic Fuzzy Clustering algorithm by Krishnapuram and Keler (1993) and the Fuzzy Learning Vector Quantization (FLVQ) algorithm by Bezdek and Pal (1995), which could well be applied to these problems.

Application of fuzzy clustering in the decision-making rule for classifying segments in the continuous time series of a biological signal, to be amplified further on in this chapter, was first proposed by Gath and Bar-On (1980) for classifying quasi-stationary segments in the human EEG during sleep. Data reduction was performed by choosing up to 9 descriptive features, including the spectral powers of several frequency bands and parameters derived from the standard deviations of the signal and its first and second derivatives. Arguing that EEG pattern changes (probably reflecting brain state transitions) are not sharp, each segment, defined by an autoregressive-model-based adaptive segmentation, was assigned degrees of membership in several fuzzy clusters formed in the 9-dimensional feature space.

Attempts at correlating other brain states with "EEG states" as defined by the above method, were later made both during wakefulness (Gath et al. 1983) and during anaesthesia (Bankman and Gath, 1987). In the first instance, "alpha" segments were associated with a lower vigilance performance, measured through auditory choice reaction times while in the latter case, depth of halothane anaesthesia could be correlated with EEG features. As the number of EEG states (exemplified by sleep stages) and their characteristics could be determined for the population as a whole but may vary considerably in individual subjects, an unsupervised version of fuzzy clustering of bio-potential time series was called for.

The Unsupervised Fuzzy Clustering Algorithms

The goal of unsupervised fuzzy clustering algorithms is to classify a given array of M data patterns into K fuzzy sets of similar patterns, where K, the number of clusters and their centroids location are unknown *a priori*. The result of a fuzzy partitioning of M data points into K fuzzy clusters is a $K\times M$ matrix, $\mathbf{U}$, of the degree of memberships, $0 \le u_{k,i} \le 1$, of each data point, i, in each cluster, k, such that $\sum_{k=1}^{K} u_{k,i} = 1$.

Following are three ascending levels of these algorithms:

The weighted fuzzy K-mean (WFKM) algorithm

The weighted version of the fuzzy *K*-mean algorithm, is derived from the minimization with respect to **P**, a set of *K* cluster centers, $\mathbf{p}_1,\ldots,\mathbf{p}_K$, and **U**, a $K\times M$ membership matrix, of a weighted fuzzy version of the least-squares function:

$$J_q(\mathbf{U},\mathbf{P})=\sum_{i=1}^{M}\sum_{k=1}^{K} w_i\cdot u_{k,i}^{q}\cdot d^2(\mathbf{p}_k,\mathbf{x}_i), \qquad (1)$$

where $\mathbf{x}_i$ in the *i*-th pattern, the *i*-th column in the **X** data matrix, $\mathbf{p}_k$ is the center of the *k*-th cluster, $u_{k,i}$ is the degree of membership of the data pattern $\mathbf{x}_i$ in the *k*-th cluster, w_i is the weight of the *i*-th pattern (as if w_i patterns which are equal to $\mathbf{x}_i$ were included in the data matrix **X**), $d^2(\mathbf{p}_k,\mathbf{x}_i)$ is the square of the distance between $\mathbf{x}_i$ and $\mathbf{p}_k$, *M* is the number of data patterns and *K* is the number of clusters in the partition. The parameter *q* (commonly set to 2) is the weighting exponent for $u_{k,i}$ and *q* controls the "fuzziness" of the resulting clusters (Bezdek, 1981). The pseudocode of the weighted fuzzy *K*-mean clustering algorithm with the modified centroids initialization (Gath and Geva 1989b, Geva 1998, Geva and Kerem 1998, Geva and Kerem 1999) is presented below:

The WFKM algorithm

$(\mathbf{U},\mathbf{P}_K)=\mathrm{WFKM}(\mathbf{X},\mathbf{w},K,\mathbf{P}_{K-1})$:

1) Use the final centroids (prototypes) of the previous partition, $\mathbf{P}_{K-1}$, as the initial centroids for the current partition: in step **3a** of the WUOFC algorithm (see textbox 2) use the *K*-1 (*) final centroids of its previous stage and for step **3b** use all the *K* final centroids, $\mathbf{P}_K$, of step **3a;**

2) repeat Calculate the degree of membership $u_{k,i}$ of all data pattern in all clusters:

for $k \leftarrow 1$ to K (*)
 do for $i \leftarrow 1$ to M
  do

$$u_{k,i}=d^2(\mathbf{x}_i,\mathbf{p}_k)^{1/(1-q)}\Big/\sum_{j=1}^{K}\left[d^2(\mathbf{x}_i,\mathbf{p}_j)\right]^{1/(1-q)} \qquad (2)$$

(*) Only for $k = K$ and i the first iteration of the step **3a** of the WUOFC algorithm use the following distance:

$$d^2(\mathbf{x}_i,\mathbf{p}_k) = 10\%\mathrm{Sum}(\ \mathrm{Diagonal}(\ \mathrm{Covariance}(\mathbf{X})\ )\ ),\quad i=1,\ldots,M.$$

Otherwise use the Euclidean distance in step **3a** (Eq.4) or the Exponential distance (Eq.5) in step **3b** of the WUOFC algorithm (see textbox 2).

Calculate the new set of cluster centers:

for $k \leftarrow 1$ to K

do $$\mathbf{p}_k = \sum_{i=1}^{M} u_{k,i}^{q} \cdot w_i \cdot \mathbf{x}_i \Big/ \sum_{i=1}^{M} u_{k,i}^{q} \cdot w_i \qquad (3)$$

4) until $$\max_{k,i} \left| u_{k,i} - \left(previous \; u_{k,i} \right) \right| < \varepsilon$$

The weighted unsupervised optimal fuzzy clustering (WUOFC) algorithm

This algorithm has been previously presented as implemented in the analysis of electroencephalographic and evoked potential signals (Gath and Geva 1989b, Geva and Pratt, 1994, Geva 1998, Geva and Kerem 1998, Geva and Kerem 1999). Basically the WUOFC algorithm is a simple modification of the UOFC algorithm(Gath and Geva 1989a) where each point in the data set is weighted according to previous knowledge about its relative importance. The latter may allude, for instance, to members representing data segments of variable length, to cluster centroids found by prior analyses (extra weight), or, in case of an on-line analysis, to favor newly over old appearing members (forgetting function).

The advantage of the UOFC algorithm is the unsupervised initialization of cluster prototypes, and the criteria for cluster validity using fuzzy hypervolume and density functions. The weighted version of the UOFC algorithm, shown below, is iterated for an increasing number of clusters in the data set, calculating a new partition of the data set, and computing performance measures in each run, until the optimal number of clusters is obtained.

The WUOFC algorithm

$(\mathbf{U}, K_{opt}) = \text{WUOFC}(\mathbf{X}, \mathbf{w})$:

1) Choose a single initial centroid, $\mathbf{P}_0$, at the weighted (by $\mathbf{w}$) mean of all data patterns and set $K \leftarrow 1$

2) while K K_{max}, the maximal feasible number of clusters in the data;

3) do Calculate a new partition of the data set by two phases:

a) Cluster with the weighted fuzzy K-means with the Euclidean distance function:

$$(\mathbf{U}, \mathbf{P}_K) = \text{WFKM}(\mathbf{X}, \mathbf{w}, K, \mathbf{P}_{K-1})$$

b) Use the final centroids $\mathbf{P}_K$ from the previous step as the initial centroids for the weighted fuzzy K-means with the Exponential distance function; a fuzzy modification of the maximum likelihood estimation (FMLE):

$$(\mathbf{U},\mathbf{P}_K)=\mathrm{WFKM}(\mathbf{X},\mathbf{w},K,\mathbf{P}_K)$$

4) Calculate the cluster validity criteria of the Kth partition.
5) Add another centroid equally distant (with a large number of standard deviations) from all data points (see step **2** in the following modified fuzzy K-means algorithm),

$$\text{set } K \leftarrow K+1 \text{ and go to the above step } \mathbf{2};$$

6) Use the cluster validity criteria for $K=1,\ldots,K_{max}$, to choose and **return** the optimal number of cluster K_{opt}, and the corresponding partition **U**

In the first phase **3.a** of the WUOFC algorithm, the fuzzy weighted K-mean algorithm is performed with the Euclidean distance function:

$$d^2(\mathbf{p}_k,\mathbf{x}_i)=\left[(\mathbf{p}_k-\mathbf{x}_i)^T\cdot(\mathbf{p}_k-\mathbf{x}_i)\right]. \tag{4}$$

The final cluster centers of the first phase **3.a** are used as the initial centroids for the second phase. In the second phase **3.b**, a fuzzy modification of the maximum likelihood estimation is utilized, by using the following exponential distance function in the weighted fuzzy K-mean algorithm:

$$d^2(\mathbf{p}_k,\mathbf{x}_i)=\frac{[\det(\mathbf{F}_k)]^{1/2}}{a_k}\cdot\exp\left[(\mathbf{p}_k-\mathbf{x}_i)^T\cdot\mathbf{F}_k^{-1}\cdot(\mathbf{p}_k-\mathbf{x}_i)/2\right], \tag{5}$$

where $a_k=\sum_{i=1}^{M}u_{k,i}\Big/\sum_{i=1}^{M}w_i$ is the sum of memberships within the k-th cluster, which consist of the *a priori* probability of selecting the k-th cluster and

$$\mathbf{F}_k=\sum_{i=1}^{M}u_{k,i}\cdot w_i\cdot(\mathbf{p}_k-\mathbf{x}_i)\cdot(\mathbf{p}_k-\mathbf{x}_i)^T\Big/\sum_{i=1}^{M}u_{k,i}\cdot w_i \tag{6}$$

is the fuzzy covariance matrix of the k-th cluster.

By applying these two phases, the fuzzy K-mean algorithm with the Euclidean distance function is used to find a feasible initial partition, and the fuzzy modification of the maximum likelihood estimation is utilized to refine the partition for normally distributed clusters with large variability of the covariance matrix (shape, size and density) and the number of patterns in each cluster. Note that other distance functions can be used according to the intrinsic characteristics of the data.

The hierarchical unsupervised fuzzy clustering (HUFC) algorithm

Single step classification algorithms may fail when the data include complex structures with a large variability of cluster shapes, variances, densities, and number of data points in each cluster. In the case in question, rare arrhythmias or combinations of beats could form very small clusters, which may be missed as such and be lumped into bigger ones by the original algorithm. On such occasions, we have reverted to a newly presented hierarchic version of fuzzy clustering (Geva, 1999).

The basic notion is a re-examination of each cluster formed by a primary process of fuzzy clustering, as a candidate for fuzzy sub-classification. In the first call to the procedure all data points have an equal weight (of one) in the partitioning. In the next level of the recursive process the same partitioning procedure is applied on each of the formed fuzzy clusters, composed of all *i*'s with non-zero membership values in it. These memberships are used to weigh the *i*'s, before submitting them to re-partitioning. Thus, the genealogy of the degree of membership of *i* in the evolving process is preserved by serial multiplication such that in each classification step, *n*, the actual degree of membership of *i* in a daughter cluster, *l*, is $u_{l,i}{}^{n} \times u_{k,i}{}^{n-1}$ where the multiplier is its weight (or degree of membership in the mother cluster, *k*).

The optimal number of clusters in each stage is determined by adapted cluster validity criteria, based on the hyper-volume measurement. Sub-classification is terminated when the optimal number of daughters comes out as one, or when the number of data points in a proposed daughter is smaller than some predetermined constant multiplied by the number of features. The combined memberships of each data point in all final fuzzy clusters is maintained at one. One may note that in contrast to crisp hierarchical clustering, the final decision about each data point's affiliation is made only at the termination of the algorithm. Data points may share membership in more than one cluster of the final generation as well as in clusters of previous generations, which did not sub-divide.

The main part of the algorithm is a recursive procedure HUFC(**X**,**w**), where its inputs are an $N \times M$ data matrix, **X**, composed of M columns of (in our case, 2 or 3) data patterns, $\mathbf{x}_j \in \Re^N, j = 1,\ldots,M$, and a column vector, $\mathbf{w} \in \Re^M$, of M weights of each data pattern in the partitioning. The weight of each pattern, w_i, i=1,.,M, is treated by the clustering algorithm as if w_i patterns, which are equal to i-th pattern, $\mathbf{x}_i$, were included in the data matrix **X** (for details see Geva (1999) and Geva and Kerem (1999)). The HUFC algorithm is initiated by setting the global matrix U^g to an empty matrix and the global number of clusters K^g to zero, and executed by calling HUFC($\mathbf{X}_0$,$\mathbf{w}_0$), where $\mathbf{X}_0$ is the matrix of the M_0 original data patterns and

$\mathbf{w}_0$ is a column vector of M_0 ones. The pseudocode of the HUFC procedure includes the following steps:

The HUFC algorithm

FC(**X**,**w**):

1. If the sum of the patterns' weights $\sum_{j=1}^{M} w_j > (Constant \times N)$

2. then $(\mathbf{U}, K_{opt})$ = WUOFC(**X**).

Apply the Weighted Unsupervised Optimal Fuzzy Clustering algorithm, which finds the optimal number of clusters (by means of some validity criterion) in the given data K_{opt}, and the $K_{opt} \times M$ memberships matrix **U** of the M given patterns in these K_{opt} clusters.

3. **else** $K_{opt}=1$

4. **If** $K_{opt} > 1$

5. **then** for $k \leftarrow 1$ to K_{opt}

6. **do** HUFC(**X**, $\mathbf{w} \times \mathbf{u}_k$)

recursive call to the main procedure where $\mathbf{u}_k$ is the vector of the memberships of all M patterns in the k's cluster, and $\mathbf{w} \times \mathbf{u}_k$ denotes a vector whose j-th component is:

$$w_j \times u_{k,j}, \quad j=1,\ldots,M.$$

7. **else** append the column vector **w** to the global memberships matrix $\mathbf{U}^g$

8. $K^g \leftarrow K^g + 1$, increase the global number of clusters by one.

9. **return**

When the algorithm has terminated, $\mathbf{U}^g$ contains the final memberships of all the data patterns in all the K^g final clusters.

The Fuzzy Hypervolume Cluster Validity Criteria

In Step **4** of the WUOFC algorithm the following criteria for cluster validity are calculated:

1. The fuzzy hypervolume criterion (HPV):

$$V_{HV}(K) = \sum_{k=1}^{K} h_k \,, \tag{7}$$

where the hypervolume of the k-th cluster is defined by $h_k = [\det(\mathbf{F}_k)]^{1/2}$.

2. The partition density (PD):

$$v_{PD}(K)=\sum_{k=1}^{K}b_k \Big/ \sum_{k=1}^{K}h_k \text{ ,} \tag{8}$$

where $b_k = \sum_{i\in \mathbf{I}_k} u_{k,j}\cdot w_j$, and I_k is a set of indices of the "central members" in the k-th cluster:

$$\mathbf{I}_k=\left\{i : \left[(\mathbf{p}_k-\mathbf{x}_i)^T\cdot \mathbf{g}_j^k\right]\cdot (p_{k,j}-x_{i,j})<1 \;\; \forall j=1,\dots,N,\;\; i=1,\dots,M \right\},$$

where the N-dimensional column vector $\mathbf{g}^k_j$ is the j-th column of the matrix $\mathbf{G}_k=\mathbf{F}_k^{-1}$, the inverse of the k-th cluster covariance matrix. Note that a pattern $\mathbf{x}_i$ is a "central member" in the k-th cluster only if **all the projections** of the Mahanalobis distance between the pattern $\mathbf{x}_i$ and the k-th centroid $\mathbf{p}_k$ are smaller then one.

3. The average partition density (APD):

$$v_{AD}(K)=\frac{1}{k}\sum_{k=1}^{K}\left[b_k / h_k\right] \text{ ,} \tag{9}$$

4. The normalized (by K) partition indexes criterion:

$$J_q^K(\mathbf{U},\mathbf{P})=K\cdot\sum_{i=1}^{M}\sum_{k=1}^{K}u_{k,i}^q\cdot w_i\cdot \mathrm{d}^2(\mathbf{p}_k,\mathbf{x}_i). \tag{10}$$

The UOFC algorithm is terminated when the performance measures for cluster validity reach their best value. The choice of the criterion or combination of criteria to be the performance measure is driven by the specific distribution of the data. One of the main constraints on a validity criterion for the HUFC algorithm is its efficient applicability for *one* cluster (compared to more than one cluster), remembering that the recursive procedure is halted when the "partition" to one cluster is the best of all partitions. This constraint precludes the use of any validity criterion which involves the distance between clusters.

Detailed Examples

As detailed examples on the use of the clustering algorithms in the mining of medical data, we will focus on two aspects: classification of heart-rate fluctuations and the forecasting of epilepsy from the electroencephalogram (EEG) and electrocardiogram (ECG) records and from the time series of heart rate inter-beat intervals.

Classifying heart rate fluctuations - background

Two types of information may be obtained from the ECG signal: Information relating to the form and temporal relationship of the component waves and complexes of each or any individual heart-beat event, and information focusing on the time series of the intervals between consecutive heart-beat events, the so called heart rate variability (HRV). While the former is the principal reflection and diagnostic tool of the various potential-generators of the heart, HRV mirrors the important impingement of the autonomic nervous system efferents on the cardiac sinus pace-maker (Malik and Camm 1995).

Global time domain measures of HRV are based on various statistical descriptors of the distribution of inter-beat intervals (usually measured between one QRS complex peak to the next and termed RR-intervals) or of the differences between successive intervals. However, a major component of heart rate variability is generated by intrinsic cycles with a wide range of discrete periods, such as the well known respiratory-entrained sinus arrhythmia, slower waves which follow blood pressure oscillations and diurnal cycles which may also modulate the faster rhythms. As the parasympathetic and sympathetic autonomic nervous systems modulate the basic sinus rhythm at different parts of this range – spectral analysis of the time series of RR intervals, as introduced in 1981 by Akselrod et al. has become a major tool of HRV quantification, aimed at assessing physiological as well as pathological changes in the balance of the two inputs.

Human HRV power spectral density (PSD) distribution refers to three main frequency components: a very-low-frequency (VLF) < 0.04 Hz component arising from ill understood long-term (thermoregulatory, hormonal) regulation, a low-frequency (LF) component ranging between 0.04 and 0.15 Hz which mainly mirrors sympathetic influence and a high-frequency (HF) > 0.15 Hz component, which shifts with the respiratory frequency and is a specific marker of parasympathetic activity. Thus, for instance, an abrupt passive 90^0 head-up tilt from the supine position, termed orthostatic challenge, causes a distinct shift in the relative magnitude of the sympathetic and parasympathetic components of HRV in favor of the former. This shift is usually expressed as an increase in the ratio of the normalized power of the low and high frequency components: LF/HF, (Lipsitz et al. 1990).

A distinct drawback of frequency analysis methods of HRV lies in the interval time series being an event series which is by definition discontinuous and as such either requires interpolation in order to create a function that may be sampled at constant time increments or else, special mathematical manipulations to address this problem (Pahlm and Sornmo 1984). Other disadvantages are their inadequacy in dealing with instances of a globally depressed power spectrum (Malik 1996) and their sensitivity to independent changes in respiratory pattern (Brown et al. 1993).

A more recent analytic tool employed for HRV quantification, stems from the field of non-linear dynamics. It has been stressed that HRV rather than being truly periodic or truly random, has a fractal nature and very often behaves as if governed by a low-dimensional chaotic generator. The trajectories on a phase plane projection of a time series of RR-intervals (with the amplitude of successive RR-intervals plotted on the x-axis and its rate of change on the y-axis), reveal strange attractors which diminish their complexity and even converge into point attractors, in antecedence of sudden cardiac death (Goldberger and West 1987). This tool uses the discrete intervals as such and circumvents the need to interpolate.

The shortcoming of both approaches is the inability to deal with non-stationary states and transients, short-lasting rhythm disturbances and single aberrations, either spontaneous or intentionally induced by certain maneuvers. Such transients may have direct diagnostic value as well as a use to detect and possibly forecast extra-cardiac pathology, especially in cases where the ECG is the only monitored signal. Cases in question include sleep apnea and, as illustrated in our second example, acute global CNS pathology (which also involves the autonomic nervous system) such as epilepsy.

Several methods of time-varying PSD estimations such as short time Fourier transform (STFT) spectrograms, recursive autoregressive techniques or other time-frequency distributions (wavelet analysis), have been used to partly overcome this problem (Cerutti et al.1995, Harel et al. 1997) and their ability to detect and sometimes predict transients such as ischemic (anginal) episodes has been demonstrated (Vila et al, 1997, Wilkund et al.1997). Yet, even those methods will miss single events such as exceptional RR-intervals or exceptional Δ RR-intervals (instantaneous rate changes), occurring now and then. Indeed, ectopic beats and arrhythmic events may interfere with the spectral estimation of HRV and are often edited out or interpolated. Attractors and correlation dimensions, on their part, do offer global quantification of the complexity of state space but do not give a structural description of this space, as shaped by the various underlying heart-rate modulators.

The clustering approach

A natural way to describe and quantitate the template structure of the HRV state space is by clustering of the points occupying it. A pure, low dimension, chaotic system bifurcating into widely divergent states (ectopies etc.) has a definite pattern in state space, with dense areas and empty "forbidden zones". The latter may be invaded by harmonic and/or random Gaussian fluctuations as well as by continuous "DC" trends in the basic heart rate. This will cause the centroids of any existing clusters to continuously shift positions and the Gaussian clusters themselves, to smear and overlap as they enlarge with time. The final product from a conventional 24 hour record of normal subjects usually appears as a single, comet or torpedo shaped cluster (Malik 1995). Shorter records, separated in space by a proper choice of the number and nature of its feature dimensions and all records which include conspicuous, recurrent and reproducible rhythm disturbances, yield more detail which lends itself to either crisp or more often, to fuzzy partitioning.

In the following examples we will demonstrate the outcome of subjecting an N-dimensional feature space of RR-intervals or their differentials to either a single step or to a hierarchic unsupervised fuzzy clustering. We will try to convince the reader that this method is particularly useful for identifying and classifying rare aberrant beats and steep rate changes on a background of a fluctuating sinus rhythm, but also in bringing out detail bearing on other heart-rate modulations. It should be mentioned that fuzzy classification has been used for the detection of ventricular arrhythmias based on features derived from spectral parameters of the raw ECG signal (Cabello et al. 1991). A supervised approach with a training set and test sets was used with a trial and error algorithm optimization, set to minimize classification differences between the computation method and an expert cardiologist. A 10% error rate could be achieved, with the Fuzzy Covariance significantly out-performing the Fuzzy C-Means algorithm (ibid.).

Data sources

Digitized (360 Hz), ECG records of cardiac patients were extracted from the MIT Arrhythmia Database (Biomedical Engineering Center of the Harvard-MIT Division of Health Sciences and Technology, Cambridge, Ma, USA, 1992). Analog ECG records from human subjects, resting and performing several physiological maneuvers, were obtained in the laboratory disposable disk electrodes in the bipolar XYZ orthogonal lead system (Anon. 1989). Resting records were digitized at 400 and exercise records at 1000 Hz. ECG records of resting, unrestrained rats were obtained by means of three thin-wire loop electrodes, two on both sides of the chest and one on the lower back, inserted sub-cutaneously for the period of recording. Records were digitized at 1000 Hz.

Data analysis

The chosen digitized sections of the ECG are then subjected to a QRS-peak detection software with adaptive time, amplitude and rise-rate thresholds incorporated into the decision rule (see Pahlm and Sornmo (1984) for recommendations). The software allows user interaction in editing the detection results. The latter include displays of the original record, tick-marked on each identified peak, as well as a list of RR interval durations, graphed for each successive heartbeat, at time increments equal to the mean series interval, known as a tachogram. Other than verifying that all detected peaks were indeed QRS complexes and that no complexes were missed, all ectopies and other pathological beats are retained in the analyzed series. The final output of the software is a filed list of m consecutive RR-intervals (RRi). The list is converted into a point array in an N-dimensional space, the axes being either durations (lag plots):

$RRi(n), RRi(n+1), \ldots, RRi(n+N\text{-}1)$, $n=1,\ldots,M\text{-}N+1$ or differentials (phase plots):
$RRi(n)$, $diff[RRi(n)]$, $diff^2[RRi(n)]$, ... , $diff^{(N-1)}[RRi(n)]$, $n=1,\ldots,M\text{-}N+1$ or
$RRi(n)$, $|diff[RRi(n)]|$, $|diff^2[RRi(n)]|$, ... , $|diff^{(N-1)}[RRi(n)]|$, $n=1,\ldots,M\text{-}N+1$.

The point array is then subjected to the HUFC algorithm.

Examples of performance

Pathological cardiac arrhythmias

Three arrhythmic heart beat interval series, with increasing complexity and diversity of rhythm aberrations, on which the algorithm has been applied, are presented below. The first two are included for methodological reasons, to lead into the last example where fuzzy clustering may have a real advantage.

The first record is an analysis of a 20 minutes stretch from a rat, which inadvertently was found to exhibit a 2nd degree (intermittent) sino-atrial block. This terminology describes a condition where some of the impulses originating in the sinus pacemaker find problems in exciting the atrial cells, resulting in a prolonged PP (and thus RR) interval (type I) up to a point where one or more beats are skipped altogether (type II). The overall preponderance of this arrhythmia is evident from the compressed tachogram depicted in Figure 1_A. It shows a dominant pattern of alternation between two basic intervals: that of 0.185 s, corresponding to the normal resting rat heart rate of 335 beats per minute and a longer one lasting 0.275 s, less than twice as long, suggesting a type I (incomplete) block.

Figure 1_B shows a simple 4-cluster partitioning of RR intervals in an $RRi_{(n)}$, $RRi_{(n+1)}$ plane (otherwise known as a return map, Poincare map or Lorenz plot). This rather crisp clustering shows all 4 combinations of normal/normal, normal/long, long/normal and the much less frequent two adjoining long intervals (upper right). A closer look will show that in accordance with the underlying pathology, the interval preceding or alternating with the long one is actually slightly longer than the normal mean, i.e. 0.192 s.

The assignment of the cluster in which a point has the highest degree of membership can now be made for each consecutive temporal pattern in the series. Figure 1_C shows such labeling on a short section of the original tachogram. The normal sinus rhythm is seen to sometimes persist for a few seconds before giving way to the block pattern.

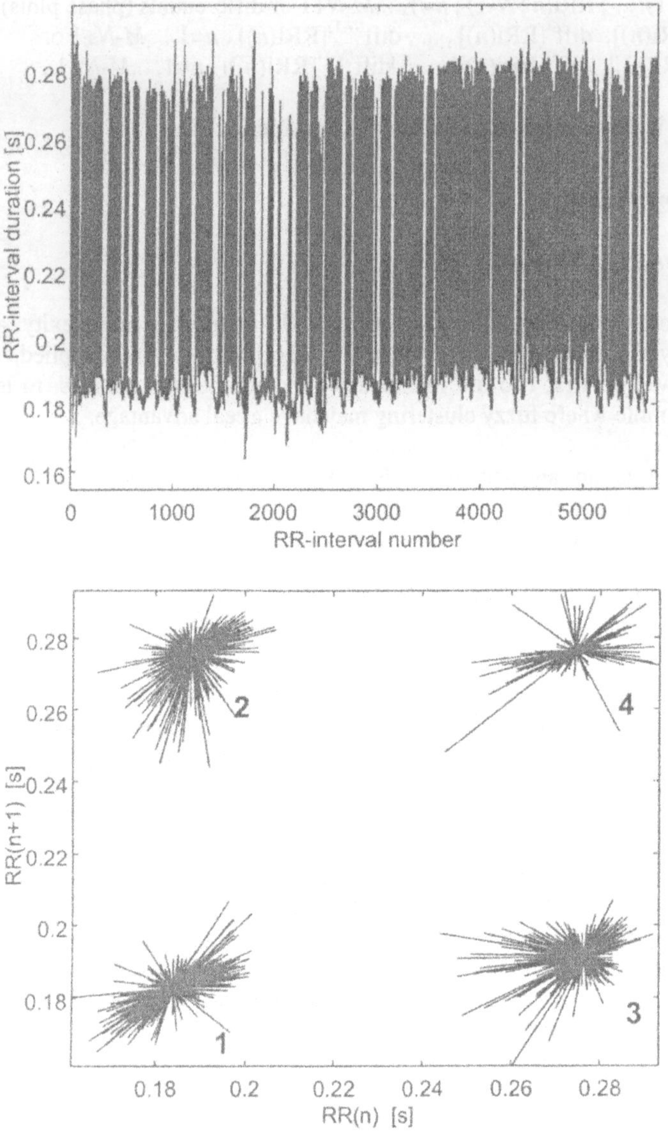

Figure 1$_{A,B}$: Clustering of RR-intervals of an arrhythmic rat:
A – Raw tachogram.
B – Clustering results in a 2-D lag plot. Points in this as well as in all similar later figures, are connected by lines to the centroids of clusters in which they have the highest degree of membership.

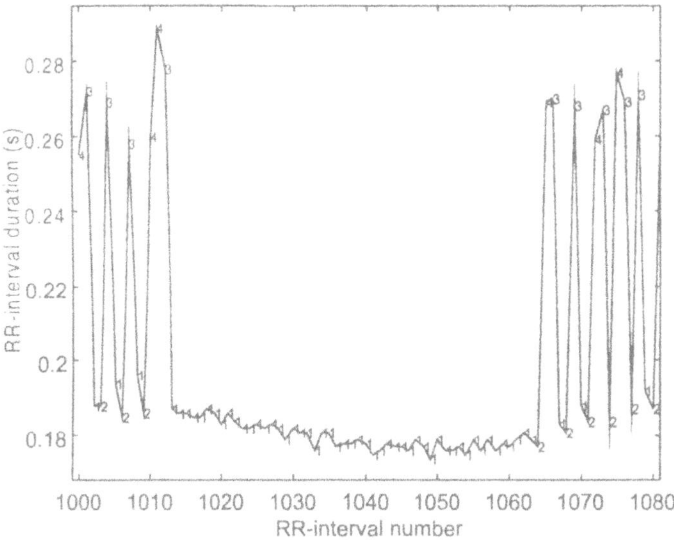

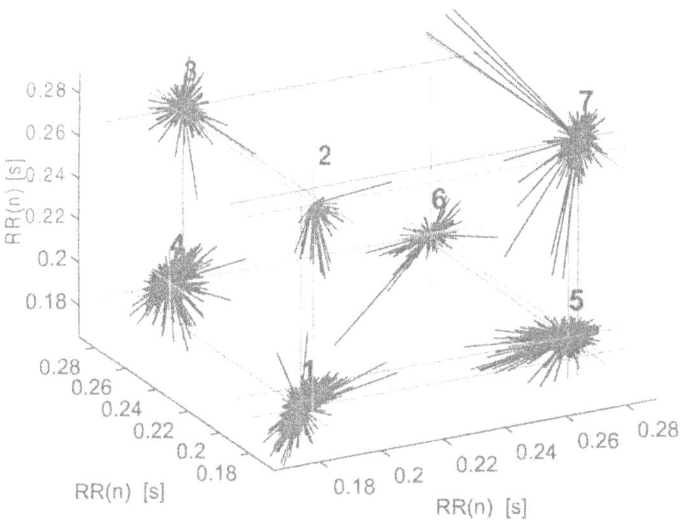

Figure $1_{A,B}$: Clustering of RR-intervals of an arrhythmic rat
C – Section of **A** with each RR-interval labeled by the results of **B** (label is on the first interval of each successive pair).
D – Clustering results in a 3-D lag plot. In order to enhance 3-dimensionality, Centroids are connected to the 3 planes by lines paralleling the axes. Lines do not overlap because of the slightly longer interval preceding the block.

To find out whether the long interval too occurs more than twice in a row and how often (one such instance shown in 1_C), we need to partition in a 3 dimensional space (Figure 1_D). If this combination exists, one would expect a partitioning to 8 clusters at the vertices of a cube. Actually, there are only 4 instances of three adjoining long intervals (furthest from observer) which are wrongly grouped within another cluster. In this case, a hierarchic reclassification of sufficient resolution to separate the 4-point cluster, results in further fragmentation of the mother cluster as well as other clusters. This sub-classification may be wholly or partly (patho)physiologically justified but does not serve this point of the presentation.

Apart from size and global variance, the actual shape of a cluster holds further indirect information on the importance of processes contributing to it. This is particularly true of the cluster representing normal sinus rhythm. Focusing on it in the 2-dimensional plot (lower left), its diagonal spread towards and away from the axes origin (variance), mirrors either the extent of slow trends in sinus rate variation, or else, abrupt but long lasting changes, associated with a variable sinus rhythm. Conversely, its spread perpendicular to this direction (covariance), reflects short-term fluctuations (next interval much different from the present one) such as may arise from pronounced respiratory sinus arrhythmia.

The second example is a 30 minute recording from a cardiac patient, which is dominated by premature ventricular complexes (PVCs), isolated as well as in sequences of bigemini (alternating premature beats and pauses) and trigemini (alternating normal, premature beats and pauses) rhythms. Unlike the rat example, we are now dealing with 3 basic intervals, that of the normal sinus rhythm, the short one of the premature beat and the longer than normal following pause. Thus, the 2-dimensional return map of this record shown in Figure 2A(top), may basically be viewed as that of paired combinations of the three mean RR intervals: the normal, of 0.9 s, the short PVC of 0.55 s and the (compensatory) pause of 1.3 s ($0{,}55+1.3 \cong 2*0.9$). The partition shows that only 5 of the 9 possible combinations actually occur.

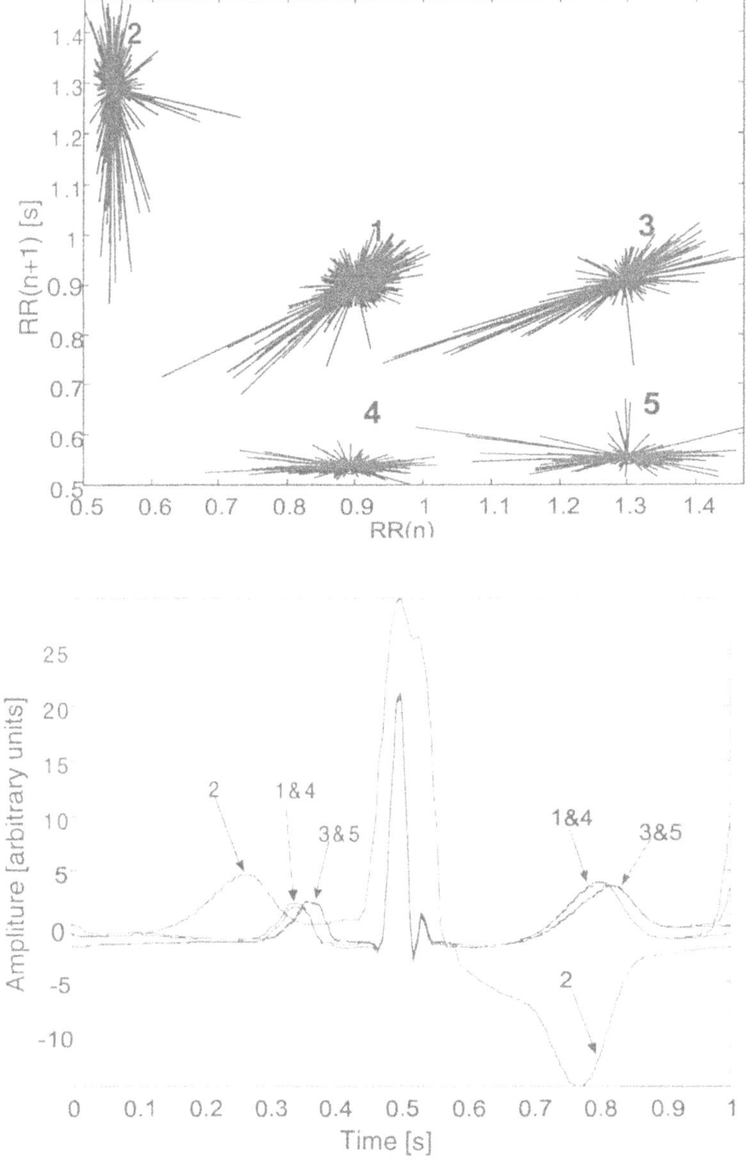

Figure 2_A: Clustering RR-intervals in a cardiac patient with moderate pathology
A – Top: Clustering results in a 2-D lag plot. Five of 9 possible combinations of three basic intervals occur. The rest are either not feasible (such as a normal beat followed by a pause) or else, not present in this stretch (such as couplets, which are two PVCs in a row). Bottom: Average PQRST complex forms of members in each of the five clusters in A.

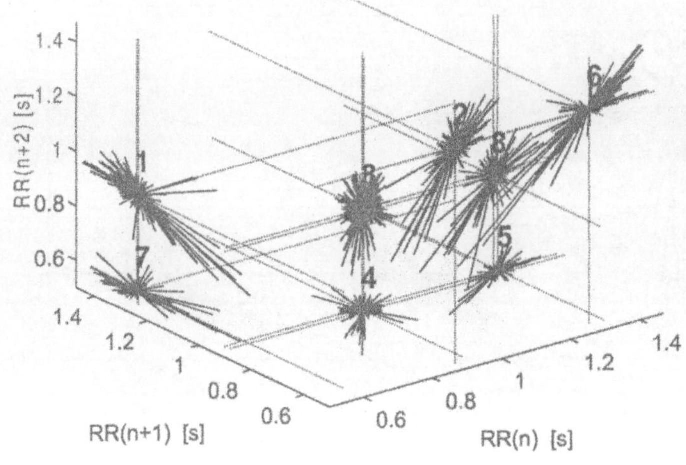

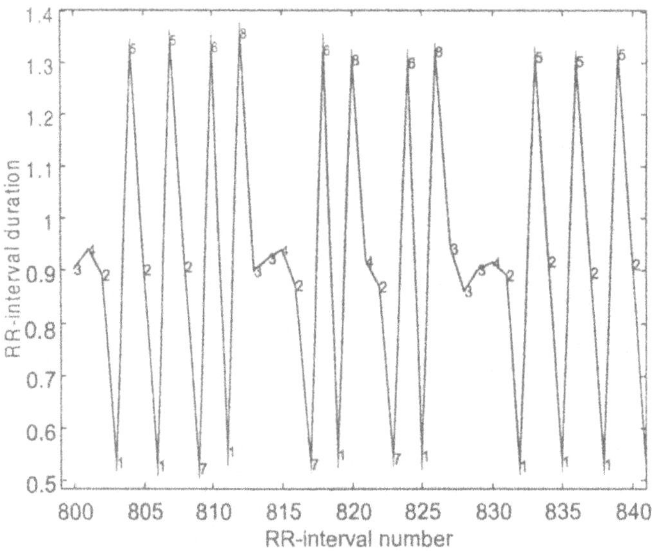

Figure $2_{B,C}$: Clustering RR-intervals in a cardiac patient with moderate pathology
B – Clustering results in a 3-D lag plot. Lines as in 2_D.
C – Portion of the tachogram labeled with results of **B**.

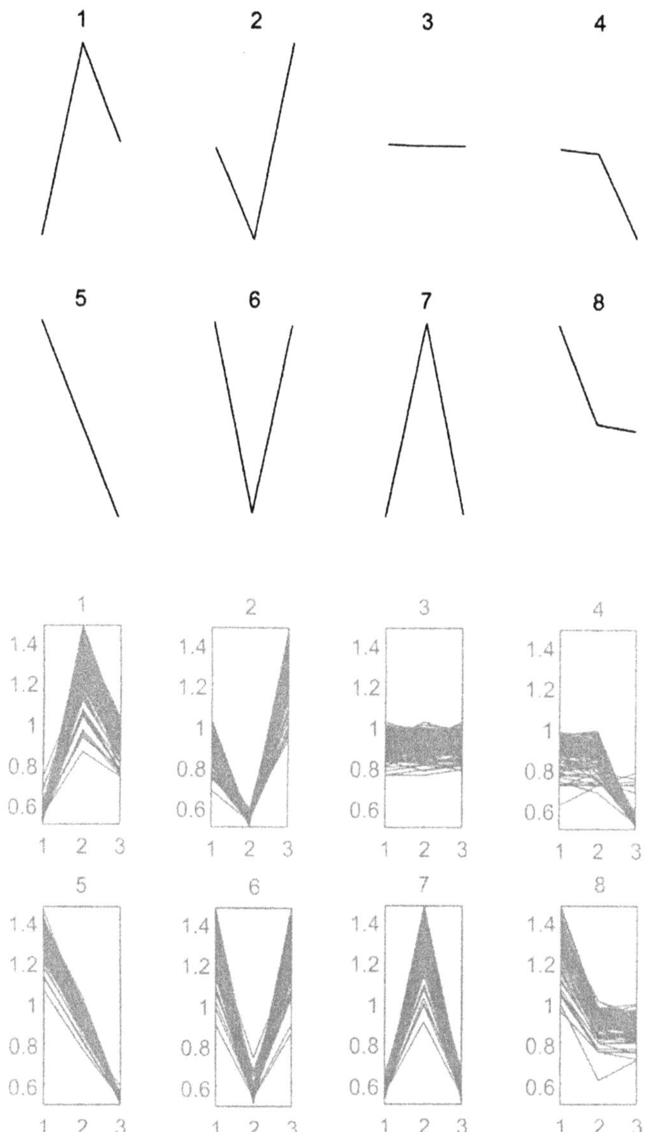

Figure 2$_{D,E}$: Clustering RR-intervals in a cardiac patient with moderate pathology
D – The 8 pattern prototypes (mean coordinates of each cluster) of **B**.
E – The pattern members belonging to each of the prototypes in **D**.

A short reflection will reveal cluster 1 to represent normal sinus rhythm, clusters 4, 2 and 3 (in sequential order), isolated PVCs and/or trigemini rhythm, while cluster 5 specifies the bigemini rhythm (4 and 3 at its start and termination, respectively). The down and/or leftward smearing of cluster 1 and other clusters are the result of an increased heart rate (shorter RR intervals) developing in the latter part of the record. Since the segments of the original ECG record around each identified peak are sequentially stored by the software, the individual shapes of the entire PQRST complex belonging to members of various clusters may be inspected to ascertain the nature of the arrhythmia. Figure 2A (bottom) shows the superimposed (by the point of peak-identification) average forms of the second of the 3 complexes in each of the 5 clusters. Two basic forms, that of the sinus-originated beat (clusters 1-4) and that of the ventricular beat (#2), originating soon after the preceding T-wave, are apparent. In addition, one may notice that compensatory sinus beats (# 3&5) have slightly shorter P-Q segments and slightly longer S-T segments.

The trigemini rhythm may be distinguished in a 3-D projection (Fig 2_B), embodied in cluster 5, the members of which have a long-normal-short sequence specific to this rhythm. In this partitioning (where 8 of the possible 27 combinations are actually occupied by clusters), cluster 3 hosts members of the normal sinus rhythm, cluster 4 heralds an isolated PVC or one of the aberrant rhythms and cluster 8 is the termination and return to normal rhythm (always from the pause). Clusters 6 and 7 are bigemini while 1 and 2 are PVCs, trigemini and several transitions between rhythms. The above apportionment is confirmed and realized in the section of the labeled tachogram shown in Figure 2_C.

The actual mean pattern of each of the 8 combinations of 3 successive beats is shown in Figure 2_D and the individual patterns of all class members in Figure 2_E. One may see that some classes, such as the trigemini thythm of #5, are rather compact with minimal variation from the mean, while the fuzziness of others (#4) is evident from the inclusion of members not even sharing the basic form. Close inspection of figure 2_D shows other detail, such as that upon return to sinus rhythm, the first normal interval is slightly longer than the mean while when switching out of sinus rhythm, the last normal beat is slightly shorter than the mean.

Table 1 lists some relevant descriptive statistics of the eight clusters. Out of 2000 intervals, 666 are sinus rhythm, 336 ($168 \cdot 2$) bigemini, 357 ($119 \cdot 3$) trigemini, 314 (161+153) are starts and ends and the rest are isolated PVCs and transitions. Noting the variances, as expected, they are higher the larger the basic interval. Yet, comparing the trigemini sequence of cluster 5 with the bigemini sequences of clusters 6 and 7, one can see that the long pause is twice as variant and the short premature beat 5 times as variant in the latter. The coherence of the trigemini rhythm is also evident from its co-variance. Thus, the sequence long-normal (cov 1-2) in cluster 5 has a half the co-variance of the same sequence in cluster 8.

Table 1. The fuzzy number of members and the co-variance matrices of each of the final classes of Figure 2_B.

Class	# Mem	Var 1	Var 2	Var 3	Cov 1-2	Cov 1-3	Cov 2-3
1	275.00	0.51	6.50	2.36	-0.25	-0.02	3.08
2	274.00	2.06	0.18	6.28	-0.05	2.74	-0.12
3	666.10	1.26	1.14	1.10	0.62	0.45	0.58
4	160.90	3.35	3.09	1.48	2.39	-1.22	-1.07
5	119.00	3.44	1.37	0.15	1.72	0.02	0.00
6	168.00	6.61	0.73	7.50	0.02	6.20	-0.31
7	168.00	0.38	7.17	0.56	-0.21	0.03	-0.10
8	153.01	6.62	3.04	2.12	3.62	3.08	2.02

The last example is from a patient expressing a variety of abnormal rhythms as well as a variable sinus rhythm. It is presented mainly to stress the effectiveness of unsupervised fuzzy classification, unavailable with conventional Holter softwares. A glance at the 2-D return map of a 20 min RR-interval series, reveals a very undefined and smeared array, although quite a few fuzzy point concentrations are apparent (Figure 3_A). Forced-partitioning to a large number of clusters may help us decide on the optimum number, by inspecting the peaks in the graphs of the validity criteria values versus number of classes (Figure 3_B). One can see that after an initial high at 1-2 classes (which would be the choice of an unsupervised run), several criteria have a distinct peak at 15 clusters. Re-clustering to15 (Figure 3_C) and labeling the results on a particularly problematic portion of the time series (Figure 3_D), should convince the observer that the division is indeed a faithful representation of the reality with its sudden changes in basic heart rate and its diverse arrhythmias.

The presented method which focuses on rhythm rather than on the shape of the original ECG record, might be dismissed by cardiologists accustomed to interpret Holter records. Yet, the information it conveys is intended to complement rather than to replace shape-related information. Also, as shown above, the average PQRST shape for each cluster is readily available for consideration. Signal averaging of long sections of the ECG record are often used to obtain otherwise obscure shape details such as late potentials which are considered risk factors for cardiac pathology (Schlactman and Green, 1990). Differential signal averaging of cluster members may yield completely new shape detail (Figure 2A (bottom)). This approach has been successfully applied in increasing signal-to-noise ratio by fuzzy-clustering-based selective averaging of evoked responses (Zouridakis et al. 1997).

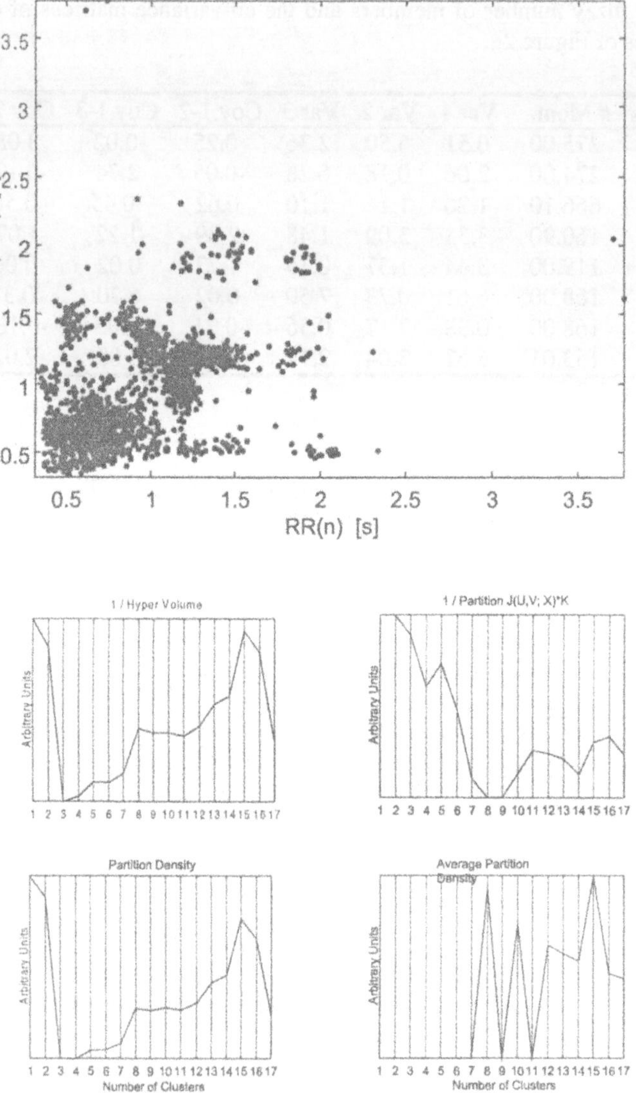

Figure 3$_{A,B}$: Clustering of RR-intervals in a cardiac patient with severe pathology
A – The fuzzy point array obtained by projecting the RR-interval time series in a 2-D lag plot.
B – Validity criteria values versus cluster number, obtained by forcing the algorithm to partition to a high number of clusters. A distinct peak at 15 is seen in 3 of the 4 criteria.

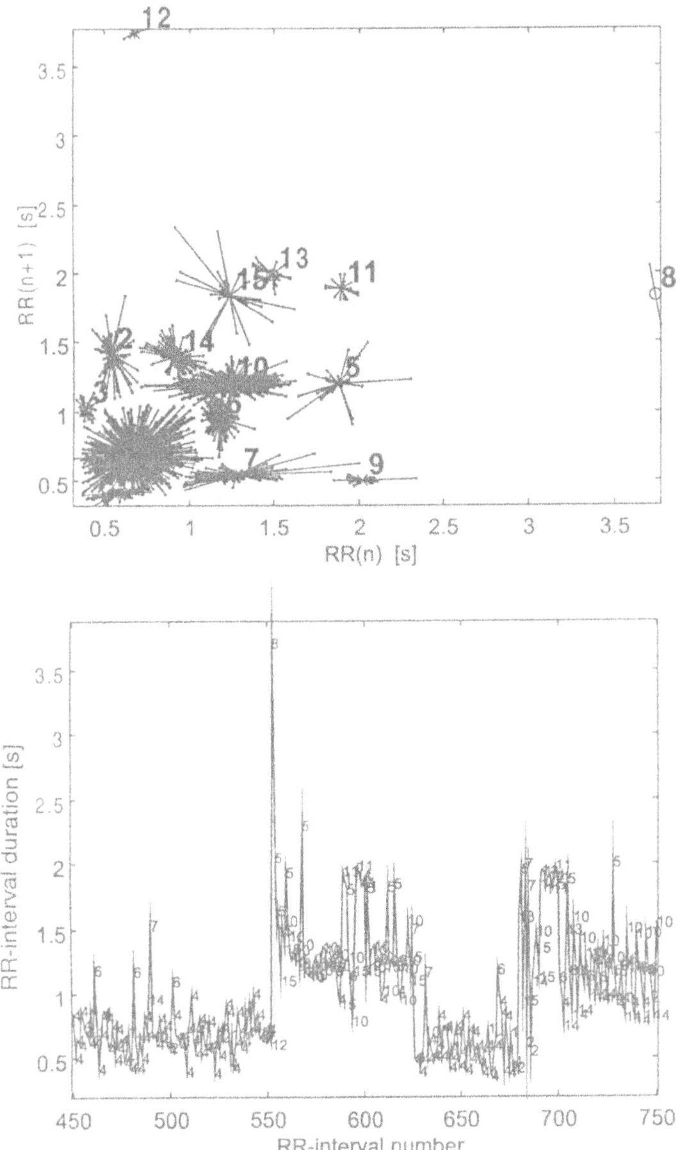

Figure 3$_{C,D}$,: Clustering of RR-intervals in a cardiac patient with severe pathology
C – Results of a 15-cluster partitioning.
D – A portion of the tachogram, labeled with the results of **C**. Three different sinus rates with RR-intervals of 0.7 (cluster 4), 1.25 (cluster 10) and 1.8 (cluster 11) seconds, with riding ectopies, including an atrio-ventricular block lasting several beats (clusters 8&12).

Maneuver-provoked heart rate fluctuations

The source of this example is a 7 minutes long record from a resting supine subject, who on four occasions was asked to rapidly assume the erect standing position for about 15 seconds before lying down again. Applying the hierarchic algorithm on a 3-D phase plot, resulted in a 3-cluster fuzzy partitioning (Figure 4_A) which, as seen in the labeled tachogram (figure 4_B), identify the resting rhythm, the four maneuvers by the transient heart rate acceleration induced by the abrupt vertical shift and a third group of beats with large rate swings, mainly upon reassuming the horizontal state and also during some pronounced respiratory fluctuations.

In this particular example, since ortho-static shift is a classic example of a transient provocation of the sympathetic branch, time-variant spectral analysis would also be expected to detect it. Figure 4_C shows a cascade presentation of a 12-order model AR spectrogram, performed on a sliding window of 32 intervals with a 50% overlap. It may be seen that the maneuvers involve transient flattening of the HF peak (in this instance of a slow breather, at an uncharacteristically low frequency of 0.15 Hz) and a coinciding increase in the low and very low frequency, partly as a result of the modulation in heart rate introduced by the maneuver itself.

The panels of Figure 4_D , from bottom up, show the mean heart rate and SD and the LF/HF ratio, calculated for the same sliding window. While mean RR-interval is directly modified by the maneuvers, they hardly influence SD. Although peaks in the LF/HF ratio roughly parallel the 4 maneuvers, the very low respiratory rate, which places the wave outside the HF range, causes the 1 to 1 correspondence not to be perfect.

Summary

To summarize this aspect, the unsupervised operation of the method avoids the use of universal thresholds or templates, currently used in automated identifiers of rhythm disturbances such as Holters. Still, it should be realized that the method does "train itself" on the subject's own pattern and is thus sensitive to changes that need not be specified beforehand. One training mode may consist of an *a priori* feeding in of long signal stretches in order to establish the range of the its "normal" structure, in anticipation of incoming changes during a planed provocation or a suspected pathology. On the other hand, educated supervision of some aspects (use of the hierarchic version, number of clusters) on specific occasions such as arrhythmic example 3, may prove mandatory for a meaningful operation.

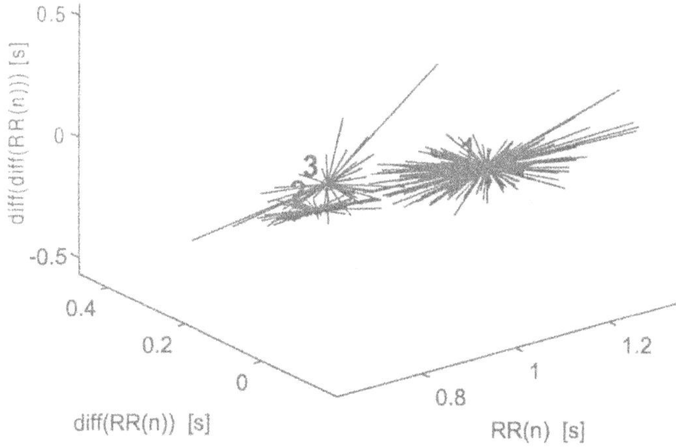

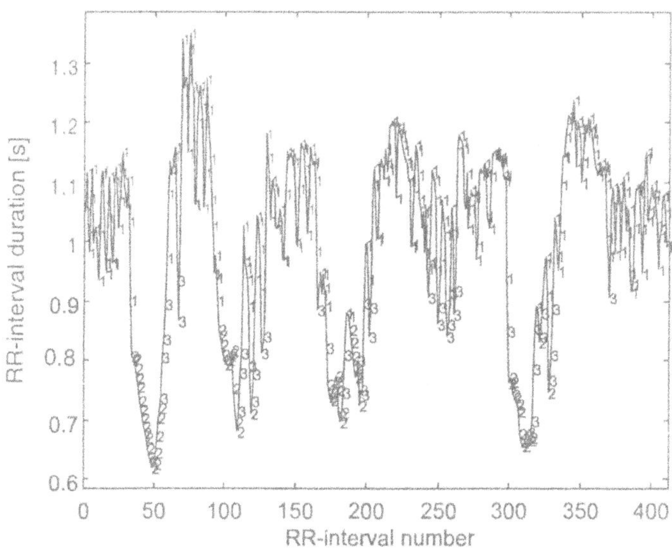

Figure 4$_{A,B}$: Clustering of HRV in a subject performing ortho-static shift maneuvers.

A – Three-class partitioning results applied on a 3-D phase plot.

B – The labeled 7 min tachogram, with the four 15 s-long maneuvers identified mainly by the emergence of cluster 2, hosting successive rapid beats and no respiratory fluctuations.

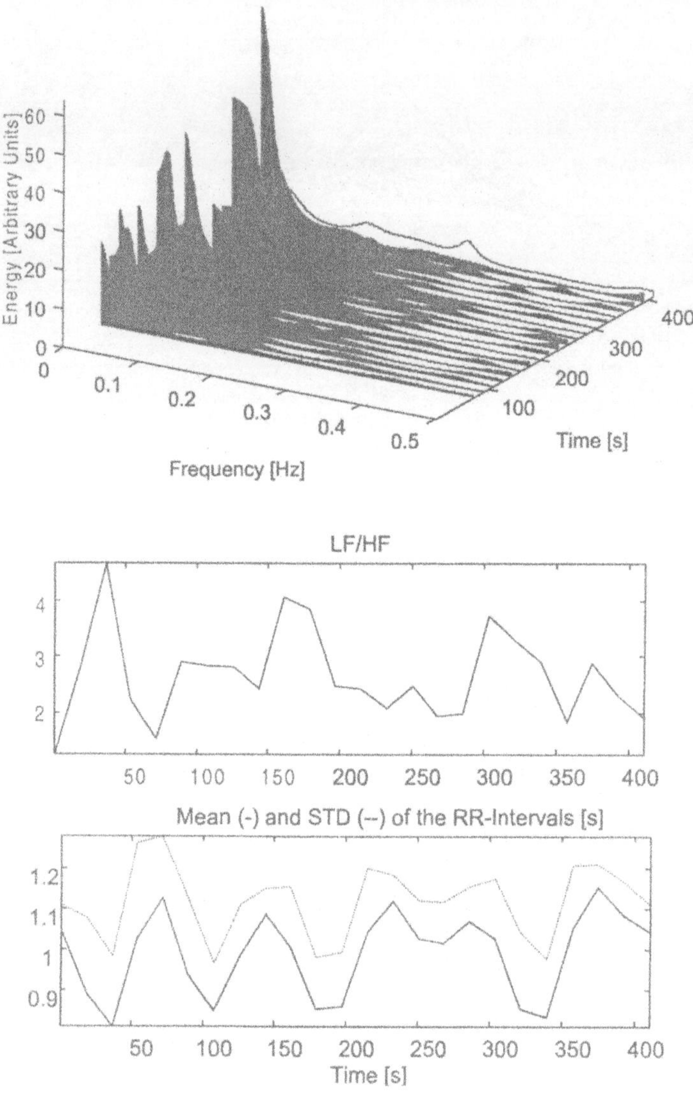

Figure 4$_{C,D}$: Clustering of HRV in a subject performing ortho-static shift maneuvers.

C – The same 7 min in a cascade presentation of a time-variant, 12-order model, AR spectrogram. Sliding time window of 32 intervals with a 50% overlap. Waxing and waning of the 0.15 Hz respiratory wave mark the maneuvers.

D – Maneuver identification by other HRV estimators, calculated for the same sliding time window as in **C**.

The use of this method to identify and describe the results of provocative maneuvers such as abrupt orthostatic shift may supply other comparative parameters of the response to supplement the currently used ratio of the longest to the shortest interval following the provocation (Andersen, Brugemanne, Behrens and Ehlers, 1995).

Forecasting Epilepsy

Background

Many biomedical phenomena are observed and treated in terms of a non-stationary time series of a monitored signal (Weigend and Gershenfeld, 1994). State recognition (*diagnosis*) and event prediction (*prognosis*) are important tasks in biomedical signal processing. Examples of the latter are the soon to be discussed prediction of an epileptic seizure from the EEG signal, prediction of atrial fibrilation from the ECG signal, and foretelling of drowsiness in vehicle drivers from both signals. The problem generally addresses a set of ordered measurements of the monitored system's behavior and seeks the recognition of temporal patterns or the transition to a new state of the system which may forecast an ominous event.

Common methods model the series generators by a set of states that the system traverses, where in each of these states the system outputs a stationary segment of distributed observations or samples, that is longer than an assumed minimal length. For each one of these states a specific probability distribution function (PDF) is estimated (Hamilton,1994). The subject is usually titled 'changes in regime'(Weigend and Gershenfeld,1994) and handled by several algorithms, which are generally related to the framework of Hidden Markov Models (HMM), see Deller et al, 1987 for a general description.

In numerous applications, however, the assumption of consecutive stationary periods is not accurate. One example is when the switching periods between regimes are of non-negligible length. In that case we encounter a considerable number of observations which are related to transient periods and may deteriorate the performance of a HMM-motivated PDF estimation algorithm. Moreover, in some cases it is of great importance to analyze the drift between any two states and to detect that such a drift is underway.

The importance of alerting epileptic outpatients (as well as the attending staff of patients in the ward) to an impending seizure, several minutes before its outset, should be obvious even to non-clinicians. A prime harbinger candidate is the EEG signal, which switches into a very distinct and characteristic pattern, dramatically different from the baseline pattern, as though a chaotic system reaching a bifurcation has veered into a new, notably more synchronous state. The epileptic seizure may involve a discrete part of the brain (partial), at which case its arisal may be traced to a defined location or focus, or the whole cerebral mass (generalized). In the latter instance, seizures or ictal states are recurrent, with inter-ictal periods ranging from several minutes to many days. Ictal EEG is characterized by repetitive high amplitude activity, either fast (spikes) slow (waves) or spike-and-wave (SPW) complexes. This activity may take the form of 2-60 second periods of very regular and symmetric 3 Hz SPW discharges in *absence* or *petit mal* epilepsy. The *tonic-clonic,* or *grand mal* epilepsy, has 40-60 second seizures, starting with fast, 6-12 Hz, poly-spike activity, gradually decreasing in frequency and increasing in amplitude (tonic phase) interrupted by slow waves (clonic phase) and followed by post-ictal general EEG depression (Loiseau, 1995).

The EEG in the inter-ictal periods ranges from normal, through isolated epileptic activity (single events or brief bursts) riding on a normal background, to an abnormal background (usually slow) with or without riding isolated epileptic activity. As regards the few minutes constituting the immediate pre-seizure period (PSP), in selected patients there is obvious transient pathological activity heralding the seizure. This, in principle, could be taught to automated pattern-recognition devices such as neuronal nets, but, in practice, a high patient-specificity of such patterns precludes a universal system. Furthermore, since more often than not the electric seizure seems to strike unheralded, coincidental with the motor involvement, a state of affairs remains where an early and reliable universal forecaster is yet to be found.

To this effect, the individual subject's PSP should be searched for unique abnormal isolated activity and/or non-paroxysmal changes in background activity. Indeed, a gradual change in the state of the cortex may be required for single events (normally suppressed) to evolve into a full-blown seizure (Lopes da Silva et al. 1996). During this gradual shift, the EEG might be expected to diverge only slightly and infrequently from the normal waking pattern, which may explain why even the expert eye fails to notice specific changes in the PSP. Also, the sought-after changes may only be apparent from information contained in two or more channels, which show coherent activity (or become "entrained") prior to the seizure. Preictal EEG changes, manifested in single channels or as entrainment of pairs of channels, have recently been described. Non-linear dynamic changes in both deep (intracerebral) as well as scalp electrodes were detected a few minutes prior to seizures in patients with focal epilepsy (Sackellares and Iasemidis (1999), Van Quyen et al. (1999a,b)).

Another candidate signal is the ECG, mainly on account of its being a readily obtained signal in both in and outpatient scenarios, but also by the rational that generalized epilepsies might also affect either or both branches of the autonomic system and possibly in the PSP. Both shape and rhythm changes may be expected. Indeed, ictal tachicardia is a known phenomenon, occurring in the vast majority of partial seizures. As a seizure detector, it has been shown to be overall less sensitive than EEG-based detection, but more sensitive in some patients and with less false positives (Long et al.1999). An example of human ictal tachicardia is shown in Figure 5, where the upper panel depicts a single-channel EEG trace containing a seizure, and the lower panel, the simultaneous tachogram.

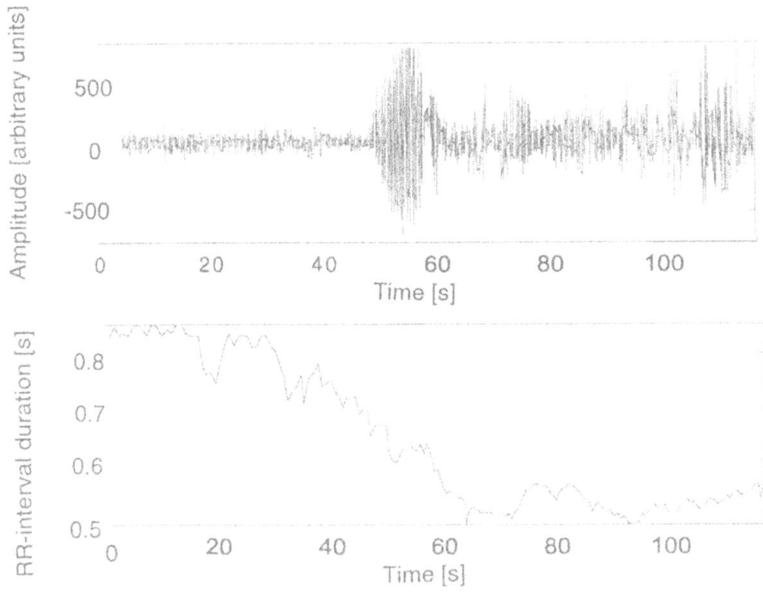

Figure 5: Ictal tachicardia during a complex partial seizure in a 23-year-old female patient.

The fuzzy clustering approach

The use of the UOFC algorithm in conjunction with features extracted from the EEG by the wavelet transform has been described (Geva and Kerem 1999). Briefly, the transform is applied on segments which are long enough to convey even the slowest rhythms but short enough so as not to dilute the contribution of single events which are deemed important. Next, the values of a selected list of extracted features are assigned to each segment. If the values of a properly chosen combination of parameters, so produced over time, are pooled and fed to the fuzzy clustering procedure, they would be expected to be naturally classifiable into fuzzy clusters representing EEG states. Then, if the results of the procedure (degree of membership in each cluster/state of each segment) are reproduced as a time-series, EEG states will stand out as strings of segments sharing one dominant cluster or a unique membership partitioning among several clusters. Transients and drifts may be defined by periods of altered membership sharing in one or

more clusters. The evolution of states, the gradual (as well as sharp) transitions between states and the emergence of abnormal (warning) states, may then all be followed. The resulting time-projected membership functions will also reveal the probability of appearance of each cluster, which can be periodic, increasing or decreasing through time or any other.
In the case of the ECG, fuzzy clustering of features derived from the RR-interval series as presented above, may also prove predictive by identifying abnormal intervals in the PSP.

Data sources

Hyperbaric-oxygen-induced generalized epileptic seizures were obtained by exposing laboratory rats implanted with chronic surface cortical electrodes to pure oxygen at 5 atmospheres in a pressure chamber. Details of this procedure can be found in Geva and Kerem, 1998. One-time electrocardiographic electrodes were attached just prior to exposure. The ECG and two bipolar EEG channels were amplified, filtered to pass between 1-1000 and 1-100 Hz, respectively (-6 db/octave), notch-filtered at 50 Hz (-20 db/octave), displayed and recorded on tape.

After 10 minutes of accustoming to the chamber, recording started and the rat was compressed at a rate of 1 atm/min and held at pressure until the appearance on one or both EEG channels of the first major (>20 s) ictal discharge which prompted decompression. At this pressure the resting rat will experience the first seizure after a delay of 13-55 min. On rare occasions rats will escape a seizure for the longest exposure time of 60 min. In order to exclude possible effects of compression and early effects of pressure, we chose to analyze the section from 5 min at pressure, up to and including the seizure. For control sections, we analyzed the period between 5-25 minutes, in rats that escaped seizing. The selected sections were digitized at a sampling rate of 1000 Hz.

Data analysis

ECG

Data was analyzed in the same manner as described above for the heart rate fluctuation analysis.

EEG

The digitized time series of each channel of the EEG record is divided into M consecutive epochs $S(n),\ n=1,\ldots,(M-1)\cdot D+N$, which are arranged as the columns (pattern vectors) of an NxM matrix $\mathbf{S}$, where N is the length (number of samples) of each pattern vector, and D is the delay between patterns:

$$\mathbf{S} = \begin{bmatrix} S(1) & S(D+1) & \cdot & \cdot & S((M-1)\cdot D+1) \\ S(2) & S(D+2) & \cdot & \cdot & S((M-1)\cdot D+2) \\ \cdot & \cdot & \cdot & & \cdot \\ \cdot & \cdot & \cdot & & \cdot \\ S(N) & S(D+N) & \cdot & \cdot & S((M-1)\cdot D+N) \end{bmatrix}$$

In our realization, N=1000 samples (1 second) and D=N/2 (overlap of half of the samples between consecutive pattern vectors), making $M \approx 2400$ for 20 min sections. The short time window and the overlap are chosen to ensure that all transient events will be completely captured and dominant in at least one of the patterns. Yet, the window is long enough to represent the main "rhythms" (between 2 and 30 Hz) of the on-going EEG signal. Details of feature extraction leading to the feature matrix on which the clustering algorithm is applied can be found in Geva and Kerem (1999). Also, in accordance with findings detailed in that reference, the wavelet coefficients picked to be fed to the clustering procedure were the combined variances (energies) of the 4th to 8th wavelet scales.

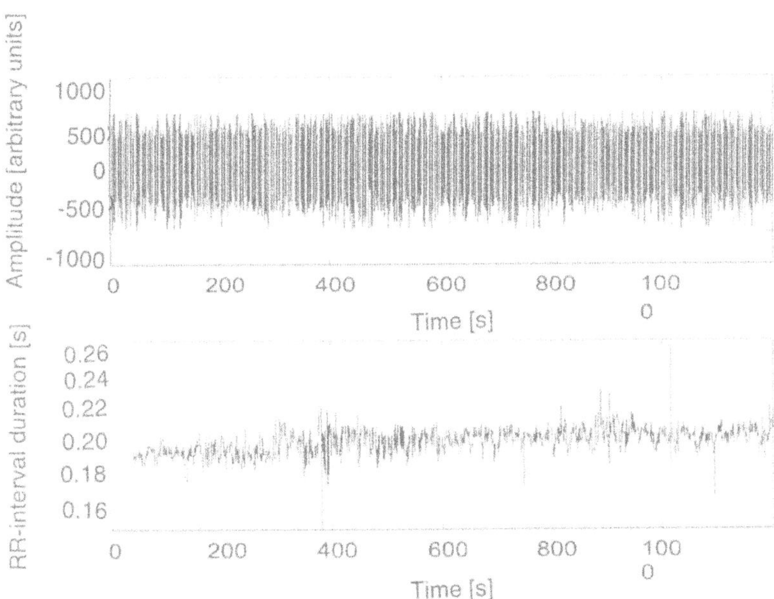

(Figure $6_{A,B,C}$ - continued on next page)

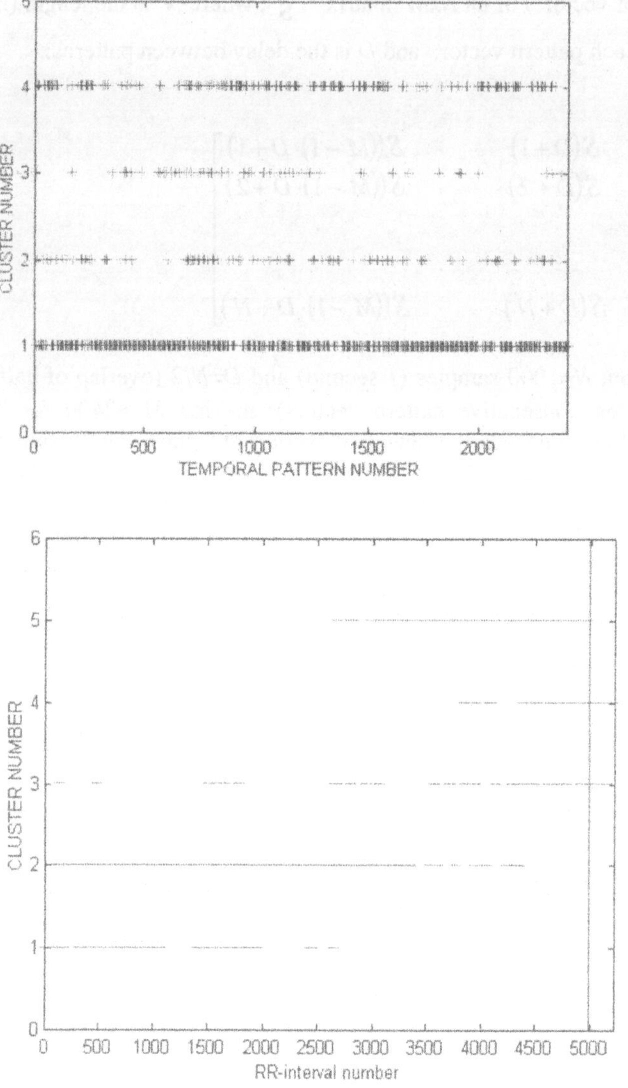

Figure 6$_{A,B,C}$: Clustering of HRV in a rat which resisted epilepsy.
A – Raw 20 min EEG signal and tachogram.
B – Assignment of consecutive temporal patterns (2400, 50%-overlapping, 1 s patterns) of the EEG time series to the cluster in which they the highest degree of membership.
C – Assignment of consecutive RR-intervals in the tachogram to the cluster in which they the highest degree of membership.

As a control, the analysis of HRV in minutes 5-25 at pressure, in a rat that escaped the seizure for an exposure of 50 min, is shown in Figure $6_{A\text{-}C}$. The raw EEG and tachogram are seen in the upper and lower panels, respectively. Some apparently seizure-unrelated effects of the exposure such as progressive heart rate slowing and a few dispersed divergent RR-intervals are evident. The assignment of temporal patterns to each of four clusters found by the UOFC algorithm for the EEG data and by the HUFC algorithm for the RR-interval series, is respectively presented in Figures 6_B and 6_C. Points in both time series are rather uniformly distributed between the clusters, with no apparent trend with time. The same analysis in another rat, which seized after 22 min, is shown in Figure $7_{A\text{-}C}$. In this case, the EEG record appears uniform until the eruption of the seizure at 960 s, while a considerable increase in HRV is seen to ride on top of the progressive heart rate slowing. The evolution of the seizure is forecasted and followed by a progression of 6 out of 9 clusters, into which EEG features were classified, starting 4 min prior to its onset (Figure 7_B). The 5-cluster RR-interval partitioning (Figure 7_C), shows one clusters (#4) to emerge and another (#3) to become prominent in the same four minutes leading to the seizure as well as throughout its duration. Investigation of the temporal and structural content of cluster 4, shows it to contain isolated episodes of both abnormally large and abnormally short (grouped together by the absolute value differential partitioning) sinus-originating beats as well as complementary pairs. So far, the specificity of forecasting by both signals seems good, as none of 4 control rats showed warning clusters. The sensitivity in 12 rats that seized was only 60%, roughly the same for the two signals.

Concluding Remarks

The clustering method hereby proposed for electrophysiological signal analysis, offers a unified procedure for state recognition and event prediction. In the case of the ECG, it deals with the basic sinus rhythm and its overall variability, with pathological rhythms, with transient changes and with the advent of imminent pathology. In case of the EEG it can define both background changes as well as group various types of short transients or single complexes. We have demonstrated the potential usefulness of the method in both quasi-stationary states where the current importance of an underlying mechanism is mirrored in the current size of its representative cluster(s) or in the rate at which members are added to it, and for dynamic states where the number and location of clusters are ever changing. While in the first instance the current size and rate of growth of a given cluster would determine the probability of an incoming pattern to belong to it, in the second, prediction can only be based on a hindsight identification of warning or heralding clusters.

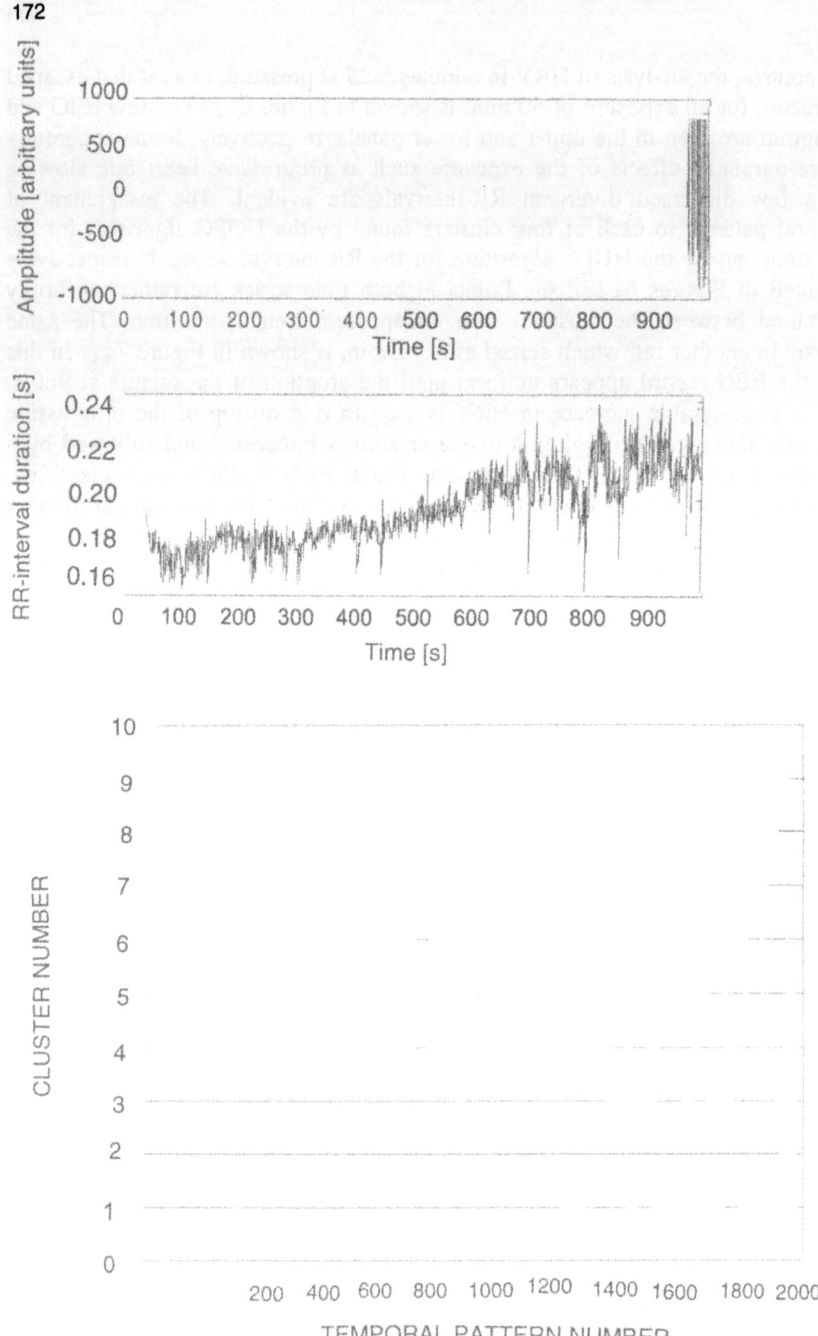

(Figure 7$_{A, B, C}$ continued on next page)

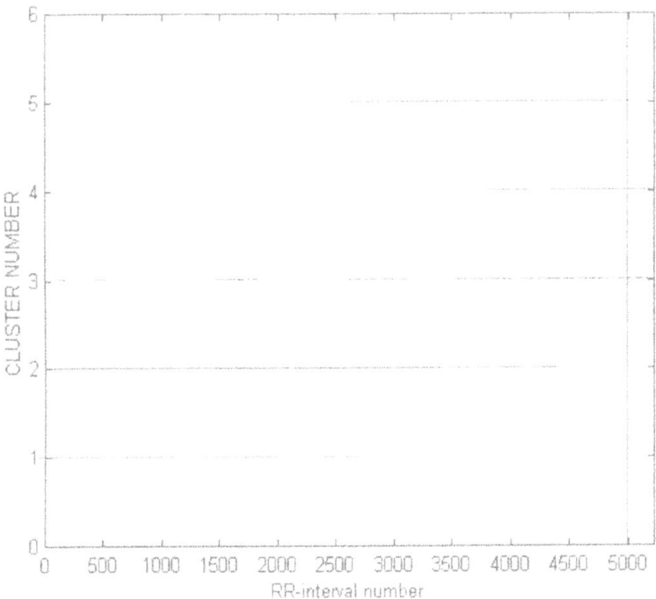

Figure 7$_{A,B,C}$: Clustering of HRV in a rat which suffered a generalized electric seizure.
A-C – As in Fig 6, but with a 17 min long recording. Vertical line in B & C marks the onset of the seizure at 960 s.

Universal merging rules should be used to compact the partition into the minimal number of clusters representing all governing mechanisms. Candidates for merging are clusters of same size and rate of growth, which by nature of the generator, by choice of clustering features, or both, are most likely redundant.

The mere fact that a generalized epileptic seizure may, at times, be forecasted by a few minutes from HRV changes alone (a possible evidence of an early deviant involvement of the central autonomic nervous system) is a novel finding with mechanistic as well as practical implications. Apart from the emergence of new clusters and major shifts in degrees of membership between clusters, changes in centroid locations, variance, covariance etc. are all candidates for forecasting, which could enhance the sensitivity of a forecasting device. Adding information from the EEG and possibly from stimuli-evoked responses, may further improve forecasting The potential use of this method in being incorporated into such and other warning devices (drowsiness, heart attack) based only on HRV or in conjunction with other biological signals may be pursued.

References

Andresen D, Bruggemann T, Behrens S, Ehlers C (1995) Heart rate response to provocative maneuvers. In: Malik M, Camm AJ (eds) Heart rate variability. Futura Publ., Armonk, NY.

Bezdek JC (1981) Pattern Recognition with Fuzzy Objective Function Algorithms. Plenum Press, New York, pp 228.

Bezdek JC, Pal NR (1995) Tow Soft Relatives of Learning Vector Quantization. Neural Networks 8(5):729-743.

Bezdek JC, Hall LO, Clark MC, Goldgof DB, Clarke LP (1997) Medical image analysis with fuzzy models. Stat. Methods Med. Res. 6:191-214.

Bankman I, Gath I (1987) Feature extraction and clustering of EEG during anaesthesia. Med. & Biol. Eng. & Comput. 25:474-477.

Bianchi, A. M., Mainardi, L. T., Signorini, M. G., Mainardi, M. And Cerutti, S. (1993) Time variant power spectrum analysis for the detection of transient episodes in HRV signal. IEEE Trans. Biom. Eng. 40:136-144.

Brown TB, Beightol LA, Koh J, Ecckberg DL (1993) Important influence of respiration on human R-R interval power spectra is largely ignored. J. Appl. Physiol. 75:2310-2317.

Cabello D, Barro S, Salceda JM, Ruiz R, Mira J (1991) Fuzzy K-nearest neighbor classifiers for ventricular arrythmia detection. Int. J. Biomed. Comput. 27:77-93.

Cannon RL, Dave JV, Bezdek JC (1986) Efficient implementation of the fuzzy-c-means clustering algorithm. IEEE trans. Pattern Anal. & Mach. Intell. 8:248-255.

Cerutti S, Bianchi AM, Mainardi LT (1995) Spectral analysis of the heart rate variability signal. In: Malik M, Camm AJ (eds) Heart rate variability. Futura Publ., Armonk, NY.

Clark MC, Hall LO, Goldgof DB, Velthuizen R, Murtagh R, Silbiger MS (1998) Unsupervised brain tumor segmentation using knowledge-based fuzzy techniques. In: Teodorescu Hn, Kandel A, Jain LCJ Fuzzy and Neurofuzzy Systems in Medicine. CRC International Series on Computational Inteligence, CRC Press, Boca Raton, Florida, pp 137-169.

Deller JR, Proakis JG, Hansen JHL (1987) Discrete-time processing of speech signals. Prentice-Hall,

Gath I, Bar-On E (1980) Computerized method for scoring of polygraphic sleep recordings. Comput. Progr. Biomed. 11:217-223,.

GATH I, GEVA AB (1989 a) Unsupervised Optimal Fuzzy Clustering. IEEE Trans. on Pattern Anal. Machine Intell. 7:773-781.

Gath I, Geva AB (1989 b) Fuzzy clustering for the estimation of the parameters of the components of mixtures of normal distributions. Pattern Recognition Letters 9:77-86.

Gath I, Hoory D, (1995) Fuzzy clustering of elliptic ring-shaped clusters. Pattern Recog. Let. 16: 727-741.

Gath I, Lehman D, Bar-On E (1983) Fuzzy clustering of EEG signal and vigilance performance. Int. J. Neurosci. 20: 303-312,

Geva AB (1998) Feature extraction and state recognition in biomedical signals with hierarchical unsupervised fuzzy clustering methods. Medical & Biological Engineering & Computing 36: 608-614.

Geva AB, Pratt H (1994) Unsupervised clustering of evoked potentials by Waveform. Medical & Biological Engineering & Computing 32:543-550.

Geva AB, Pratt H, Zeevi YY (1997) Multichannel wavelet-type decomposition of evoked potentials: model-based recognition of generator activity. Med. & Biol. Eng. & Comput. 95:40-46.

Geva AB, Kerem DH (1998) Forecasting generalized epileptic seizures from the EEG signal by wavelet analysis and dynamic unsupervised fuzzy clustering. IEEE Trans. Biomed Engin. 45:1205-1216.

Geva AB, Kerem DH (1999) Brain state identification and forecasting of acute pathology using unsupervised fuzzy clustering of EEG temporal patterns. In: Teodorescu HN, Kandel A, Jain LC (eds) Fuzzy and Neurofuzzy systems in Medicine. CRC International Series on Computational Inteligence, CRC Press, Boca Raton, Florida, pp 57-93.

Goldberger Al, West B J (1987) Applications of nonlinear dynamics to clinical cardiology. Ann. NY Acad. Sci. 504:195-213.

Hamilton D (1994) Time Series Analysis. Princeton University Press, pp. 677-699.

Harel T, Gath I, Ben-Haim S (1997) High resolution estimation of the heart rate variability signal. Med. & Biol. Eng. & Comput. 35:1-5.

Kamath MV, Fallen EL (1995) Correction of the heart rate variability signal for ectopies and missing beats. In: Malik M, Camm AJ (eds) (1995) Heart rate variability. Futura Publ., Armonk, NY.

Krishnapuram R, Keller J (1993) A possibilistic Approach to Clustering. IEEE Transactions on Fuzzy Systems 1(2):98-110.

Le Van Quyen M, Martinerie J, Baulac M, Varela F (1999) Anticipating epileptic seizures in real time by a non-linear analysis of similarity between EEG recordings. Neuroreport 13: 2149-2155.

Le Van Quyen M, Martinerie J, Navarro V, Adam C, Varela F, Baulac M (1999) Evidence of pre-seizure changes on scalp EEG recordings by non linear analysis. Epilepsia 40 suppl 7: 174.

Loiseau P (1995) Epilepsies. In: Guide to clinical neurology. Churchill, Livingstone NY, pp 903-914.

Lopes da Silva FH, Pijn JP, Veli DN (1996) Signal processing of EEG: evidence for chaos or noise. An application to seizure activity in epilepsy. In: Advances in processing and pattern analysis of biological signals. Plenum Press, New York, pp 21-32.

Lipsitz LA, Mietus J, Moody JB Goldberger AL (1990) Spectral characteristics of heart rate variability before and during postural tilt. Relations to aging and risk of syncope. Circulation 81:1803-1810.

Long TJ, Robinson SE, Quinlivan LS (1999) Effectiveness of heart rate seizure detection compared to EEG in an epilepsy monitoring unit (EMU). Epilepsia 40 suppl. 7:174.

Malik M (1995) Geometrical methods for heart rate variability assessment. In: Malik M Camm AJ (eds) Heart rate variability. Futura Publ., Armonk NY, pp 47-62.

MALIK, M. (chairman) (1996) Heart rate variability: standards of measurements, physiological interpretation and clinical use. Task Force of the European Society of Cardiology and the North American Society of Pacing & Electrophysiology. Circulation 93:1043-1065.

Malik M, Camm AJ (eds) (1995) Heart rate variability. Futura Publ., Armonk, NY.

Masulli F and Schenone A (1999) A fuzzy clustering based segmentation system as support to diagnosis in medical imaging. Artif. Intell. Med. 16:129-147.

O'Malley MJ, Abel MF, Damiano DL, Vaughan CL (1997) Fuzzy clustering of children with cerebral palsy based on temporal-distance gait parameters. IEEE Trans. Rehabil. Engin. 5: 300-309.

Pagani, M., Malfatto, G., Pierini, S., Casati, R., Masu, A.M., Poli, M., Guzzetti, S., Lombardi, F., Cerutti, S., and Malliani, A. (1988) Spectral analysis of heart rate variability in the assessment of autonomic diabetic neuropathy. *J. Auton Nerv Syst.* **23**: 143-153.

Peters RM, Shanies SA, Peters JC (1998) Fuzzy cluster analysis – a new method to predict future cardiac events in patients with positive stress tests. Jpn. Circ. J. 62:750-754.

Sackellares C, Iasemidis LD (1999) Detection of the preictal transition in scalp EEG. Epilepsia 40 suppl 7:174.

Schlactman M, Green JS (1991) Signal-averaged electrocardiography: a new technique for determining which patients may be at risk for sudden cardiac death. Focus. Crit. Care 18: 202-221.

Schmidt G, Morfill GE (1995) Nonlinear methods for heart rate variability assessment. In: Malik M, Camm AJ (eds) Heart rate variability. Futura Publ., Armonk, NY.

Skinner JE, Carpeggiani C, Landisman CE, Fulton KW (1991) The correlation-dimension of the heartbeat is reduced by myocardial ischemia in conscious pigs. Circ. Res. 68:966-976.

Skinner, J. E. , C. M. Pratt And T. Vybiral (1993) Reduction in the correlation dimension of heartbeat intervals precedes imminent ventricular fibrilation in human subjects. Am. Heart J. 125:731-743.

Suckling J, Sigmundsson T, Greenwood K, Bullmore ET (1999) A modified fuzzy clustering algorithm for operator in dependent brain tissue classification of dual echo MR images. Magn. Reson. Imaging 17:1065-1076.

Tolias YA, Panas SM (1998) A fuzzy vessel tracking algorithm for retinal images based on fuzzy clustering. IEEE Trans. Med. Imaging 17:263-273,

Vila J, Palacios F, Presedo J, Fernandez-Delgado M, Felix P, Barro S (1997) Time-frequency analysis of heart-rate variability: an improved method for monitoring and diagnosing miocardial ischemia. IEEE Eng. Med Biol. 16:119-126.

Weigend AS, Gershenfeld NA (eds) (1994) Time Series Prediction: Forecasting the Future and Understanding the Past. Addison-Wesley,

Wilkund U, Akay M, Niklasson U (1997) Short-term analysis of heart-rate variability by adapted wavelet transforms. IEEE Eng. in Med. & Biol. 16:113-118.

Zouridakis G, Boutros NN, Jansen BH (1997) A fuzzy clustering approach to study the auditory P50 component in schizophrenia. Psychiatry Res. 69:169-181.

Acknowledgements

Research reported in this chapter was supported by The Israel Science Foundation; founded by the Israel Academy of Sciences and Humanities. The authors thank Professor M. Neufeld from the Neurology Department in Ichilov Hospital for the epileptic patient data. Rat EEG and ECG data were collected by the second author while serving at the Israeli Naval Hyperbaric Institute, IDF Medical Corps, Haifa, Israel.

Fuzzy Logic in a Decision Support System in the Domain of Coronary Heart Disease Risk Assessment

Alfons Schuster, Kenneth Adamson and David A. Bell

Faculty of Informatics
School of Information and Software Engineering
University of Ulster at Jordanstown
Shore Road
Newtownabbey, Co. Antrim BT37 0QB
Northern Ireland
E-mail: {a.schuster, k.adamson, da.bell}@ulst.ac.uk

1. Introduction

Every day humans are confronted in numerous occasions with tasks that include the management and the processing of information of various degrees of complexity. Regardless of what the actual information consists of, its degree of complexity, or simplicity, can be associated with the number of recognised parts and the extent of their interrelationship (Klir and Folger 1988). The capability to manage such information considerably depends on the actual understanding of the person(s) involved. The more experienced the person the better the understanding and the information management. Further, although different persons may approach the same problem differently a solution is very often based on a combination of different strategies. This paper has a focus on two strategies:

- First, a very common way of managing complex information for domain experts, or humans in general, is to reduce the complexity of the information by allowing a certain degree of uncertainty without loosing the actual content of the original information. In a very natural, but also radical way, complexity reduction occurs when humans summarise information onto vague linguistic expressions. For example, a clinician may say to a person: "Your blood pressure is *ok*, your heart rate is *just fine*, and your cholesterol values are *normal*". Note that despite the availability of precise values for blood pressure, heart rate and cholesterol the clinician uses the vague linguistic terms *ok, just fine* and *normal* to describe the person's state of health. These terms however are expressive and satisfactory for further decision-making (Ross TJ 1995). Fuzzy logic is a technique that, in many situations, may provide a solution for the modelling of such situations (Zadeh 1996).
- A second strategy many problem solvers apply is to try to get reminded of similar situations they have solved in the past (Riesbeck and Schank 1989).

Whenever such prior solutions are available experts apply (possibly adapt) these solutions or the plans that led to a successful problem solving of these old situations to fit the needs of the new situation. For example, a treatment regime suggested by a clinician could be largely based on the experience the clinician encountered within previous, similar situations. Case-based reasoning (CBR) is a problem solving technique in which the processes of reminding and adaptation, amongst others, play a fundamental role (Brown 1992), (Kolodner 1993).

Fuzzy logic and CBR are cornerstones of the DSCHDRA system and therefore are central in this paper. The paper particularly emphasises the mutually supporting character of these techniques. For example, CBR uses abstract entities referred to as cases for the modelling of past situations. Very frequently a single case is described by a set of primitive and complex attributes, where the complex attributes are composed of a set of primitive attributes. This paper for example, introduces a general method for the generation of complex case attributes. In many situations attributes can be described by imprecise or vague linguistic expressions, for example a *high* systolic blood pressure in the CHDRA domain. It therefor can be advantageous for a system to have facilities that allow to deal with the vagueness pertained in such linguistic expressions. In DSCHDRA this task is realised by a fuzzy expert system (FES). A further study presented here relates to a sub-problem in FESs' building, namely the rule weight assignment in such a system. The paper therefore includes a section where a genetic algorithm is used to determine the rule weights for the FES. To evaluate the applicability and usefulness of our approaches we have undertaken a number of tests in the domain of coronary heart disease risk assessment (CHDRA). The results established in these tests are carefully analysed and discussed in the paper.

The remainder of the paper is organised as follows: Section 2 describes the medical domain and the available data. The DSCHDRA system and its components are introduced in the same section. Section 3 reports on a FES study we have undertaken in a sub-field of the wider CHDRA domain, the task of cholesterol assessment. Section 4 presents the results of a case retrieval study that is largely based on fuzzy case attributes. The genetic algorithm component and its use in DSCHDRA are the content of Section 5. Section 6 ends the paper with a discussion and future work.

2. Medical Domain and DSCHDRA Prototype System

Coronary Heart Disease (CHD) is generally acknowledged to be a multi-factorial disease. It results from a condition termed atherosclerosis. Atherosclerosis refers to the loss of elasticity and thickening of coronary artery walls resulting in partial or complete obstruction of blood supply to the heart, ultimately provoking death (Ross R 1986). Despite major advances in the understanding of the disease and its management CHD remains the leading cause of morbidity and mortality in western society (Hopkins and Wiliams 1981), (Levy 1993). For example, CHD continues to be the cause of the greatest number of deaths among adult Americans. Due to this fact a lot of effort has been put into comprehensive and very often long-term epidemiological studies to identify factors associated with increased CHD risk (Dawber et al. 1951), (Kannel et al. 1979). Based on the data of such studies statistical analysis has been used to derive algorithms and strategies that can help in the identification and management of individuals at high risk of CHD (Shaper et al 1987), (Tunstall-Pedoe 1991), (Anderson et al. 1991). One result of such analysis is that among other factors increased blood cholesterol levels have been identified to be main risk factors for myocardial infarction and subsequent sudden death. Cholesterol assessment and the identification of increased blood cholesterol levels is a difficult and complex subject in its own right. This is one of the reasons why the applications presented here are restricted to this sub-problem of the wider CHDRA domain.

2.1. Cholesterol assessment

Increased blood cholesterol levels, or hypercholesterolaemia, to use the correct medical term, is a main risk factor for CHD. It is treated primarily by correction of overweight, careful reduction of cholesterol levels through a lipid-lowering diet, and removal of underlying causes (e.g. suggestions to exercise regularly, and to be more active). Cholesterol travels in the blood in distinct particles called lipoproteins. The two major types of lipoproteins are low-density lipoproteins (LDL) and high-density lipoproteins (HDL). LDL, often called 'bad cholesterol', delivers the cholesterol to the arterial walls with the ultimate consequence of narrowing the arteries (Slyper 1994). HDL, often called 'good cholesterol', protects against heart disease by removing excess cholesterol from the blood (Gordon et al. 1989). In a fasting blood test, a clinician first finds out what a person's TOTAL cholesterol level is. If the TOTAL cholesterol level is too high then additional measurements of LDL and HDL are required (note: a *high* HDL value compensates a *high* TOTAL cholesterol value, and therefore, a person's cholesterol can still be described as *normal*). The two cholesterol type ratios TOTAL/HDL and LDL/HDL are also important because they provide more meaningful indicators of coronary heart disease risk than TOTAL cholesterol per se (Kinosian et el. 1994). In terms of CHD risk very simple rules for the two ratios are that high ratio values are bad for a person and low ratio values are good for a person. So, for example, having the following five values of a person in front of him <TOTAL, 5.30 mmoll^{-1}>, <LDL, 3.82 mmoll^{-1}>, <HDL, 0.63 mmoll^{-1}>, <TOTAL/HDL, 8.40> and <LDL/HDL, 6.10>, a clinician might say that the person's cholesterol is *normal*. Clearly, the linguistic term *normal* used by the clinician to describe the person's cholesterol is a summary that is derived by an aggregation of different cholesterol type values and cholesterol type ratio values (Figure 1). Note that from now on in a general discussion the term 'cholesterol' is used, whereas the term 'CHOLESTEROL' is used for the overall aggregated cholesterol.

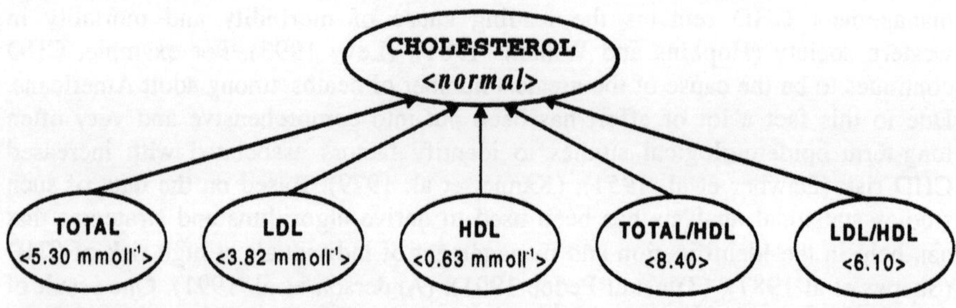

Figure 1: Aggregation of cholesterol type values and ratios onto a single, vague linguistic expression.

The previous example illustrates very well that a very common way for humans to reduce the complexity of many decision-making situations is to aggregate available pieces of information into bigger lumps of information. The point of such an aggregation process is to establish a trade-off between reducing complexity by increasing the degree of uncertainty without loosing the actual content of the original information. The capability to manage such aggregation processes considerably depends on the actual understanding of the person(s) involved. The more experienced the person the better the person will understand and master the prevailing situation. Very frequently it is not possible to obtain a crisp, numeric value for an aggregated piece of information. For example, it is not possible to 'measure' a person's CHOLESTEROL. In situations like this humans often use vague linguistic terms to describe such entities (e.g. *normal* CHOLESTEROL). Even in situations where precise numeric values are obtainable humans often fall back upon the use of vague linguistic terms. For example, a clinician might describe a LDL value of 2.50 mmoll^{-1} simply as *normal*, and one of 5.10 mmoll^{-1} simply as *abnormal*. Naturally, the question arises: Where exactly is the boundary between a *normal* and an *abnormal* LDL value? Categories are typically expressed in intervals. For example, a TOTAL/HDL ratio between 4.00 and 4.50 is considered as *good*, and one below 4.00 is regarded to be even *better* (Pyorala et al. 1994). Such a representation however is not intuitive to a human's understanding of the problem. In a human's understanding the transition from *good* to *better*, or from *normal* to *abnormal* should be gradual or fuzzy rather than abrupt (Zadeh 1973). Before this idea is elaborated in more detail we use the next section to introduce the medical data that is used in this study.

2.2. Medical data

The available data is derived from 83 middle-aged men between 30 and 65 years of age who undertook standard screening tests in 1993 and again in 1996 in order to identify selected CHD risk factors (Lopes et al. 1994), (Lopes et al. 1997). A series of qualitative and quantitative information were collected including: age, height, weight, body fat percentage, personal and family medical history, smoking, nutrition habits, blood pressure, cholesterol, stress, and physical activity levels. The data also contains information on a subject's management and treatment between the two measurements. The individual CHD risk of a person relies on a point scoring system proposed by Anderson (Anderson et al. 1991). Risk values range in the interval [1 ≤ risk value ≤ 32] and correspond to a person's 10-year CHD risk. For example, a risk score of 29 is corresponding to a predicted 10-year CHD risk of 36%. In DSCHDRA the data is organised and referred to by attributes. Table 1 illustrates the format and the representation for some of these attributes.

Table 1

No.	Attribute	Type	Range	Explanation
1	Age	Integer	[30, 65]	Age in years.
2	Smoking	Yes/No	[Yes, No]	Is the person smoking?
4	LDL	Real	[1.5, 8.0]	Low density lipoprotein cholesterol.
-	-	-	-	-
24	SoClass	Integer	[1, 2, 3, 4, 5]	Social class and education of the person.

2.3. The DSCHDRA prototype system

It was already mentioned that one of the motivations for this research was to have an application in a real world environment (CHDRA) in which the benefit and the advantages, but also the disadvantages of advanced computer science techniques could be applied, tested, and evaluated. Figure 2 illustrates a simplified view of the DSCHDRA system.

Figure 2 also identifies the main building blocks of the system, a CBR component, a FES component, and a genetic algorithm (GA) component. Although the different components are discussed in more depth in forthcoming sections their basic functionality and purpose is briefly discussed here:

- The CBR component has been integrated to allow a more person/case oriented approach to CHDRA, as opposed to mere statistical approaches to the problem (Schuster et al. 1998a). For example, the DSCHDRA case base contains 83 cases (Base Case 1, ..., Base Case 83 in Figure 2). Each case holds the personal and medical data for a person collected in the underlying studies (Section 2.2). In the CBR reasoning and decision-making process a new person, depicted as a query case in Figure 2, is compared against this library and the nearest neighbours that most closely match the query case are retrieved. Given that the CHD risk and a treatment regime of these subjects are known, DSCHDRA promises to be useful in providing information about

(a) the CHD risk of the person, and (b) information about a possible treatment for the query case/person.

- The FES component is used to generate abstract summaries. So far the component is employed on a sub-problem in the CHD domain, the identification of increased blood cholesterol levels. For example, instead of using values for TOTAL, HDL, LDL, TOTAL/HDL, and LDL/HDL cholesterol a clinician may use a summary like '*normal* CHOLESTEROL'. The FES component simulates such an aggregation process. DSCHDRA further uses these summaries for various tasks. For example, they are used in the CBR component for the description of a case via complex case attributes (Schuster et al. 1997). They are also utilised in the processes of case retrieval and case interpretation, which are both central issues in CBR research (Schuster et al. 1999).
- The GA component finally is used to approach a general problem related to the building process of rule based systems, and hence FESs. Namely the weight assignment on the rule base of such a system. For example, the domain expert involved in the project found it quite difficult to come up with a weight assignment for the rules that are used in the FES component. The GA paradigm has been successfully applied to similar tasks in the past and therefore is utilised in DSCHDRA to attack the problem. First results indicate the value of this approach. The results are also encouraging from the point of view of a possible enhancement for the CBR component, because weight assignment for case attributes is another important issue in CBR.

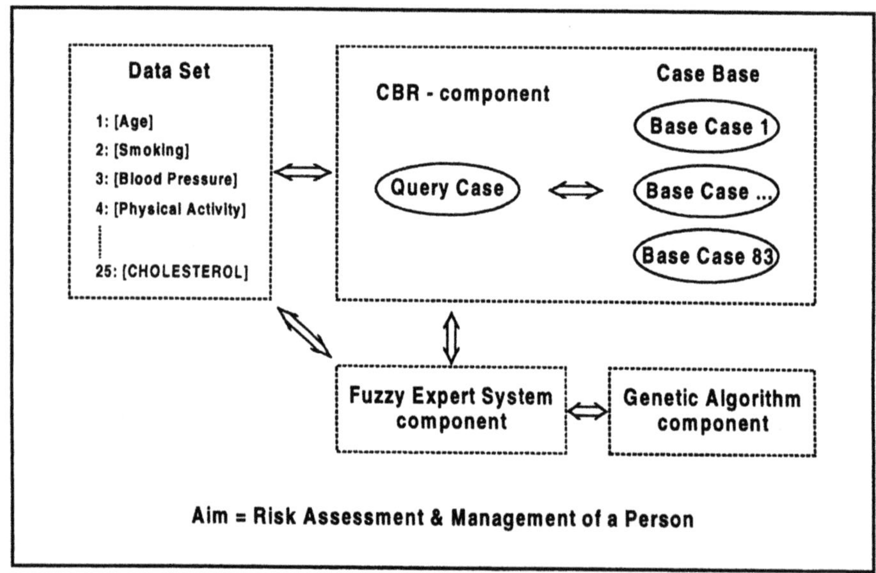

Figure 2: Simplified view of the DSCHDRA system.

3. Cholesterol Assessment and the DSCHDRA Prototype System

To repeat, the main aim of the FES is to aggregate lower level information (TOTAL, HDL, etc., cholesterol) onto bigger junks of information (CHOLESTEROL). In general such a process increases the uncertainty, but reduces the complexity of the available information. The basic requirements therefore are:

- The transition between CHOLESTEROL categories, for example between *good* and *normal* CHOLESTEROL should be gradual or fuzzy rather than abrupt.
- The aggregated CHOLESTEROL values should be intuitively appealing to an expert's understanding of the problem in question.
- The use of aggregated CHOLESTEROL values in further decision-making process should lead to meaningful, justifiable and consistent results.

The building process of the FES involved the normal steps of knowledge acquisition, knowledge representation and the design of an inference engine (Schuster et al. 1998b). Within knowledge acquisition a knowledge engineer and a domain expert were involved in order to extract the domain knowledge for its use in the FES. The bases for the knowledge acquisition were 166 data records. The 166 records include 83 records obtained from the first measurement in 1993, and 83 records obtained from the same persons measured in 1996 (see Section 2.2). Each record initially held the TOTAL, HDL, LDL, TOTAL/HDL and LDL/HDL values of a person's cholesterol. In a first step the domain expert was questioned to provide his expertise about the CHOLESTEROL of a person. The expert therefore was asked to indicate one of the fields *normal*, *borderline*, *abnormal*, or *at risk* for each data record (Table 2).

Table 2

No.	TOTAL, LDL, HDL, TOTAL/HDL, LDL/HDL					Expert CHOLESTEROL* N	B	A	R
1	7.25	5.49	0.91	8.00	6.00	-	-	X	-
2	6.22	4.14	1.46	4.26	2.83	-	X	-	-
-	-	-	-	-	-	-	-	-	-
166	4.82	3.17	1.22	3.97	2.59	X	-	-	-

*N = normal, B = borderline, A = abnormal, R = at risk.

For example, the domain expert interpreted the CHOLESTEROL of the first data record in Table 2 to be *abnormal* (A), the second to be *borderline* (B) and the last record as *normal* (N). The domain expert was also asked to establish fuzzy sets for the inputs and the output of the FES. Figure 3 illustrates the fuzzy sets for two inputs (TOTAL, LDL), and also those used for the output (CHOLESTEROL) of the FES.

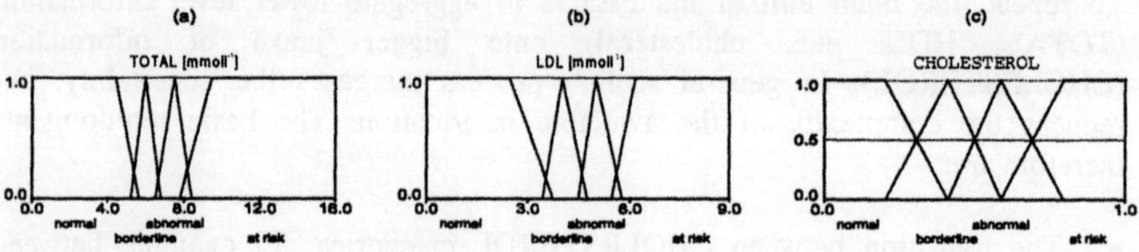

Figure 3: Input and output fuzzy sets.

Note that from now on a collection of fuzzy sets used to describe a cholesterol type, a cholesterol ratio, or the aggregated CHOLESTEROL is termed a 'frame'. For example, the TOTAL frame in Figure 3a consists of the fuzzy sets *normal, borderline, abnormal* and *at risk.* The next task of the domain expert was to express the association between input fuzzy sets and output fuzzy sets in the form of IF-THEN statements, where the IF-part of a rule corresponds to a system input and the THEN-part to a system output. There exist many different ways to obtain rules from data. Statistical methods, the C4 algorithm, the fuzzy-C-means algorithm, or neural networks are some examples. Further, the available data can be comprehensive, but it can also be limited to the extreme of only a few examples as in CBR for example (Schuster 1999). A domain expert has provided the rules in this study, and so the rules are based on the expert's background in medicine and his personal experience in the field of CHD research. Once established however rules are regarded to represent so-called domain knowledge. Very frequently however some rules are more important than other rules, and so a further task for the domain expert was to provide a weight assignment for the rule base of the FES. The weight assignment was restricted by the requirements that a weight value (w_i) had to be drawn from the interval $w_i \in [0, 1]$, and that the distributed weight values should sum up to one, thus $\Sigma w_i = 1$. Note that there are different ways to generate a weight assignment. It is possible to choose weight values from an arbitrary interval (e.g. the interval [1, 20]). Application specific these values then may or may not be normalised. In the presented study however a weight value can not exceed the value 1. This is because in the FES a weight value is actually multiplied with a membership degree (μ) obtained from a fuzzy set. A membership degree is always smaller or equal to one ($\mu \leq 1$). The second requirement therefore basically prevents a situation where the product $w_i \cdot \mu > 1$. It is also important mentioning that the weight assignment in this study is an intuitive assignment given by the domain expert on the basis of his experience. In other applications weights might be derived statistically for example. Table 3 illustrates the weight assignment given by the domain expert. In forthcoming sections such a weight assignment is going to be referred to as a 'weight vector'.

Table 3

	TOTAL	LDL	HDL	TOTAL/HDL	LDL/HDL	Σ
Weight	0.40	0.15	0.20	0.125	0.125	1.00

So, a typical system rule has the form: [(weight) **IF** (input **is** A) **THEN** (output **is** B)], where 'input' is an input frame (e.g. TOTAL), A is an input fuzzy set (e.g. *borderline*), 'output' an output frame (e.g. CHOLESTEROL) and B an output fuzzy set (e.g. *borderline*). A crucial concept of FESs is that all rules apply at all times (Cox 1995). If more than one rule applies then the separate responses have to be combined to a composite output. FES decision-making therefore usually comprises the sub-processes: fuzzification, inference (combination) and defuzzification. There exist different methods for these processes and it is part of the knowledge engineer's work to select appropriate methods for a given problem (Ross TJ 1995). For the information aggregation process fuzzification was undertaken via the 'correlation-product' encoding, inference and combination via 'sum-combination' and finally, defuzzification via the 'centre of gravity' method.

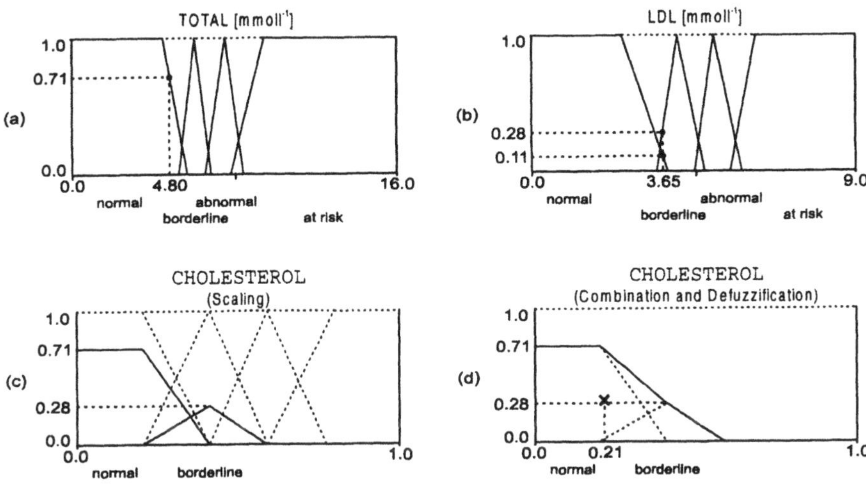

Figure 4: Generation of a CHOLESTEROL summary.

To ease the explanation of the information aggregation process we disregard the weight assignment on a rule for the moment, and also only use the cholesterol types TOTAL and LDL (Figure 4). For example, in the TOTAL frame in Figure 4a the value <TOTAL, 4.80 $mmoll^{-1}$> intersects the fuzzy set *normal*, scoring a membership degree of 0.71 (fuzzification). On the other hand in the LDL frame in Figure 4b the value <LDL, 3.65 $mmoll^{-1}$> intersects the fuzzy sets *normal* and *borderline*, scoring membership degrees of 0.11 and 0.28. The inference process of the FES applies the activation via the rules to the fuzzy sets of the output (CHOLESTEROL). For example, imagine the following rule: [**IF** LDL is *borderline* **THEN** CHOLESTEROL is *borderline*]. According to this rule the output fuzzy set *borderline* in Figure 4c is scaled down to the degree 0.28. The situation is slightly different when the same output fuzzy set is activated by more than one input fuzzy set. In this case the separate responses need to be combined. The FES in this study uses an operation where the output fuzzy set is scaled according to the maximum activation. Although many other possibilities exist this is a very common implementation of a so-called fuzzy **or** operator (Ross TJ 1995). For example imagine the two rules [**IF** LDL is *normal* **THEN** CHOLESTEROL is *normal*], and [**IF** TOTAL is *normal* **THEN** CHOLESTEROL is *normal*] in the scenario illustrated in Figure 4. Both rules apply to the same output fuzzy set. The output fuzzy set *normal* is activated by two inputs (<TOTAL, 4.80 mmoll^{-1} = 0.71, and <LDL, 3.65 mmoll^{-1}> = 0.11>), and according to the maximum method it is scaled down to max[0.71, 0.11] = 0.71 (Figure 4c). So far the weight assignment has been neglected. A weight value would simply be multiplied with an input fuzzy set activation and the resulting value would be used for scaling. Imagine the rule [**IF** TOTAL is *normal* **THEN** CHOLESTEROL is *normal*] again. The fuzzy set TOTAL/*normal* is activated to a degree of 0.71. The weight value for TOTAL cholesterol is 0.40. Hence the value propagated for scaling would be 0.71*0.40 = 0.284. After scaling the sum-combination method is used to calculate the point-wise maximum of the fuzzy sets *normal* and *borderline* to generate a combined output (Figure 4d). The centre of gravity method finally defuzzifies the combined output. In Figure 4d this process generates the final outcome 0.21. Here it has to be mentioned again that the design of a FES is very much of a trial and error process. There exist many different methods for fuzzification, inference (combination) and defuzzification. We have tested many different approaches. Many of them performed equivalently well. The approach presented here is selected on the basis of achieving the best results.

3.1. Interpretation of a system output

There exist different methods to interpret a FES output. One possibility is to simply take the label of the output fuzzy set that is activated by the highest membership degree. In this case the output would be <0.21 = CHOLESTEROL/*normal*>. Such an interpretation would be sufficient and meaningful. For example, a clinician might say: "Don't worry your CHOLESTEROL is *normal*". In this study such an interpretation is considered to be an oversimplification, because the explicit use of the sum-combination and the centre of gravity method for combination and defuzzification provide the means for a more precise interpretation. According to Figure 4d both fuzzy sets, the fuzzy set *normal* and the fuzzy set *borderline* in the CHOLESTEROL frame should be considered in the final decision-making process. To overcome this difficulty here the so-called *tendency* of an output value is introduced. The tendency of an output value is indicated by the *tendency interval* an output value belongs to. The original CHOLESTEROL frame is therefore divided into the eight tendency intervals N+, N-, B+, B-, A+, A-, R+ and R- (Figure 5).

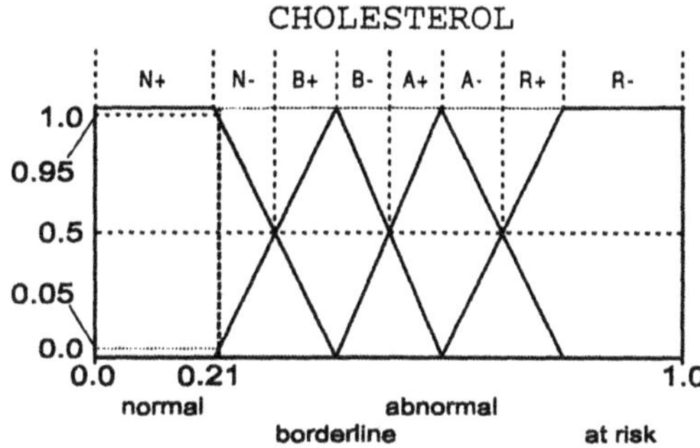

Figure 5: Interpretation of an output.

The system output 0.21 in Figure 5 obviously is falling into the N- tendency interval, intersecting the fuzzy sets *normal* and *borderline* to a degree of 0.95 and 0.05, respectively. Based on the idea of a tendency interval, the system output now would look like <0.21= CHOLESTEROL/N->, and should be interpreted as: "The CHOLESTEROL of the person is *normal* with a tendency to *borderline*". Such a result is intuitively appealing and close to an expert's explanation in such a situation.

3.2 Results generated by the FES

The assessment process was utilised for all 166 data records. The FES outcome of each record was then compared with the expert's judgement of the record in question (Table 4).

Table 4

No.	Cholesterol Data					Expert* N	B	A	R	FES* COG	CHOL
1	7.25	5.49	0.91	8.00	6.00	-	-	X	-	0.67	A–
2	6.22	4.14	1.46	4.26	2.83	-	X	-	-	0.24	N–
-	-	-	-	-	-	-	-	-	-	-	-
166	4.82	3.17	1.22	3.95	2.59	X	-	-	-	0.16	N+

*N = normal, B = borderline, A = abnormal, R = at risk, COG = center of gravity, CHOL = CHOLESTEROL.

Table 4 is similar to Table 2, but also contains the columns COG and CHOL for the FES output. Column COG displays the centre of the gravity generated by the

FES and column CHOL holds the FES's decision on the CHOLESTEROL for the corresponding record. The results have been evaluated in two steps. The first step computes the number of 'direct matches', and the second step the number of 'tendency matches'. A direct match was considered to be the case when the expert and the FES classified a data record into the same category. For example, the first and the last record in Table 4 are direct matches. The expert and the FES classify the first record to be *abnormal* (expert = A, FES = A–), and the last record to be *normal* (expert = N, FES = N+). On the other hand, the second record in Table 4 represents a tendency match. The expert considers the CHOLESTEROL of this record to be *borderline* (B), whereas the FES's outcome is N–. However, this is a meaningful result as Figure 5 illustrates. A rational thought supports this argument. Even in situations where the domain expert found it difficult to classify a person's CHOLESTEROL he was forced to choose one of the four categories for such an in-between value. It is therefore more than convenient to have a method for the identification of such values available. It is also understandable that there are not only 'exact' tendency matches or 'exact' direct matches. It is more appropriate to assume that the cholesterol values cover the complete extent of their domain, especially when the number of records increases. So, it makes sense to use the plus (+) and minus (–) indicators for both, direct matches and tendency matches. Table 5 holds the results generated by the FES.

Table 5

Direct Match	Tendency Match	Meaningful Results
101 = 60.8%	59 = 35.5%	160 = 96.3%

Table 5 shows that a direct match happened 101 times that is in 60.8% of the sample, and a tendency match 59 times equalling 35.5% of the sample. In total the FES derived 160 meaningful results, which is equivalent to 96.3% of the sample. This result is quite satisfactory, especially when considering that for several reasons the information aggregation approach was not expected to establish 166 (100%) meaningful results. Firstly, asked about the same situation or problem twice (e.g. repeated after some weeks), even a single expert's decision-making diverges very often. Secondly, when several experts are available it is very likely that they will disagree in some cases. Thirdly, during knowledge acquisition the expert was enforced to chose one of the four categories (*normal*, *borderline*, *abnormal*, or *at risk*) for a record, invoking one of the weaknesses of a discrete choice; very often it is not possible to express intermediate values. From this perspective the results established in this sections can be summarised as meaningful and valuable. There is however one more issue that needs addressing. There are 166 data records. Ideally there should be as many *normal* records as there are *borderline*, *abnormal*, or *at risk* records. This however was not the case. There have been more *normal* and *borderline* records than *abnormal* or *at risk* records. The data set therefore is not exhaustive. The FES therefore needs additional testing whenever more data records of these classes are available. From a positive viewpoint this indicates an advantage of a rule-based approach. Rules are able to represent knowledge on a high level and so it is possible to establish classifiers even in situations where only few samples are available. This applies in particular to techniques such as CBR, which are particularly designed from this position. The following sections report how aggregates like CHOLESTEROL are further applied in DSCHDRA as possible solutions to some of the central issues in CBR research.

4. Case-Based Reasoning in the DSCHDRA System

The CBR component aims to provide information about the CHD risk and a possible treatment regime for a subject. The decision for the inclusion of the component is also based on some of the advantages CBR has over other problem solving approaches:

- For example, CBR does not require causal models or a deep understanding of a domain and therefore it can be used in poorly defined domains, situations where information is incomplete or contradictory, or where it is difficult to get sufficient domain knowledge.
- It is often easier for experts to provide cases rather than to provide precise rules.
- Cases in general are a rather uncomplicated and familiar problem representation scheme for many domain experts.
- Cases provide the ability to explain by example (retrieved cases) and to learn (adding a case to the case base). Past solutions and steps involved in the problem-solving process can be reused and also provide valuable help in preventing repetition of previous errors.
- An increasing CBR knowledge base is frequently easier to maintain rather than a growing rule based knowledge base. For example, adding or deleting cases is easier opposed to changing rules, which often implies a lot of reorganisation work in rule based systems.

The advantages presented above are given from a very general perspective. CBR applications are usually very specialised and what was as an advantage earlier may give birth to other problems. Maintenance of a CBR knowledge base via the addition or deletion of cases seems simple enough for example. On the other hand, the issue of consistency of memory that can be associated with it sometimes might be easier in a rule-based system. This is one of the reasons however why many systems are hybrids (like CHDRA) in which the strengths of different techniques is used complementary. From the CHDRA perspective it is important to mention that a lot of effort has been directed towards, very often long-term, epidemiological studies to identify CHD risk factors. Based on the data of such studies statistical analysis has been used to derive algorithms and strategies that can help in the identification and management of individuals at high CHD risk (Tunstall-Pedoe 1991), (Shaper et al. 1987).

Some of the disadvantages of such long-term epidemiological studies and underlying statistical analysis are as follows:

- Statistical analysis is data driven and precludes the use of available domain knowledge.
- The performance of statistics largely depends on the amount of available data (samples, records). Crudely speaking, the more data the better statistics performs.
- At a later stage of a study it can be difficult if not impossible to add factors into an existing statistics-based model that were not considered during data collection. Thus, a need for systems exists where expert knowledge can be added at any stage.
- There are other factors associated with increased CHD risk, but data on the benefits of their management are still lacking. For example, none of the statistics-based models incorporates a wider range of factors such as physical activity levels, stress, etc., which are known to contribute to CHD risk (Theorell 1992), (Lopes et al. 1994).
- Studies, for example in medical domains, quite frequently demand a considerable amount of time and therefore there is a need for more efficient learning methods.

CBR is a large research field with many unanswered questions. The presented study can only deal with some of them. This chapter therefore has a focus in investigating the potential aggregated summaries provide for some of the fundamental CBR issues. Figure 6 illustrates the context in which these issues are going to be dealt with.

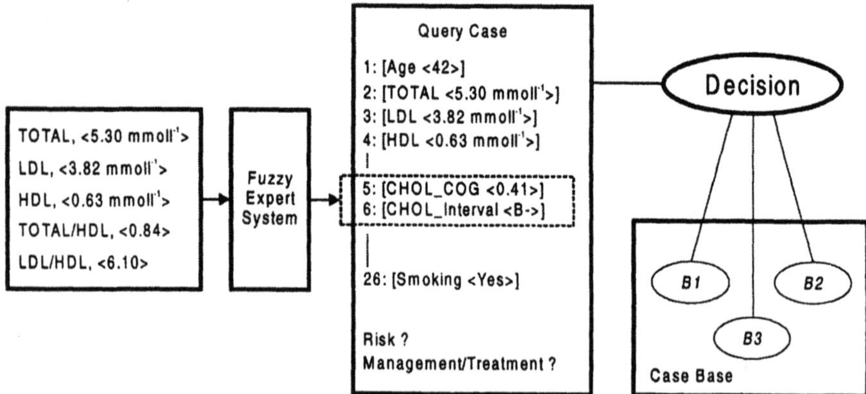

Figure 6: DSCHDRA-CBR environment.

Figure 6 illustrates a query case (person) and a case base. The query case indicates that we are interested in the CHD risk and also in a possible treatment regime for a subject. Both, risk and treatment regime is known for the base cases B1, B2 and B3 in Figure 6. Further, the query case and each base case are described by a set of attributes. So, suppose the query case in Figure 6 enters the system. Then, according to the recorded data (attributes) the system retrieves the cases most similar to the query case out of the case base. The underlying assumption is that the information that is available through the retrieved cases is useful for the query case. CBR is a model for human reasoning. Such reasoning is very often based on abstract summaries. In CBR abstract summaries are often referred to as complex attributes. Complex attributes are often composed from a set of primitive attributes. For example, Age, TOTAL, LDL, HDL and Smoking in Figure 6 are primitive case attributes, whereas CHOL_COG, and CHOL_Interval are complex attributes, generated by the FES. The attribute CHOL_COG holds the value for the centre of gravity for the summary CHOLESTEROL and CHOL_Interval holds the value of the tendency interval (Section 3.1).

The following sections investigate the potential of complex case attributes in the CBR areas of: uncertainty management, time performance, case retrieval, and case evaluation:

- **Time performance:** Complex attributes address time performance by their mere capability of reducing the number of case attributes. Case retrieval is based on an attribute to attribute comparison between cases. The number of attributes therefore significantly determines the retrieval time of a CBR system, especially large systems (Aamodt and Plaza 1994), (Jones and Roydhouse 1995).
- **Uncertainty management:** As the number of case attributes decreases so does the complexity of the system. The price paid for a less complex system however is on an increase in the uncertainty prevailing in the system. For example, a meteorological phenomenon can be described in terms of primitive attributes like pressure, temperature, relative humidity and wind speed. Alternatively the same phenomenon might be described by one of the complex attributes low-pressure system, jet stream, or frontal region (Jones and Roydhouse 1995). Useful complex attributes therefore should establish an efficient complexity reduction without loosing the original information content.
- **Case retrieval:** The retrieval time advantage was already mentioned. Complex attributes further allow the performance of a two-step retrieval process, in which the first step retrieves a set of candidate cases on the bases of complex attributes (less complexity but increased uncertainty). Step 2 then performs a refined similarity assessment on the pre-selected candidate cases but uses primitive attributes instead of complex attributes. This strategy is especially useful for large case bases (Jones and Roydhouse 1995).
- **Case evaluation:** Another advantage of complex attributes can be found in the problem area of case evaluation. Suppose that for the query case in Figure

6 a certain number of base cases has been retrieved from the case base. The problem-solving potential of **all** of these cases then has to be evaluated. This is done by an attribute to attribute comparison between each retrieved case and the query case, and is usually undertaken by a system user. Consequently case evaluation can be time consuming and difficult. Experts commonly undertake evaluation tasks via the use of summaries. It therefore would be helpful to have a mechanism for the identification and generation of prominent characteristics and summaries of retrieved base cases and to make this information accessible for the system user. Unfortunately there is not enough space here to report in detail on the work we have undertaken in this area. We therefore here only provide a reference under which further information can be found (Schuster et al. 1999).

4.1. A case-based reasoning study based on complex case attributes

The following sections present the results of an extensive case retrieval study in which the complex attributes CHOL_COG and CHOL_Interval play an important role. Three types of retrieval, referred to as *Retrieval 1*, *Retrieval 2* and *Retrieval 3*, are employed in the study. Common to each retrieval is the utilisation of the nearest neighbour method for twenty query cases. The three retrievals however are significantly different in using (a) a complete set of primitive case attributes (*Retrieval 1*), or (b) a reduced set of primitive and complex case attributes (*Retrieval 2* and *Retrieval 3*). Table 6 illustrates which cholesterol attributes are included in the different retrievals.

Table 6

Retrieval	*Retrieval 1*	*Retrieval 2*	*Retrieval 3*
Included attributes	TOTAL, LDL, HDL	CHOL_COG	CHOL_Interval

For example, *Retrieval 1* uses the complete set of primitive attributes including TOTAL, LDL and HDL cholesterol, and therefore runs on twenty-four case attributes (Figure 6). On the other hand, *Retrieval 2* uses the complex attribute CHOL_COG instead of the primitive attributes TOTAL, LDL and HDL. A *Retrieval 2* search therefore uses only twenty-two attributes (Figure 6). The same applies for *Retrieval 3*, which utilises the complex attribute CHOL_Interval in its search. The aim of the study is to examine how successful *Retrieval 2* and *Retrieval 3* are in extracting from the DSCHDRA case base those same cases as returned by *Retrieval 1*. To answer that question, *Retrieval 2* and *Retrieval 3* are evaluated by four measures (Measure 1, Measure 2, Measure 3 and Measure 4):

- **Measure 1:** *Retrieval 1*, *Retrieval 2* and *Retrieval 3* retrieve the five most similar base for twenty query cases. The success in Measure 1 is determined by registering the total number of *Retrieval 2* and *Retrieval 3* cases matching those returned by *Retrieval 1*.
- **Measure 2:** Measure 2 narrows Measure 1 by investigating the success of *Retrieval 2* and *Retrieval 3* in matching one, two, three, four, or all five *Retrieval 1* returns.
- **Measure 3:** Measure 3 emphasises the similarity degrees of retrieved cases, and determines how many times the most similar, the two most similar, the three most similar, the four most similar, or all five most similar cases in *Retrieval 1* were returned by *Retrieval 2* and *Retrieval 3*.
- **Measure 4:** Measure 4 computes the total degree of dissimilarity (ΔSim) between cases retrieved by *Retrieval 1* and those **same** cases recalled by *Retrieval 2* and *Retrieval 3*.

Before these measures can be derived one more issue needs to be addressed. The question of weight assignments on case attributes in general and the weight assignment for complex case attributes in DSCHDRA in particular. Case retrieval is based on a similarity assessment between case attributes. A similarity assessment establishes a similarity score for a case. In many situations the computation of this score includes the use of attribute weights, where a weight reflects the importance of the attribute. A final similarity score (**S**) may be generated as follows $\mathbf{S} = (w_{A1}{*}S_{A1} + w_{A2}{*}S_{A2} + \dots + w_{An}{*}S_{An})$, where **S** is the final score, n the total number of attributes, w_{An} the weight for attribute n, and S_{An} a similarity score for attribute n. Weights can be derived statistically. They can also be assigned subjectively by domain experts, reflecting their experience and domain knowledge. However, the influence of weights and consequently problem-solving is vast. DSCHDRA relies on the experience of a domain expert who was involved in the development of the system. The expert was asked to express the relevant importance of a risk factor through a weight value w_i, where $w_i \in \{1, \dots, 20\}$. Table 7 illustrates the expert's assignment for the attributes used in the CBR study.

Table 7

Attribute (Weight), physical activity (20), TOTAL, HDL, LDL, blood pressure, smoking, age (18), history of CHD, stress (13), personal history of diabetes (11), body fat in %, body mass index (8), alcohol consume (3), social class (1)
CHOL_COG, CHOL_Interval = ?

For example, the weights twenty on the physical activity attribute, and eighteen on the attributes TOTAL, HDL, LDL, blood pressure, smoking and age reflect the relative importance of these factors in the DSCHDRA system. Table 7 also indicates the problem of weight value assignment to the aggregated complex case attributes CHOL_COG and CHOL_Interval. Common approaches would suggest the use of the average weight of the TOTAL, LDL and HDL cholesterol weights: w = ($Weight_{TOTAL}$ + $Weight_{LDL}$ + $Weight_{HDL}$)/3 = (18+18+18)/3 = 18, or to use the sum of these weights: w = 18+18+18 = 54. A third alternative would be to chose a weight between these two values, for example: w = (18+18+18)/2 = 27. The forthcoming investigations successively utilise the weight values 18, 27 and 54 for the complex attributes in *Retrieval 2* and *Retrieval 3*.

4.2. Case retrieval results

Table 8, for example, illustrates the outcome of a *Retrieval 1*-*Retrieval 2* comparison.

Table 8

QC	*Retrieval 1* (TOTAL, LDL, HDL, w = 18)					*Retrieval 2* (CHOL_COG, w = 18)					N
1	2/93	29/93	77/92	7/92	6/92	2/93	7/92	6/92	29/92	77/92	5
2	1/93	70/93	17/93	8/93	18/92	62/94	15/93	70/93	33/93	66/93	1
-	-	-	-	-	-	-	-	-	-	-	-
20	51/95	21/93	34/93	38/93	60/93	51/95	21/94	62/93	34/93	43/93	3
Σ N = Total number of cases retrieved by *Retrieval 1* and *Retrieval 2* =											60

Table 8 shows that both retrievals run on twenty (randomly selected) query cases (QC). *Retrieval 1* always includes the primitive case attributes TOTAL, LDL and HDL and also always uses the weight value 18 on each of these attributes. *Retrieval 2* on the other hand, utilises the complex attribute CHOL_COG and the weight value 18 (the average of the TOTAL, LDL and HDL weights) in its search. The table also illustrates that each retrieval comes up with the five most similar base cases for each of the twenty query cases. For example, for query case No.1 *Retrieval 1* returns the base cases, 2, 29, 77, 7 and 6. To express the closeness to a query case a retrieved case is also accompanied by a similarity degree in percent. For example, base case No.2 retrieved in *Retrieval 1* is similar to query case No.1 to a degree of 93% (note: the similarity of retrieved cases decreases from left to right). Further, for the same query case *Retrieval 2* returns the base cases number 2, 7, 6, 29 and 77. So, in this situation *Retrieval 2* recalled all five *Retrieval 1* cases, and therefore the last column (N) in Table 8 carries the value 5. There are however differences. Firstly, the case order in *Retrieval 2* is different. Secondly, in *Retrieval 1* and *Retrieval 2* case number 29 shows different similarity degrees. Indeed, these characteristics will be observed throughout the investigations. Measure 1, Measure 2, and Measure 3 can be instantly derived from Table 8 for an evaluation:

- Measure 1 is indicated by the last row in Table 8. In total, *Retrieval 1* and *Retrieval 2* each retrieved 20*5 = 100 base cases. Sixty of these one-hundred

Retrieval 1 cases have been returned by *Retrieval 2*. This is equal to 60% of the sample.

- Measure 2 describes how often in a *Retrieval 2* query only one, two, three, four, or all five *Retrieval 1* cases were included. For example, for query case No.20 *Retrieval 2* returned the three *Retrieval 1* cases 51, 21 and 34. In the twenty retrievals *Retrieval 2* returned: (only one case / 2 times), (two cases / 3 times), (three cases / 9 times), (four cases / 5 times), and (all five cases / once).
- Measure 3 recalls how many times the five, or four, or three, or two, or single most similar cases in *Retrieval 1* were returned by *Retrieval 2*. For example, according to Table 8, the five most similar *Retrieval 1* cases retrieved for query case No.20 are the base cases 51, 21, 34, 38 and 60. For the same query case, *Retrieval 2* has retrieved (a) the most similar case (51), (b) the two most similar cases (51 and 21), and (c) the three most similar cases (51, 21, and 34). In the present comparison the most similar case was included in eighteen of the twenty *Retrieval 2* retrievals, equalling 90%. The two most similar cases were included in 70%, the three most similar cases in 55%, the four most similar cases in 25%, and all five most similar cases in 5% of the *Retrieval 2* returns.

Measure 4 can't be derived from Table 8, as the total degree of dissimilarity (ΔSim) relies on the cases retrieved by *Retrieval 1* and the **same** cases recalled by *Retrieval 2*. Therefore, *Retrieval 2* runs again, however this time in a different mode. Not restricted in retrieving only five base cases, in the new mode *Retrieval 2* successively increases the number of returned base cases until all *Retrieval 1* cases are included in *Retrieval 2*. Table 9 presents the results for such a *Retrieval 1-Retrieval 2* scenario.

Table 9

QC	***Retrieval 1*** (TOTAL, LDL, HDL, w = 18)					***Retrieval 2*** (CHOL_COG, w = 18)					δSim
1	2/93	29/93	77/92	7/92	6/92	2/93	29/92	77/92	7/92	6/92	1
2	1/93	70/93	17/93	8/93	18/92	1/93	70/93	17/92	8/92	18/92	2
-	-	-	-	-	-	-	-	-	-	-	-
20	51/95	21/93	34/93	38/93	60/93	51/95	21/94	34/93	38/92	60/92	3
Σ δSim =											54
ΔSim = 1/100 Σ δSim =											0.54

Measure 4 can be derived from Table 9 in two steps. Initially, Equation (1) computes the dissimilarity per retrieval (δSim):

$$\delta\text{Sim} = \sum_{n=1}^{n=5} |\,\text{Sim}(C_n)_{RA} - \text{Sim}(C_n)_{RB}\,| \qquad (1)$$

where RA = *Retrieval 1*, RB either *Retrieval 2* or *Retrieval 3*, and Cn base cases retrieved in RA and RB. For example, for query case No.1 in Table 9, Eq. 1 works out: δSim = |93-93| + |93-92| + |92-92| + |92-92| + |92-92| = 0 + 1 + 0 + 0 + 0 = 1. The δSim values for a query case are listed in the last column of Table 9. The results of step one are used in step two to compute the total degree of dissimilarity (ΔSim) for a retrieval comparison:

$$\Delta \text{Sim} = \frac{1}{100} \sum_{n=1}^{n=20} \delta Sim \qquad (2)$$

ΔSim makes the total degree of dissimilarity equivalent to the average dissimilarity per case in percent in a retrieval comparison. For Table 9 Eq. 2 yields to: ΔSim = (1/100)*54 = 0.54. The complete results for Measure 1 to Measure 4 established in the six retrieval comparisons are illustrated in the following four tables. Table 10 illustrates Measure 1, the total number of *Retrieval 2* and *Retrieval 3* cases matching those returned by *Retrieval 1*.

Table 10

Retrieval	Matches	Retrieval	Matches
Retrieval 2 weight = 18	60	*Retrieval 3* weight = 18	58
Retrieval 2 weight = 27	62	*Retrieval 3* weight = 27	62
Retrieval 2 weight = 54	63	*Retrieval 3* weight = 54	52

Table 11 holds the results for Measure 2, the success for *Retrieval* 2 and *Retrieval 3* in matching one, two, three, four, or all five *Retrieval 1* returns.

Table 11

Retrieval	One	Two	three	four	Five
Retrieval 2 weight = 18	2	3	9	5	1
Retrieval 2 weight = 27	2	1	10	7	-
Retrieval 2 weight = 54	-	6	6	7	1
Retrieval 3 weight = 18	1	4	11	4	-
Retrieval 3 weight = 27	1	2	11	6	-
Retrieval 3 weight = 54	2	9	4	5	-

Table 12 reports on Measure 3, the success for *Retrieval 2* and *Retrieval 3* in matching (a) the most, (b) the two most, (c) the three most, (d) the four most, or (e) the five most similar *Retrieval 1* cases.

Table 12

Retrieval	(a)	(b)	(c)	(d)	(e)
Retrieval 2 weight = 18	18	14	11	5	1
Retrieval 2 weight = 27	18	15	10	3	-
Retrieval 2 weight = 54	18	14	8	4	1
Retrieval 3 weight = 18	18	14	7	1	-
Retrieval 3 weight = 27	18	13	7	1	-
Retrieval 3 weight = 54	14	7	2	1	-

Table 13 finally presents Measure 4, the total degree of dissimilarity (ΔSim) in % between cases retrieved by and the same cases recalled by *Retrieval 2* and *Retrieval 3*.

Table 13

Retrieval	ΔSim	Retrieval	ΔSim
Retrieval 2 weight = 18	0.54 %	*Retrieval 3* weight = 18	0.63 %
Retrieval 2 weight = 27	0.62 %	*Retrieval 3* weight = 27	0.85 %
Retrieval 2 weight = 54	0.80 %	*Retrieval 3* weight = 54	1.47 %

4.3. Interpretation of the results

Table 10 (Measure 1) shows that (a) *Retrieval 2* always returns more, or at least the same number of matching cases than *Retrieval 3* does, and (b) in *Retrieval 2* the best results are achieved by the weight value 54, whereas in *Retrieval 3* the best result is obtained by the weight value 27. (Measure 2) investigates the success of *Retrieval 2* and *Retrieval 3* in matching one, two, three, four, or all five *Retrieval 1*returns. Looking at Table 11 from this point of view, *Retrieval 2* has to be preferred again. Measure 1 and Measure 2 do not report on the similarity of retrieved cases. DSCHDRA however is an interpretative CBR application where the retrieval of highly similar cases is of prime importance. Measure 3 reveals that in retrieving the most, the two most, the three most, the four most, or all five most similar cases *Retrieval 2* again provides better results. Note also that retrieving all five most similar cases is of course considered to be very good; it is however not expected to be the general case. The most convincing evidence for aggregated complex case attributes is provided by Table 13 (Measure 4), where apart from *Retrieval 3* (weight = 54) all total degrees of dissimilarity are clearly below 1%. The same table also answers the weight assignment question for aggregated complex case attributes. Since the total degree of dissimilarity increases with increased weight values, the (average) weight value 18 will be put to use in DSCHDRA. The table also shows that there is hardly any difference in using the numeric CHOL_COG attribute (ΔSim = 0.54) or the symbolic CHOL_Interval attribute (ΔSim = 0.63) for case retrieval. These final results quite clearly indicate the value of aggregated complex attributes for case retrieval in CBR.

5. A Genetic Algorithm for Rule Weight Assignment

The final problem under investigation in this paper is quite common in the field of rule based systems and addresses the rule weight assignment task in such a system. In most rule based systems, and hence in FESs, some rules are more important than others are (Schneider and Kandel 1992). This importance is commonly expressed in a system via a real valued rule weight assignment. In most cases a domain expert provides the assignment. To come up with an assignment however can be a complex and difficult matter. For example, for a rule base with a large number of rules, or for domains that are not well defined. We identified this problem within the building process of the FES. The domain expert found it quite difficult to come up with a weight assignment for the rule base of the FES. In a sense, finding the 'best' weight configuration for a rule base can be viewed as an optimisation task. In the past the GA paradigm has been successfully applied to similar tasks (Goldberg 1989), (Mitchell 1996). In the following sections we therefore utilise a GA to attack this problem. To be able to compare the performance of the GA on the CHOLESTEROL assignment task the results of the FES using weights generated by the GA are compared with those results that are based on the weight assignment that was given by the domain expert. Before the results are going to be presented we first briefly describe the GA.

5.1. Brief introduction to GAs

In simple terms a GA is a search procedure modelling the mechanics of natural selection. A GA can be described as: A GA starts with the (random) generation of a *start population* (G_{ti}). The start population consists of a pre-defined number (n) of possible candidate solutions, also often termed an *organism* (e.g. n weight vectors). The performance of the organisms of a population is evaluated by a so-called 'fitness-function'. Based on the evaluation of G_{ti} the GA generates a new population G_{ti+1}. The generation of a new population is based on the modelling of genetically based selection. Common operations for such modelling are 'crossover' and 'mutation'. The GA generates population after population. Every new population is evaluated by the fitness function, and the GA stops when a satisfactory solution to the problem is found, or when a pre-defined threshold is reached (e.g. certain number of iterations).

5.2. GA and CHOLESTEROL assessment

In the CHOLESTEROL assessment task a weight vector corresponds to an organism. An organism is often represented in binary format. In the underlying study for example, the weight value 0.74 corresponds to the binary representation 1001010. A fitness proportionate selection procedure was implemented for the selection of highly fit weight vectors (Goldberg 1989). The procedure allocates areas of a roulette-wheel for the weight vectors of a population, where the size of an area is proportional to the fitness of a weight vector. The roulette-wheel is spun and the weight vector where the ball comes to rest is selected for the next generation. Crossover and mutation are employed before selected weight vectors are promoted to the next generation. As for FES there exist no predefined rules for the development of a GA. For example, there exists a wide range of possibilities for the implementation of both operations (Grefenstette 1986).

Table 14

Crossover		**Mutation**
(weight vector 1) 01**01100** (weight vector 2) 000**0110**	⇒ 010**0110**	(weight vector 1) 0000110 ⇒ 0010110

Table 14 illustrates the crossover for the CHOLESTEROL study. A new weight vector is generated from two selected weight vectors by replacing a sub-part of the first weight vector with the corresponding gene of the second weight vector. The choice of which gene has to be replaced is based on a random selection. Mutation on the other hand, works on the genes of a single record only. Mutation manipulates a gene by converting activated bits (1) into deactivated bits (0). Again, the gene(s) and the bit(s) in question are selected randomly. Finally, as for the implementation of crossover and mutation there exist many ways to utilise 'crossover rate' and 'mutation rate'. For example, we achieved satisfactorily results on the basis of only employing crossover with a crossover rate of 100%, meaning that all organisms of a new population are generated via crossover.

5.3. Results generated by the GA

For the CHOLESTEROL study the start population was seeded with n=50, randomly generated, binary weight vectors. Each weight vector and each population was evaluated by a fitness function where:

- The number of matching outcomes a single GA weight vector achieves determines the fitness of the weight vector. There are 166 records. So a single weight vector may achieve 166 correct CHOLESTEROL classifications.
- The total number of matching outcomes achieved by the complete population determines the fitness of a population. A population consists of n=50 weight vectors. The total number of matching outcomes for a population therefore can be 50*166 = 8300.
- The stop criterion for the GA was determined by a pre-defined number of 50 iterations.

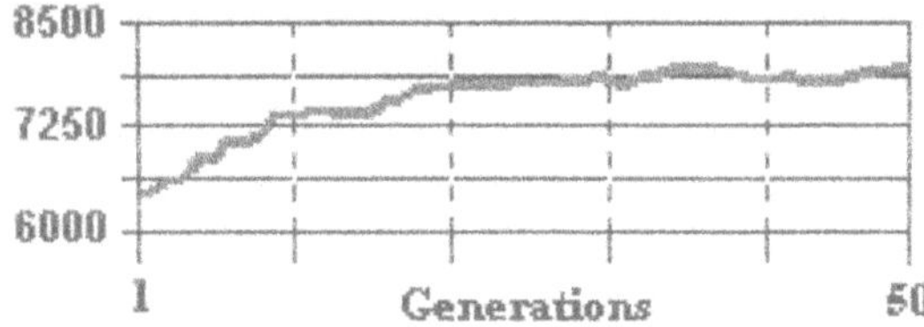

Figure 7: Total number of correct classifications per population.

Figure 7 presents the outcome of a typical GA scenario. Figure 7 illustrates how the GA climbs from 6434 (77.5%) matching outcomes for the start population to 7918 (95.4%) matching outcomes after 50 generations. Table 15 illustrates three normalised weight vectors and their individual performance on the data set after 50 generations. The last row in Table 15 also repeats the domain expert's assignment for the reason of allowing comparison.

Table 15

TOTAL	LDL	HDL	TOTAL/HDL	LDL/HDL	Meaningful Results
0.49	0.15	0.03	0.11	0.22	158 / 95.0%
0.31	0.39	0.05	0.08	0.17	160 / 96.3%
0.36	0.36	0.05	0.08	0.15	161 / 96.9%
0.40	0.15	0.20	0.125	0.125	160 / 96.3%

Compared with the domain expert's assignment (160 / 96.3%), Table 15 indicates an equally high number of matching outcomes for all three weight vectors generated by the GA (158, 160, and 161, respectively). From the point of view of performance the GA therefore can be viewed as a good solution to the problem. A comparison of the individual weight vectors in Table 15 however reveals differences. For example, according to the domain expert TOTAL cholesterol should carry the highest weight value (0.40), and HDL the second highest weight value (0.20). For weight vector two the GA assigns the highest weight value to LDL, and for weight vector three TOTAL and LDL both have the same values. Furthermore, for HDL all three GA weight vectors carry the lowest weight assignments. These are interesting results, because they contradict with the expertise the expert provided in the form of rules and fuzzy sets, and consequently have to be discussed and analysed with the domain expert. In this research the results may be interpreted as follows: The generation of a FES is very often a rather intuitive and empirical matter, and is largely influenced by the domain expert(s) involved. Although the knowledge contained in the rules should reflect the knowledge represented by the fuzzy sets, and vice versa, it may occur that a domain expert is inconsistent in his/her expertise. For example, asked about the same situation or problem twice, maybe repeated after some weeks, even a single experts decision-making diverges very often. For the DSCHDRA system this means that after a certain time the domain expert might come up with (slightly) different rules, weights, or shapes of the fuzzy sets. Nevertheless, it was the aim of this research to assist a domain expert in these tasks. One of the remaining questions to answer however is: Which of the 50 weight vectors of the final population has to be selected for the FES? One of the characteristics of the GA is that the number of identical organisms within a population increases with the number of iterations. This is basically an effect of the fitness-proportionate selection. The selection is therefore based on the frequency of identical organisms in the population after 50 iterations. For example, based on this criterion the tests underlying Table 15 established record number three as the 'best' weight vector for the FES.

6. Conclusions and Future Work

This paper provided an overview of research the authors have undertaken in the area of CHDRA. The DSCHDRA prototype system plays a central role in this research. The different components of the system and their functionality have been explained in great detail. The components work highly interrelated and DSCHDRA therefore can be classified to be a hybrid system. The research demonstrated the significant role fuzzy logic and fundamental concepts of this theory play in the system. The paper also presented the results of detailed investigations. The results have been transparent, consistent and useful, and therefore provide convincing evidence about the value of the DSCHDRA system in general and of the applied problem solving techniques in particular. Further, also we applied the presented processes to a specific problem (CHOLESTEROL assessment) we consider the solutions presented in this study to be general solutions that might be applied in many similar situations. For example, the authors are currently involved in a large-scale telecommunications project. It is already clear at this stage of the project that some of the techniques presented in this paper (probably with some modifications) are useful for similar problem constellations in the telecomms project. On a broader note future work aims towards a large scale decision support system in the telecomms area, where the experience we have gathered in the presented project is certainly very valuable and useful.

Abbreviations

CBR = case-based reasoning, CHD = coronary heart disease, CHDRA = coronary heart disease risk assessment, DSCHDRA = decision support for coronary heart disease risk assessment, FES = fuzzy expert system, GA = genetic algorithm, HDL = high-density lipoproteins, LDL = low-density lipoproteins, TOTAL = total cholesterol level.

References

1. Aamodt A and Plaza E (1994) Case-based Reasoning: Foundational Issues, Methodological Variations, and System Approaches. AICOM, (vol)7:1:39-59
2. Anderson KM, Wilson PWF, Odell PM and Kannel WB (1991) An Updated Coronary Risk Profile. Circulation (AHA Medical/Scientific Statement) (vol)83:1:356-362
3. Bonissone PP (1985) Editorial: Reasoning with uncertainty in expert systems. Int. Journal Man-Machine Studies 22:241-250
4. Brown M (1992) Case-Based Reasoning: principles and potential. AI Intelligence, January
5. Cox ED (1995) Fuzzy Logic for Business and Industry. Charles River Media, Rockland, Massachusetts
6. Dawber TR, Meadors GF and Moore FEJ (1951) Epidemiological approaches to heart disease: the framingham study. Am J Public Health 41:279-286
7. Goldberg DE (1989) Genetic Algorithm in Search. Optimization, and Machine Learning. Addison Wesley
8. Gordon DJ, Probstfield JL and Garrison RJ (1989) High density lipoprotein cholesterol and cardiovascular disease. Circulation (vol)79:8:8-15
9. Grefenstette JJ (1986) Optimization of control parameters for denetic algorithms. In: Buckles BP, Petry FE (eds) Genetic Algorithms. IEEE Computer Society Press, Los Alamos, California, pp 5-11

10. Hopkins PN and Williams RR (1981) A survey of 246 suggested coronary risk factors. Atherosclerosis 40:1-52
11. Jones EK and Roydhouse A (1995) Intelligent retrieval of archived meteorological data. IEEE Expert Intelligent Systems and their Applications, pp 50-57
12. Kannel WB, Feinleib M, McNamara PM, Garrison RJ and Castelli WP (1979) An investigation of coronary heart disease in families: the Framingham offspring study. Am J Epideniol 110:281-290
13. Kinosian B, Glick H and Garland G (1994) Cholesterol and coronary heart disease - predicting risks by levels and ratios. Annals of Internal Medicine (vol)121:9:641-647
14. Klir GJ and Folger TA (1988) Fuzzy Sets, Uncertainty and Information. Prentice Hall, Englewood Cliffs, New Jersey
15. Kolodner J (1993) Case-Based Reasoning. Morgan Kaufmann, San Mateo, California
16. Levy D (1993) A multifactorial approach to coronary disease risk assessment. Clin. And Exper. Hypertension (vol)15:6:1077-1086
17. Lopes P, White JA and Anderson J (1997) Decreased respiratory sinus arrhythmia as an indicator of coronary heart disease risk in middle-aged males. Medical and Biological Engineering and Computing (vol)35:1:578
18. Lopes PL, Mitchell RH and White JA (1994) The relationships between respiratory sinus arrhythmia and coronary heart disease risk factors in middle-aged males. Automedica, 16:71-76
19. Mitchell M (1996) An Introduction to Genetic Algorithms. MIT Press, Cambridge, Massachusetts, London
20. Riesbeck CK and Schank RC (1989) Inside Case-Based Reasoning. Lawrence Erlbaum Associates, Hillsdale, New Jersey
21. Ross R (1986) The pathogenesis of atherosclerosis: an update. New Engl. J. Med. 314:488-500
22. Ross TJ (1995) Fuzzy Logic with Engineering Applications. New York; London, McGraw-Hill
23. Schneider M and Kandel A (1992) General purpose fuzzy expert systems. In: Kandel A (ed) Fuzzy Expert Systems. CRC Press, Boca Raton, Florida, pp 23-41
24. Schuster A, Adamson K and Bell DA (1999) Generating summaries from retrieved base cases. Workshop on Data Analysis in Medicine and Pharmacology IDAMAP'99, Washington DC, USA, pp 117-122
25. Schuster A, Dubitzky W, Lopes P, Adamson K, Bell DA, Hughes JG and White JA (1997) Aggregating features and matching cases on vague linguistic expressions. 15th Int. Joint Conference on Artificial Intelligence IJCAI 1997, Nagoya, Japan, pp 252-257
26. Schuster A, Lopes P, Adamson K, Bell DA and White JA (1998a) An application of case-based reasoning in the domain of coronary heart disease risk. Int. ICSC Symposium on Engineering of Intelligent Systems EIS'98, University of La Laguna, Tenerife, Spain, pp 469-475

27. Schuster A, Lopes P, Adamson K, Bell DA and White JA (1998b) Intelligent diagnosis through fuzzy expert systems. The World Multiconference on Systemics, Cybernetics and Informatics SCI'98 and the 4th Int. Conference on Information System Analysis and Synthesis ISAS'98, Orlando, USA, pp 157-163
28. Shaper AG, Pocock SJ, Phillips AN and Walker M (1987) A scoring system to identity men at high risk of heart attack. Health Trends 19:37-39
29. Slyper AH (1994) Low-density-lipoprotein density and atherosclerosis - unravelling the connection. JAMA (vol)272:4:305-308
30. Theorell T (1992) The Psycho-Social Environment, Stress and Coronary Heart Disease. In: Marmott G, Elliot P (eds) Coronary Heart Disease Epidemiology: from Aetiology to Public Health. Oxford University Press, Oxford, UK
31. Tunstall-Pedoe H (1991) The Dundee risk-disk for management of change in risk factors. Brit Med J, September 303:744-747
32. Wilensky R (1986) Knowledge representation - A critique and a proposal. In: Kolodner J, Riesbeck K (eds) Experience, Memory, And Reasoning. Lawrence Erlbaum Associates, Hillsdale, New Jersey, pp 15-28
33. Zadeh LA (1996) Fuzzy logic = computing with words. IEEE Transactions on Fuzzy Systems, May (vol)4:2:103-111
34. Zadeh LA (1973) Outline of a New Approach to the Analysis of Complex Systems and Decision Processes. IEEE Transactions on Systems, Man, and Cybernetics, SMC (vol)3:1:28-45

A Model-based Temporal Abductive Diagnosis Model for an Intensive Coronary Care Unit*

J.T. Palma[1], R. Marín[1], J.L. Sánchez[1], and F. Palacios[2]

[1] Artificial Intelligence and Knowledge Engineering Group
Computer Science School
University of Murcia
Campus de Espinardo
30071 Murcia, Spain

[2] Hospital General de Elche
03203 Elche, Spain

1 Introduction

In current high-dependency clinical environments such as Intensive Coronary Care Unit (ICCU hereinafter), operating rooms and so on, the clinical staff is presented with a large mass of data about the patient's state. These data can be obtained from the advanced biomedical equipment (especially from electrical and hemodynamical monitors), patient's history, physical examination findings and test results. This massive flow of information can lead to some well-known problems such as data overload and missing data and misinterpretation [1,13]. In order to avoid these kinds of problems, Intelligent Patient Supervision Systems (IPSS hereinafter) have been developed. IPSSs must be developed to support the interpretation of these data and they should provide information in higher abstraction levels in order to improve the decision making process.

Diagnosis is one of the most important tasks in ICCUs and should be supported by IPSSs. The diagnosis task takes as inputs the patient's history, physical examination findings, drug administration, information from physiological signals and clinical tests and it tries to make a diagnosis about the case in question. Model-Based diagnosis has been considered the most promising method for diagnosis in medicine [5,20]. Model-Based diagnostic systems work from an explicit information source (the device model) that, in principle, can explain all possible causes of failure [4]. Thus, the manifestations acquired are compared to the device model to determine the possible causes of failure. The use of an explicit device model (the patient model in medical domains) makes the implementation of explanation facilities easier, since explanations can be built from the model. On the other hand, since

* This paper was presented as a research work carried out in the project Temporal Information Management and Intelligent Interaction in Medicine (TIC95-0604-C02-01) supported by the Spanish CICYT

its beginnings, temporal reasoning has been considered an important dimension of diagnostic systems [8,9,13,18], because most of the real world systems present a time dependent behaviour. Indeed, pathophysiological processes associated to a certain pathology have an important dynamic component, and therefore, its observable manifestations also evolve along time. Therefore the device models used in Model-Based diagnosis need to capture this temporal dimension.

It should be noted that the selected application domain (the ICCU environment) imposes some requirements on the design of such a task. Firstly, the patient may spend several days in the ICCU, so the diagnosis task must be designed to operate in a continuous mode throughout the patient's stay, and must detect and explain any complication that might appear during his or her stay. Diagnosis results (that is, the explanations provided) must be extended from the patient's admission until his or her discharge. Secondly, the diagnosis task must allow the incorporation of retrospective information since, for example, when the results of an analysis are received by the doctor, the data are referred to the time at which the analysis was made (probably some hours or days before) and, of course, this data has to be introduced into the system with the time stamp at which the blood sample was taken. This retrospective data processing may force the system to discard or reinforce the hypotheses previously made. Of course, the latter obliges us to use temporal reasoning techniques. Thus, our diagnosis task is based on conventional causal methods which have been extended to incorporate the characteristics mentioned above: continuous operation mode, retrospective data processing and temporal reasoning. Due to the complexity of the selected domain, we have restricted our diagnostic model to those patients presenting an initial diagnosis of Acute Myochardial Infarction (AMI hereinafter), with the main objective of the model being the detection and explanation of complications. Nevertheless, the principles presented in this work can easily be extended to other initial diagnosis.

The structure of the paper is as follows. In Section 2, the ontology underlying the AMI environment is put forward. The definition of a temporal pattern, which is the main elements of our diagnosis model, is presented in Section 3. A Diagnosis task based in this model is outlined in Section 4. In Section 5, tools around the diagnosis model are presented. An example of our diagnosis task is presented in Section 6. Finally, we provide conclusions, along with related and future works.

2 Ontology for AMI Domain

The AMI ontology, as in most of the diagnostic systems described so far, is comprised of diagnostic concepts and manifestations (findings) concepts. In these terms, the main objective of a diagnostic system is to determine what diagnostic concepts, that is hypotheses, explain the set of observed manifestations. It should be noted that the term "explain" admits different interpretations [11]. Basically, all the possible interpretations ranges from a consistency based explanation to a set covering based explanation, being the latter more restrictive. In a set covering based explanation, all the observed manifestations has to be covered by set of possible hypotheses without introducing any logical inconsistency. Therefore, a set covering based explanation is also consistent, but a consistency based explanation may not cover all the observed manifestations since it only requires that the selected hypotheses do not introduce any logical inconsistencies. In the model proposed here, we consider that a set of hypotheses explain the observed manifestation when the set of hypotheses covers all the observed abnormal manifestations and is consistent with the observed normal manifestations.

As developers of diagnostic systems try to approach more complex domains (such as the AMI domain) one of the main difficulties that has to be faced is the so called knowledge acquisition bottleneck, from both bibliographical sources and domain experts. The term "knowledge acquisition bottleneck" stems for the difficulties which arose when developers of the first expert systems approached the constructions of the knowledge bases extracting knowledge from experts. Since then, a great step forward in the field of knowledge acquisition has been achieved through the development of new methodologies. Nevertheless, knowledge acquisition remains as the most important difficulty in the construction of a practical knowledge base. One way to overcome this difficulty is the construction of domain ontologies. For this purpose, a generic ontology for medical diagnostic problems is presented in this section. Through the definition of this kind of ontology, we want to pursue a double objective: firstly, it can help us to organize the concepts detected through several knowledge acquisition sessions with physicians, and secondly, it serves as a generic conceptualization that can be reused in other medical diagnosis domains, through the selection of the appropriate branches of global ontology.

In our ontology manifestations (figure 1), the inputs of the diagnosis task can be classified into different types, depending on their nature or how they are acquired:

- **Administrative Data** are composed of those items in the patient record, relevant to the domain considered, such as age, sex, habits (such as smoking, sport practice, etc.), previous clinical history, and so on.
- By **Signal manifestations** we understand those manifestations which are directly acquired from electrical and hemodynamic monitoring equipment such as ECG, temperature, blood presure and so on.
- **Clinical manifestations** concepts are used to classify those manifestations that are obtained directly from patients by the physician without the intervention of any monitoring equipment. These manifestations can be divided into the following subconcepts:

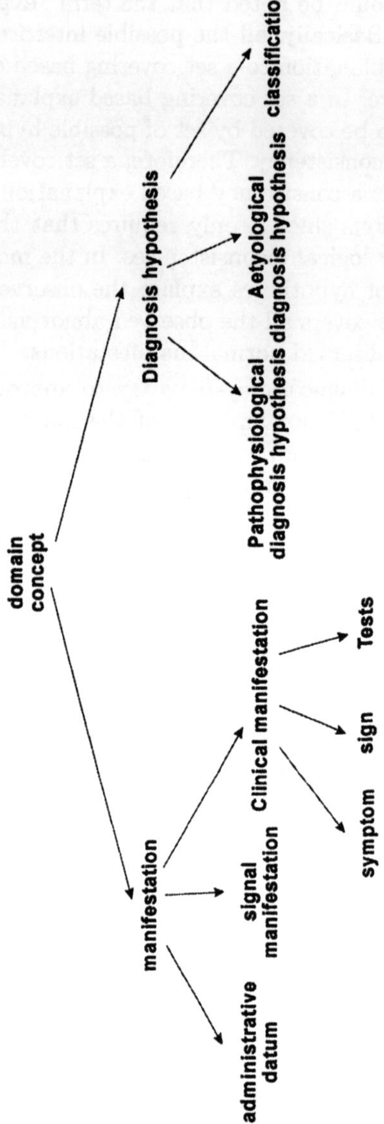

Fig. 1. Ontology for a medical diagnostic problem

- **Symptoms** are used to represent those manifestations related with the subjective sensations expressed by patients such as pain, fatigue, sleepiness, lack of appetite, etc.
- **Signs** represent those manifestations that are observed in the patient by the physician and are not acquired by means of any monitoring system. The presence or absence of sybilants, crepitants and coughs are example of this type.
- **Tests** represent those manifestations that are acquired through laboratory tests (such as a blood assay, a glucose level analysis, etc.) or other diagnostic techniques such as interpretation of radiographs.

On the other side of the proposed ontology we can find diagnostic concepts, which play the role of output of the diagnosis task. In most diagnosis systems (see, for example,[9]) the need for different abstraction levels between diagnosis hypotheses has been emphasized so that the patient evolution can be expressed in a more precise fashion. Therefore, to make it possible for our ontology to cope with different abstraction levels of diagnostic concepts, we distinguish between the following types of diagnosis hypotheses:

- **Pathophysiological diagnostic hypotheses**, which are used to represent the different pathophysiological states which may be detected in a patient. The main objective of Pathophysiological knowledge is to acquire causal relations between pathophysiological concepts, and among theses concepts and their corresponding manifestations.
- **Aetyological diagnostic hypotheses**, which represent the final diagnostic causes of the observed patient behaviour. Of course, the patient model must include diagnostic knowledge which makes the representation of causal relations between pathophysiological states and aetyological diagnostic concepts possible.
- **Classifications**. These are a special type of diagnostic concepts which can be reached by means of a simple classification process, in contrast with pathophysiological and aetyological concepts which are reached by a more complex diagnosis process such as an abductive diagnosis. For example, in AMI domain, physician usually classify the patient state according to different scales, such as Forrester and Killip, which define different and non overlapping possibilities of patient states.

Once we have described the conceptualization underlying the AMI domain, we can define the instances of domain concepts by means of the following expression:

$$C_i((a_1 = v_1), (a_2 = v_2), \cdots, (a_k = v_k)) \quad (1)$$

In expression (1), C_i stands for an instance of a domain concept (i.e., *pain*), a_j represents the jth concept attribute with v_j being its corresponding value. In our model, the set of possible values of an attribute, $V_{C_i}(a_j)$ is comprised of the set of normal attribute values, $V_{C_i}^N(a_j)$, the set of abnormal attribute values, $V_{C_i}^A(a_j)$, and the literal $UNKNOWN$. For example, the concept *pain* has an attribute describing the intensity. The set of possible values for *intensity* is composed of $\{0,1,2,3,4,5\}$ (this scale has been defined after a knowledge acquisition session in which the physician was asked for a description of the different pain grades that can be identified in patients). In this scale the 0 value represents *no pain* and is the only normal value for pain intensity. On the contrary, the set of abnormal values for pain intensity is made up of values from 1 to 5. In the expression (2), an instance of the concept *pain* (a manifestation of symptom type) can be seen as well as the different value sets associated to its attributes, which are shown in expression (3):

$$pain((intensity = 3), (type = atypical), (location = precordial)) \qquad (2)$$

$$\begin{aligned}
&V_{pain}^N(intensity) = \{0\}\\
&V_{pain}^A(intensity) = \{1,2,3,4,5\}\\
&V_{pain}^N(type) = \emptyset\\
&V_{pain}^A(type) = \{isquemic, no_isquemic, patient_isquemic, atypical\} \qquad (3)\\
&V_{pain}^N(location) = \emptyset\\
&V_{pain}^A(location) =\\
&\qquad = \{chest, precordial, neck, epigastric, jaw, back, sup_extrem.\}
\end{aligned}$$

The next issue to be solved is the representation of the temporal dimension of domain concepts. In our model, concepts whose attribute values can change during the diagnosis process are represented by *fuzzy events*. Representing a concept by a fuzzy event allows us to specify the approximate time instant at which the value of, at least, one of its attributes changes. The precise time instant is determined by one or more fuzzy temporal constraints between different fuzzy events. To make this possible, each fuzzy event is associated with one temporal variable and a non empty set of fuzzy temporal binary constraints between the temporal variable associated to the fuzzy event and the temporal variables associated with other fuzzy events. These fuzzy temporal binary constraints define the approximate durations between fuzzy events. As should be noticed, all the temporal variables as well as their fuzzy temporal constraints conform a *Fuzzy Temporal Constraint Network* ($FTCN$ hereinafter) whose nodes represent temporal variables and whose arcs are labeled with the corresponding fuzzy temporal constraints. In order to add this temporal dimension to our domain instances, the expression (1) must be extended in the following way:

$$C_i((a_1 = v_1), (a_2 = v_2), \cdots, (a_k = v_k), t_\alpha, d(t_\alpha, t_\beta), d(t_\alpha, t_\gamma), \cdots) \qquad (4)$$

In the previous expression, t_α stands for the temporal variable associated to the fuzzy event, and $d(t_\alpha, t_\beta)$ represents a fuzzy temporal constraint where

t_α and t_β are temporal variables associated to different fuzzy events. For example, an atypical chest pain with a moderate intensity detected approximately 5 minutes after the patient is admitted at ICCU, can be re-written in the following way:

$$\begin{aligned}&pain((intensity = 3), (type = atypical), (location = chest),\\&\qquad t_\alpha, d(t_\alpha, t_0) = (2,4,6,8))\end{aligned} \tag{5}$$

In the expression (5), t_α stands for the temporal variable associated to the fuzzy event, t_0 is a special temporal variable that represents the origin of time (the time at which the patient is admitted at ICCU), and the array $(2,4,6,8)$ is a fuzzy number representing the fuzzy temporal constraint between t_α and t_0. This fuzzy temporal constraint indicates that the previous fuzzy event has been detected possibly between 4 and 6 minutes after the patient's admission, and necessarily between 2 and 8 minutes. Obviously, more fuzzy temporal constraints can be defined. A graphical representation of the fuzzy temporal constraint associated to the fuzzy event of expression (5) can be seen in figure 2, which also shows the fuzzy temporal constraint network composed of the temporal variables t_α and t_0.

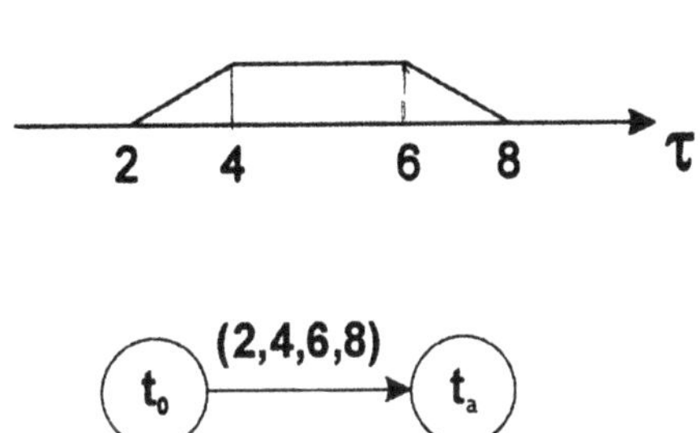

Fig. 2. Grafical Representation and FTCN for the fuzzy event $pain((intensity = 3), (type = atypical), (location = chest), t_\alpha, d(t_\alpha, t_0) = (2,4,6,8))$

The notation introduced in this section is especially suitable for representing temporal evolution of those manifestations indicated by the patient or directly observed by physicians. When expressing fuzzy events of diagnostic concepts, this notation become slightly simpler, since diagnostic concepts have only one attribute which indicates whether the corresponding diagnostic concept is present or not. For example, expression (6) can be interpreted as an indication that it is possible that the patient suffered a cardiogenic shock which might have begun between minutes 1 and 9.

$$cardiogenic\_shock((presence = TRUE), t_\beta, d(t_\beta, t_0) = (1,3,7,9)) \tag{6}$$

Similar formalisms for representation of time in medical domains have been proposed (see, for example, [14,24,5]), but the one we have presented here is simpler since it is based on fuzzy time points instead of intervals. For our purpose, the formalism presented here is very useful since our diagnostic model is intended to be integrated into a system that automatically detects qualitative events from the monitored signals ([16]). As said before, an event represents a qualitative change of, at least, one concept attribute. In a real-time environment, it is possible to detect an event when it is really produced. However, to make a prediction about the time at which the next event would appear turns out to be impossible, therefore, the temporal interval in which the new value does not change can not be predicted when the event is detected.

The management of $FTCN$ lies in what we termed *Fuzzy Temporal Constraint Logic* ($FTCL$ hereinafter) which is a logical framework that allows the generation of complex temporal queries involving fuzzy temporal concepts as well as assertion of new fuzzy events, while maintaining the temporal consistency of the network. For those interested in a deeper analysis of $FTCL$, a more detailed discussion can be found in [6,7].

3 Temporal Patterns

Temporal Patterns are the key elements in our diagnosis model. The set of temporal patterns conforms a causal model of patients. Information about cause-effect relations and temporal restriction between these relations can be found in them. A temporal pattern can be formally defined as a 4-tuple $TP_i =< H_i, IM_i, IH_i, R_i >$ where:

- H_i is the pattern's main hypothesis,
- IM_i is the set of abnormal manifestations implied by the hypothesis H_i,
- IH_i is the set of hypotheses implied by the hypothesis H_i and,
- $R_i =< L_i, X_i >$ is a temporal constraint network, where L_i stands for the set of fuzzy durations between the temporal labels (associated to the remaining temporal pattern components) defined in X_i.

The pattern's main hypothesis H_i is defined as a fuzzy event of diagnostic hypothesis type (pathophysiological or aetyological), in which the fuzzy durations are removed since they are represented in the temporal constraint network, R_i. Therefore, when a temporal pattern is instantiated, its main hypothesis can be represented by the expression:

$$\begin{array}{c} H_i((present = TRUE), t_\alpha) \\ t_\alpha \in X_i \end{array} \tag{7}$$

Hypothesis H_i represents a diagnosis that may explain the abnormal manifestations observed, without being inconsistent with the normal manifestations observed. This definition of diagnostic explanation has to be extended in order to cope with the temporal dimension since the consistency is defined not only over manifestation attributes and their values but over the pattern's temporal constraints. Of course, a temporal pattern must exist for each instance of diagnosis type (both pathophysiological and aetyological).

The set of abnormal manifestations, IM_i, is comprised of the abnormal manifestations which must be observed as a consequence of the hypothesis. The time, relative to the supposed hypothesis appearance time, at which the manifestation must appear is defined through fuzzy durations between temporal variables of the temporal constraint network, R_i). Therefore, an instantiated manifestation, m_i, can be represented by a fuzzy event of manifestation type by the expression:

$$\begin{array}{c} m_i((a_1 = v_1), (a_2 = v_2), \cdots, (a_k = v_k), t_{\alpha_i}) \\ t_{\alpha_i} \in X_i \end{array} \tag{8}$$

where, at least, one of the attribute values, v_k, must belong to the set of abnormal values, $V_{a_k}^A$, of its corresponding attribute.

Another component of a temporal pattern is the set of implied hypotheses IH_i, which is composed of pathophysiological diagnosis hypotheses that may be caused by the pattern´s main hypothesis H_i. As can be noticed, implied hypothesis are used to predict possible future complications in the patient state. Therefore, an implied hypothesis, once it has been instantiated, can be represented by the expression:

$$\begin{array}{c} ih_i((present = TRUE), t_{\alpha_i}) \\ t_{\alpha_i} \in X_i \end{array} \tag{9}$$

The last component of a temporal pattern is a fuzzy temporal constraint network, $R_i =< X_i, L_i >$, where the elements of the set L_i are binary constraints among temporal variables defined in X_i. The set of temporal variables X_i is composed of the temporal variables defined in the implied manifestations IM_i, the implied hypotheses IH_i and the hypothesis h_i, i. e., $X_i = \{t_i, t_1^m, t_2^m, \cdots, t_1^h, t_2^h, \cdots\}$. The set of binary constraints among temporal variables, L_i, is comprised of fuzzy durations which are defined over each possible pair of temporal variables in X_i. As we will see in following sections, it is not necessary to define all the possible durations among the pattern's elements, since the remaining durations can be obtained by applying a constraint propagation algorithm over the defined durations [23]. Therefore, $L_i = \{d(t_\alpha, t_\beta), t_\alpha, t_\beta \in X_i\}$, where $d(t_\alpha, t_\beta)$ represents the fuzzy duration between t_α and t_β. These constraints are defined during the knowledge acquisition process. Once the constraints are defined, the $FTCN$ is reduced to a minimal network and its temporal consistency is tested. The constraint network of a temporal pattern does not necessarily impose a sequential order on events. For example,one of the possible temporal orders among pattern elements is shown in the bottom panel of figure 3. In fact, the temporal constraint network implies a set of possible sequences of events.

In order to facilitate the definition of temporal patterns, a graphical tool which automatically checks the consistency of the acquired knowledge will be presented in section 5.

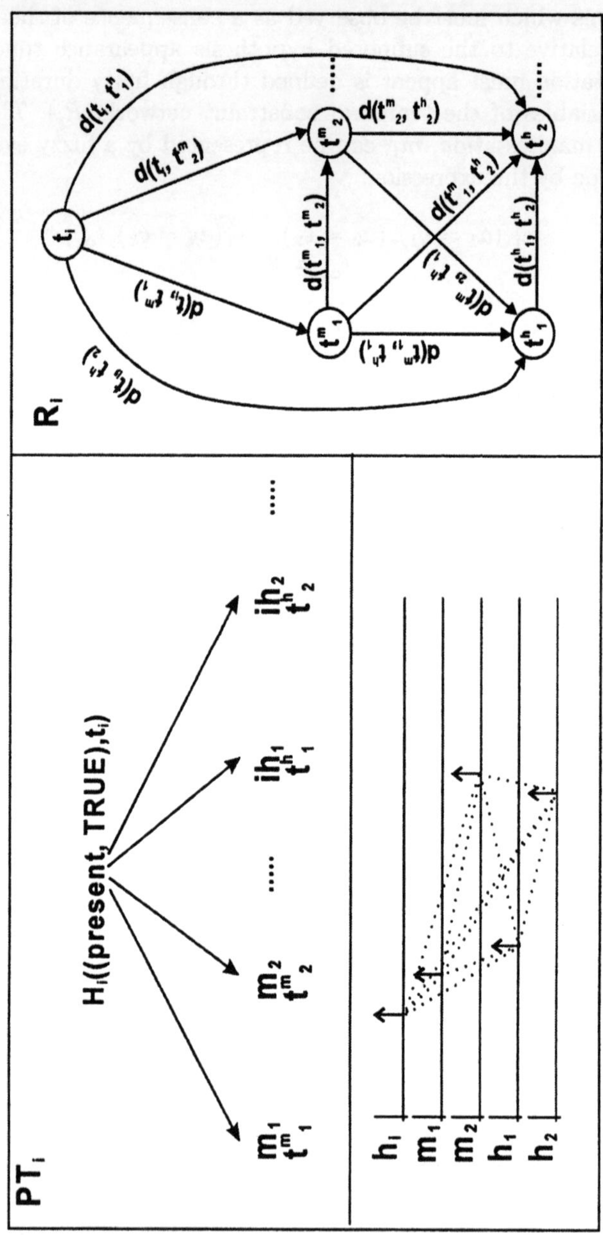

Fig. 3. Graphical representation of a temporal pattern

The pattern's implied manifestations capture knowledge about relations between the diagnosis hypothesis (cause) and manifestations (effect). Thus, this type of causal relation is termed *m-relation* or *evidential causal relation*. For example, from the *retrograde cardiac insufficiency* pattern we can deduce that the hypothesis *retrograde cardiac insufficiency* can be suggested by the presence of some effects such as *st-changes* or *murmur*. This abductive hypotheses construction process conforms the abductive phase of our diagnosis model.

Pattern's implied hypotheses represent another type of causal relations which connect the pattern's main hypothesis (pathophysiological or aetyological) with other pathophysiological diagnostic hypotheses. Thus, this kind of relation allows us to represent both pathophysiological knowledge (describing the cause-effect relations of pathophysiological states) and diagnostic knowledge (relating pathophysiological hypotheses with aetyological hypotehses). These types of relations are termed *h-relations* or *non-evidential causal relations*, in contrast with those defined in the previous paragraph. For example, a *cardiogenic shock* which is a diagnosis hypothesis (which must be defined by its corresponding temporal pattern) can be caused by a *retrograde cardiac insufficiency*, which is another diagnosis hypothesis. In our diagnosis method, non-evidential causal relations will help us to foresee new diagnoses, following the relation under question from the main hypothesis (pathophysiological ones) to implied hypotheses(either pathophysiological or aetyological ones), as well as to build explanations for the hypothesis already generated (reaching the implied manifestations for the implied hypothesis under question). The latter allows the diagnosis process to reach an aetyological diagnosis from pathophysiological ones. In most cases, aetyological diagnosis hypotheses cannot be confirmed by the observed evidence until reliable data, such as clinical analysis data, information about echography, radiography, etc., are received but they are generated as a possible alternative explanation of the hypothesis, in the same way as the hypothesis from which they are implied are evoked.

As can be deduced, the structure underlying the causal relations defined in a temporal pattern conforms a tree structure. These trees can be combined via their implied manifestations (one manifestation can be presented in two different temporal patterns) and their implied hypotheses (figure 4), with this new structure resulting in an acyclic directed graph termed *Causal Knowledge Network* (which should not be confused with an *Instantiated Causal Network*, which will be introduced in the following section). This Causal Knowledge Network describes the causal and temporal structure underlying the selected domain. Taking into account all of the above, the *Causal Knowledge Network* can be formally defined in the following way, $CKN = \{TP_i\}$, i. e., as being composed of all temporal patterns defined for a specific application domain.

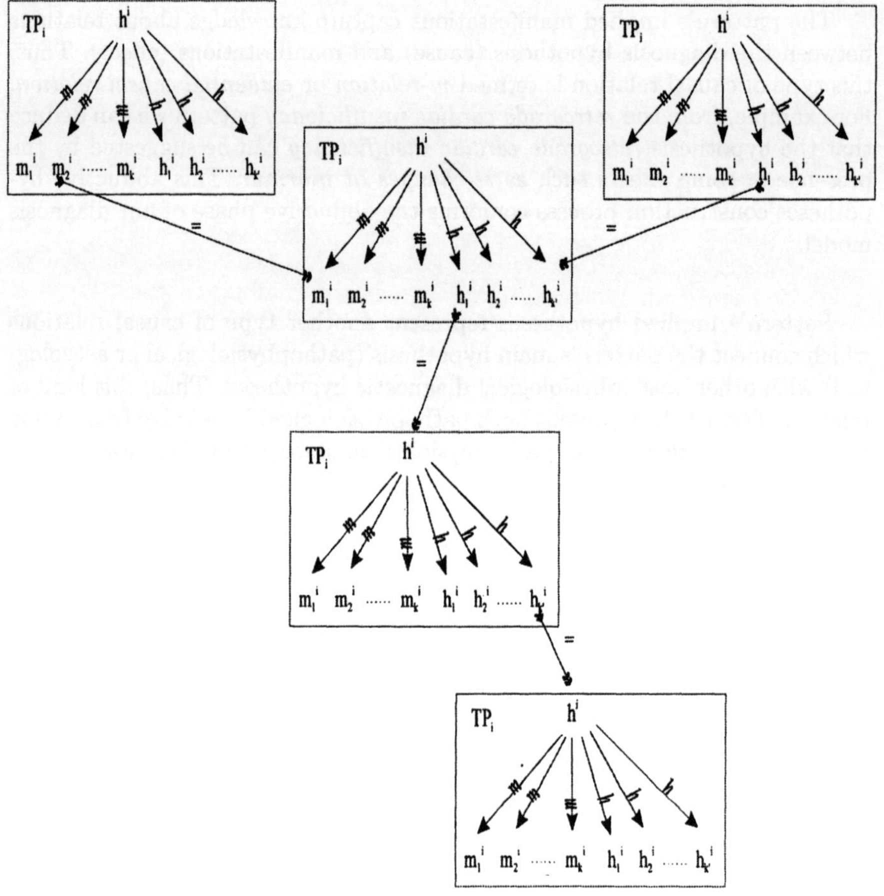

Fig. 4. The causal network of temporal patterns

4 Diagnosis Tasks

First of all, before the execution of the *Diagnosis* task, the model starts with the *Manifestation Detection* task, which is complementary to the *Diagnosis* task. This task gathers the set of new manifestations, M_{new} (i. e., the new events), which have been received after the last execution of the task, and classifies them into the sets:

- **Normal Manifestations,** M_{new}^n, which contains those manifestations whose values correspond to normal values of behaviour.
- **Abnormal Manifestations,** M_{new}^a, for the events whose values correspond to abnormal values of behaviour. These two classifications are made via the comparison with an abnormal behaviour model represented in the temporal patterns set.

- **Discriminant Manifestations,** M^d_{new}, for those manifestations which can help in the refining of the explanation obtained in the last diagnosis cycle. This set will be created in the *Differentiate* task which will be explained in the following paragraphs.
- **Non Discriminant Manifestations,** M^{nd}_{new}, for those manifestation which have nothing to do in the refining of the explanations.

It should be noticed that a manifestation cannot belong to M^n_{new} and M^a_{new} at the same time. Of course, the same property can be defined in the sets M^d_{new} and M^{nd}_{new}. However, a certain manifestation could belong at the same time to, for example, M^n_{new} and M^d_{new}, in these cases, the manifestation represents a new evidence that can be used to rule out previously evoked hypotheses. Strictly speaking, the sets obtained as an output of the *Manifestation Detection* task must have the following properties:

1. $M^n_{new} \bigcap M^a_{new} = \emptyset$
2. $M^d_{new} \bigcap M^{nd}_{new} = \emptyset$
3. $(M^n_{new} \bigcup M^a_{new}) = (M^d_{new} \bigcup M^{nd}_{new}) = M_{new}$

Once the *Manifestation Detection* task has built up the sets M^n_{new}, M^a_{new}, M^d_{new} and M^{nd}_{new}, it updates the sets M^n, M^a, M^d and M^{nd}, which gather the manifestations produced from the time the patient is admitted to the ICCU.

Once the *Manifestation Detection* task is executed the model proceeds with the so-called *Diagnosis* task, the main function of which is to explain new manifestations, if any. In order to improve the performance of the *Diagnosis* tasks, and considering that the diagnosis process is carried out by repetitive execution of the *Diagnosis* task, the latter should be designed to be reactive to the presence of new discriminant or new abnormal manifestations. Therefore, each diagnosis cycle will be executed if and only if $M^a_{new} \neq \emptyset$ or $M^d_{new} \neq \emptyset$. Of course, as can be deduced from the above, the *Diagnosis* task will require the sets M^n_{new}, M^a_{new} and M^d_{new} as inputs. Another input for this task is the explanation obtained as a result of the last execution of the *Diagnosis* task (that is, the output of the last diagnosis cycle). At this point, it is important to analyse further what the structure underlying the diagnosis explanations is. In our proposal, the explanation, which is obtained through successive diagnosis cycles, conforms a causal network, which is referred to as ICN (Instantiated Causal Network), comprised of a set of temporal pattern instances which are inter-related through their implied hypotheses. Thus, our *Diagnosis* task takes as inputs the sets M^n_{new}, M^a_{new} and M^d_{new}, and the last explanation, ICN_{old}, and then produces a new explanation ICN_{new} (as a modification of the previous one) which tries to explain the new evidence received since the last diagnosis cycle.

Our *Diagnosis* task is decomposed into two subtasks (figure 5): *Hypotheses Discrimination* and *Hypotheses Generation.* The *Hypotheses Discrimination* task will try to refine ICN_{old} according to the new discriminating evidence M^d_{new}. This refinement can consist of:

- the reinforcement of some hypotheses, and/or
- the refutation of some hypotheses.

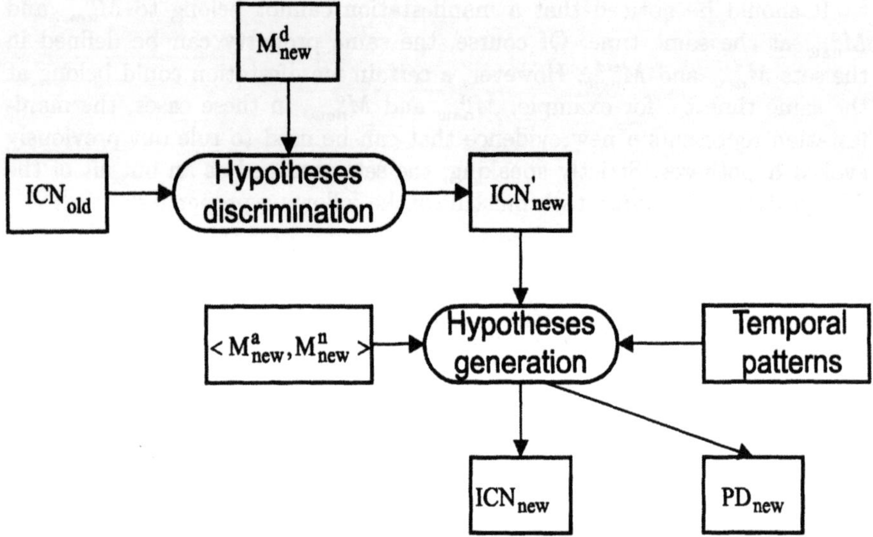

Fig. 5. Task structure for the diagnosis task

Of course, these two type of refinements produce a new explanation, named ICN'_{new}. The modus operandi of the *Hypotheses Discrimination* task is as follows (figure 6): Firstly, for each discriminant manifestation in M^d_{new}, a set of hypotheses, H_d, which can be discriminated by this manifestation, is selected from ICN_{old}. This process is guided by the discriminant parameters set PD_{old}, obtained in the last diagnosis cycle, as we will see in the following paragraphs. Secondly, the consistency of each one of these hypotheses is updated in the light of the new evidence. If the updated consistency does not exceed a previously established threshold, the corresponding hypothesis is removed from the explanation. In the contrary case, the corresponding hypothesis is not removed, but its consistency factor is updated. In both cases, updating or removal of hypotheses can induce a propagation throughout the causal explanation, following the *h-relations.*

The next task to be executed is the *Hypotheses Generation* task. This task extends the refined explanation, ICN'_{new}, which is obtained as an output of the *Hypotheses Discrimination* task, to explain all the new abnormal evidence, M^a_{new}. Of course, the *Hypotheses Generation* task must guarantee that the new hypotheses are not incompatible with the new normal evidence,

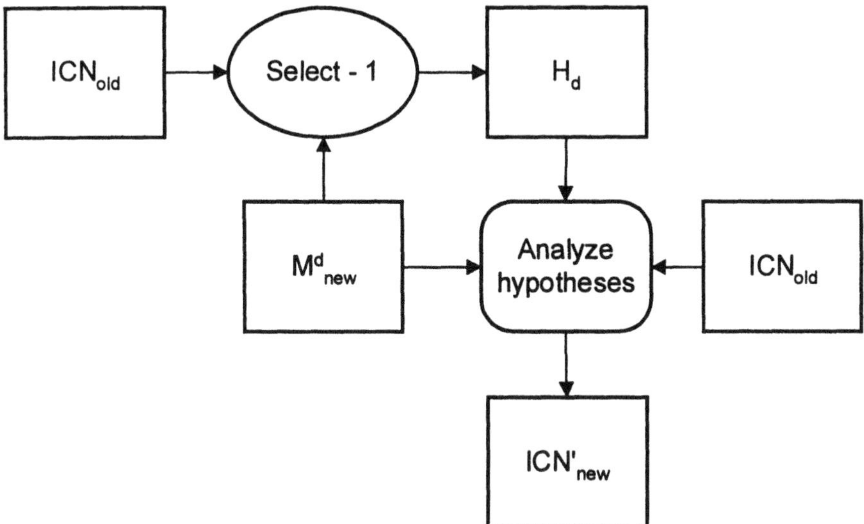

Fig. 6. Task structure for the hypotheses discrimination task

M^n_{new}. As is shown in figure 7, the *Hypotheses Generation* is based in the classical Cover-and-Differentiate approach [15,29], and therefore, the task is decomposed into two tasks: *Cover* and *Differentiate*. However, the so-called Cover-and-Differentiate approach has to be modified to cope with the temporal dimension.

The main function of the *Cover* is the extension of ICN'_{new} in the light of the new abnormal manifestation. The modus operandi of the *Cover* task is as follow: First, for each one of the new abnormal manifestations, *Cover* tries to find a temporal pattern that explains it. Once the corresponding temporal pattern has been found, the task has to instantiate it in ICN'_{new}. This step makes use of a **parsimonious instantiation** principle by which if the new manifestation to be covered can be explained by one or more hypotheses already instantiated (i. e., temporal patterns already instantiated in ICN'_{new}) and does not break the temporal consistency of the $FTCN$ corresponding to the temporal pattern, then the new manifestation under question is subsumed into the instantiated hypothesis. New hypotheses are, therefore, generated if and only if the subsumption is not possible. As a result of applying the *Cover* task, an extended instantiated causal network, ICN''_{new}, is obtained. The application of a **parsimonious instantiation** principle improves the performance of the diagnosis process and avoids an exponential blow-up in the hypotheses generation phase.

Once the causal network has been extended to explain the new abnormal manifestations, the *Differentiate* task evaluates the consistency of both the new hypotheses and those which were updated by subsumption. As in the *Hypotheses Discrimination* task, if the new hypothesis consistency ex-

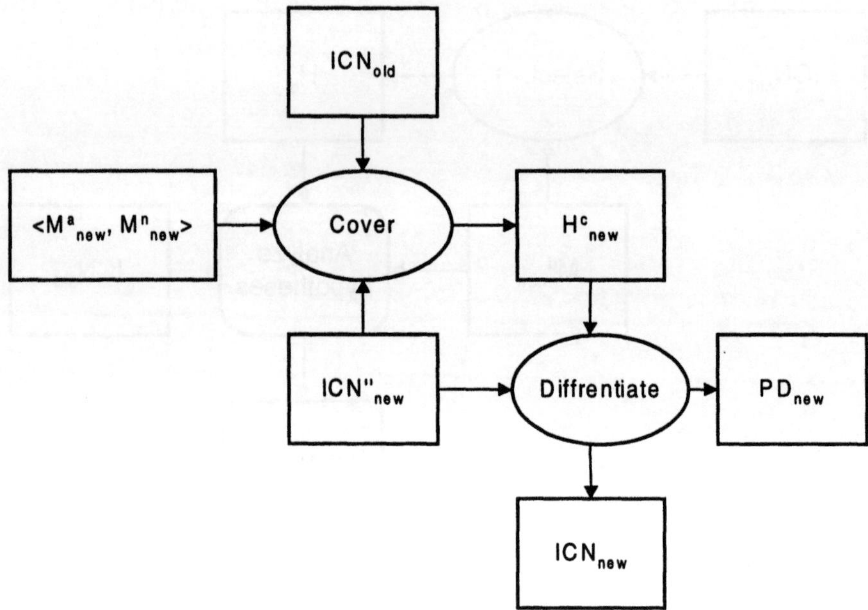

Fig. 7. Task structure for the hypotheses generation task

ceeds a previously established threshold, the hypothesis is accepted and its consistency factor updated. Otherwise, the hypothesis is removed from the explanation. It has to be taken into account that this removal of hypotheses or consistency update forces the re-evaluation of the hypotheses, which are causally connected with the hypothesis updated or removed. Therefore, the output of the *Differentiate* task is a new instantiated causal network, ICN_{new} which fully explains all the M^a_{new} and is consistent with M^n_{new}, together with a new set of discriminant parameters, PD_{new} which are comprised of the set of manifestations that can drive the refining process performed in the *Hypotheses Discrimination* task of the next diagnosis cycle.

The Diagnosis cycle ends with the execution of the *Differentiate* task. Before the execution of the next cycle the following operations has to be executed:

$$
\begin{gathered}
PD_{old} = PD_{new} \bigcup (PD_{old}/M^d_{new}) \\
ICN_{old} = ICN_{new}
\end{gathered}
\tag{10}
$$

These operations are necessary to prepare the inputs for the next diagnosis cycle. As can be deduced from the previous paragraphs, the sets PD_{old} and ICN_{old} (of course, after the previous operations) make the communication between consecutive diagnosis cycles possible as well as the extension of the explanation during the patient's stay in the ICCU.

5 Tools around the Diagnosis Task

In the previous sections, the structure underlying the domain knowledge and the abductive diagnostic model have been presented. Following this model, we have developed a first prototype implementing the diagnosis process presented here. This prototype, entirely developed in CLIPS, have been initially fed with a reduced knowledge base of temporal patterns. Currently, this initial knowledge base is being extended by the physician. Apart for this first prototype, we have developed some tools to address two specific problems.

- The temporal patterns knowledge based construction, and
- the definition of an explanation mechanism which allows the expert (the doctor) to follow the conclusions reached by the model.

In order to solve the first problem a Temporal Pattern Acquisition Tool has been developed. This tool is composed of the following utilities:

- The Browser, which allows the expert to explore the temporal patterns knowledge base.
- The Findings Editing tool, for defining new findings as being instances of concepts included in the ontology.
- The Temporal Patterns Editing Tool, for building and updating temporal patterns, which can be selected through their main hypotheses, their implied hypotheses or their implied manifestations.
- The Query Tool enables the building of simple queries such as How many patterns are defined?, Find the patterns in which a certain manifestation is present, etc.
- Finally, the acquisition tool provides an Agenda, in which the pending acquisitions tasks are registered. These tasks warn the expert about the badly defined temporal patterns as well as the causes for such a mistake. This information is saved between knowledge acquisition sessions and displayed when the acquisition tools is opened again, so the expert knows what actions should be carried out.

The main problem in the acquisition of temporal patterns is the definition of the fuzzy temporal constraints among the pattern elements. Normally, the expert only defines some of all the possible temporal relations. However, as has been explained in previous sections, in a temporal pattern all the possible temporal constraints must be defined, so a propagation process must be applied in order to complete the $FTCN$. This process can also be used to detect temporal inconsistencies in the information acquired and to inform the expert that the temporal information introduced in the pattern is inconsistent or incomplete (that is, the expert introduces an element in the pattern for which no temporal constraints are defined). In order to make the acquisition of temporal patterns easier, a tool for acquiring temporal patterns has been developed. A snapshot of the Temporal Constraints Edition Tool is shown in figure 8. In this figure, all the elements of a temporal pattern are presented:

- The main hypothesis, *retrogade cardiogenic insufficiency.*
- The manifestations associated to the main hypothesis (*dispnoea, taquipnea* and *ST Changes*) and its implied hypotheses (in this case, *cardiogenic shock*).
- The set of manifestations that can be used in the definition of new fuzzy temporal constraints.
- The defined fuzzy temporal constraints. In this case the only fuzzy temporal constraint already are defined is the constraint between the taquipnea manifestation and the main hypothesis specifying that both can appear at the same time.

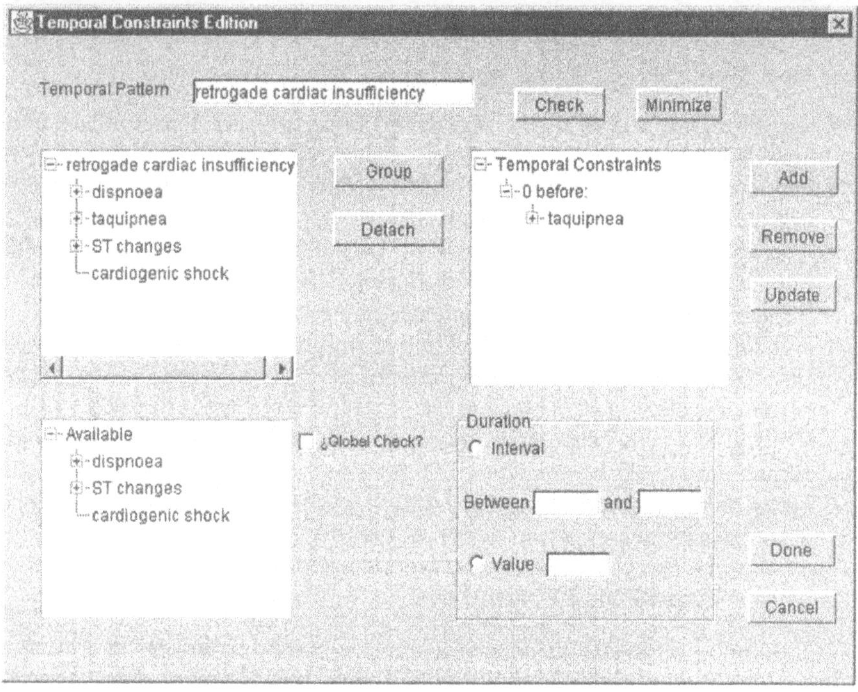

Fig. 8. Temporal constraints edition tool

A new version of this tool is under development. In this new version, it is possible to obtain a graphical view of the *FTCN*. The other issue which has not been dealt with so far is the definition of an explanation mechanism. This problem is related to how the information must be displayed to the expert. In order to make it possible for the expert to analyze the conclusion reached by the diagnostic model, the information (the causal network that the model built as a conclusion and the fuzzy temporal relation among the causal nodes) must be presented from a point of view the expert can understand.

For this purpose, an Explanation tool has been developed. Thanks to this tool, the expert can analyse the results reached by diagnostic model from different points of view. One of these views presents the evolution of the causal network as the system builds it, as shown in figure 9. The remaining views allow the graphical analysis of both the temporal sequence of events and the fuzzy temporal relations among them.

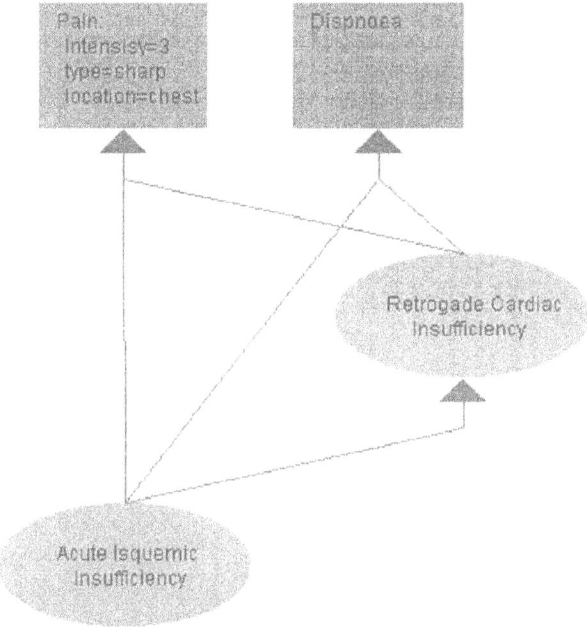

Fig. 9. Part of the causal network generated by the diagnostic process

The tools around the diagnosis task have been implemented in Java, which make it platform independent, and CORBA, allowing future interoperability with other tools under construction.

6 An Example

In this section, we will present an example of the modus operandi of our diagnosis method. The example is composed of a real case taking from the ICCU patients data base. Before describing the manifestations involved in the case under question, we have to proceed with the definition of the main elements of the diagnosis model described in previous sections. The first element to be taking into account is the temporal patterns causal network used by the diagnosis method. The part of the causal network involved in the example is shown in figure 10. It has to be noticed that causal arcs are defined through h-relations between temporal patterns. Figure 11 shows one of the temporal patterns used in this example with its corresponding $FCTN$ representing the fuzzy durations among manifestations and/or hypotheses (main or implied).

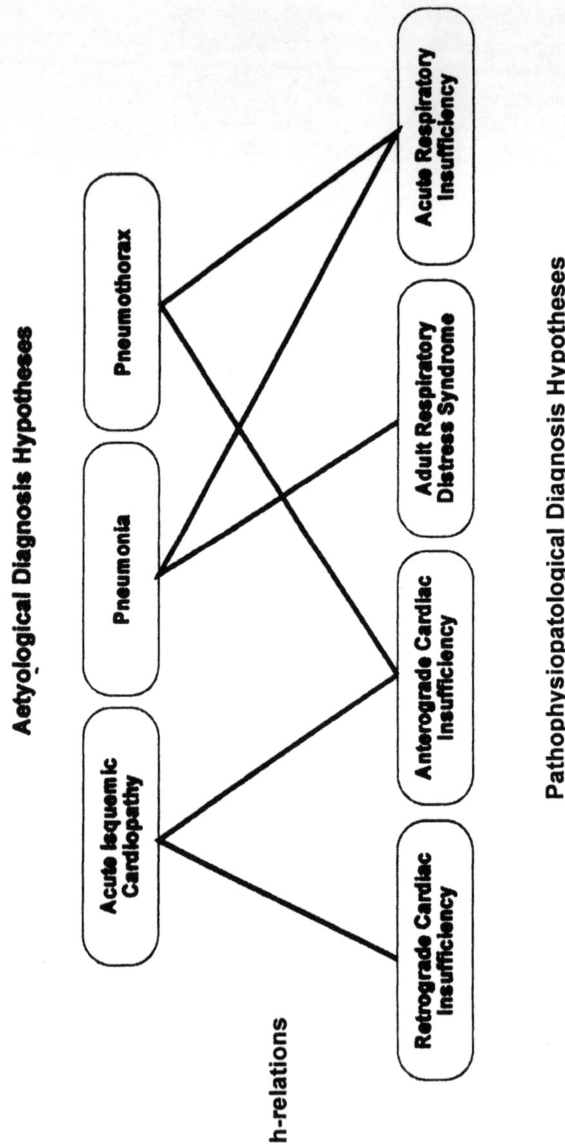

Fig. 10. Part of the causal network used in the example

Retrograde Cardiac Insufficiency((present=TRUE),t_0)

MANIFESTATIONS:

A)

Pain((present=TRUE),(intensity=3),(location=precordial),t_1)
R_vawe_grouth((present=TRUE),(grade=small),t_1)
ST_changes((present=TRUE),(rate={significant,very significant},t_1)
Fourth_heart_sound((present=TRUE),t_1)
Instersticial_alveolar_desease((present=TRUE),t_1)
Dyspnoea((present=TRUE),(intensity={moderate,serious}),t_2)
Tachycardia((present=TRUE),(type=regular),t_2)
Taquipnea((present=TRUE),(intensity={moderate,serious},t_2)
Hypoxemia((present=TRUE),(intensity=moderate),t_2)
Crepitants((present=TRUE),(intensity=basal),t_3)
SatO2_drop((present=TRUE),(intensity={moderate,serious}),t_3)
Chronic_type_changes((present=TRUE),t_3)
Alkalosys((present=TRUE),(intensity=moderate),t_3)
Cardiomegaly((present=TRUE),(intensity=moderate),t_3)
Cyanosis((present=TRUE),t_4)

IMPLIED HYPTHESES:

Cardiogenic shock((present=TRUE),t_4)

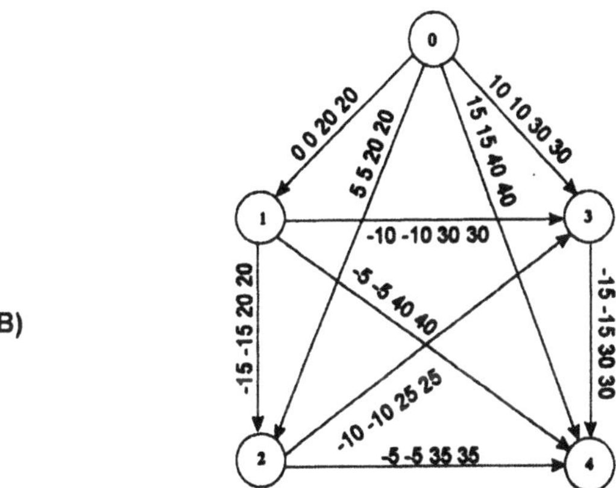

Fig. 11. Retrogade cardiac insufficiency temporal pattern (a) and its corresponding *FTCN* (b)

The case we are going to use in this example starts with a 47 years old male who arrives at emergency room with a **sharp chest pain** and signs of **dispnoea** and **fever**. Taking into account his past medical history, in which can be found antecedents of a **heart attack** three years ago, the patient is admitted in the ICCU. To enter this data into the diagnosis process we used the language described in section one. In table (11) can be seen the translation of these manifestation into the language defined in section one. As can be noticed, the temporal variable t_0 (time origin) has been assigned to all manifestations.

$$\boxed{\begin{array}{c} pain((present = TRUE), (intensity = 3), (type = sharp), \\ (location = chest), t_0) \\ dispnoea((present = TRUE), t_0) \\ fever((present = TRUE), t_0) \end{array}} \quad (11)$$

Approximately fifteen minutes later (since the arrival to the emergency room), the physician proceeds with a physical examination and detects an **oppressive chest pain** and a **periferical cyanosis**. As can be deduced from table (12), the temporal variable t_α has been assigned to the two last manifestation, with the fuzzy duration between t_0 and t_α, $d(t_0, t_\alpha)$, being the fuzzy number (12,14,16,18).

$$\boxed{\begin{array}{c} pain((present = TRUE), (type = oppressive), \\ (location = chest), t_\alpha) \\ dispnoea((present = TRUE), t_\alpha) \end{array}} \quad (12)$$

At this point (aprox. five minutes since physical examination), by a pulmonary auscultation the physician detects the presence of **alveolar sounds** located in **right hemitorax, bilateral crepitants**, symptoms of **taquipnea** and **fever** (that is, the fever at the emergency room arrival does not come down). The temporal variable associated to these manifestations is t_β, with $d(t_\alpha, t_\beta) = (3, 4, 6, 7)$ (see table 13).

$$\boxed{\begin{array}{c} alveolar\_sounds((present = TRUE), \\ (location = right\_hemitorax), t_\beta) \\ crepitants((present = TRUE), (location = bilateral), t_\beta) \\ taquipnea((present = TRUE), t_\beta)) \\ fever((present = TRUE), t_\beta) \end{array}} \quad (13)$$

Once the pulmonary auscultation finishes (approximately two minutes later), the physician proceeds with a heart auscultation which reveals a **regular tachycardia**, the presence of a **fourth heart sound**, a **murmur** and a **central cyanosis**. The temporal variable associated to these manifestations is t_γ, with $d(t_\beta, t_\gamma) = (0, 1, 3, 4)$ (see table 14).

$$\boxed{\begin{array}{c} tachycardia((present = TRUE), (type = regular), t_\gamma) \\ fourth\_heart\_tone((present = TRUE), t_\gamma) \\ murmur((present = TRUE), t_\gamma)) \\ cyanosis((present = TRUE), (type = central), t_\gamma) \end{array}} \quad (14)$$

This initial exploratory phase ends with the analysis of the ECG from which can be deduced a **small growth on R wave** and **acute changes on**

T wave as well as the presence of a **tachycardia** (manifestations that can be used as a confirmation of the tachycardia manifestation at t_δ). The temporal variable associated to these manifestations is t_δ, with $d(t_\gamma, t_\delta) = (1,2,4,5)$ (see table 15).

$$\boxed{\begin{array}{c} tachycardia((present = TRUE), (type = regular), t_\delta) \\ R\_wave\_grotwh((present = TRUE), (grade = small), t_\delta) \\ T\_wave\_chages((present = TRUE), (grade = acute), t_\delta) \end{array}} \qquad (15)$$

When the physician finishes this explanatory phase, a blood sample is taken form the patient (aprox. 7 min. later) and then he is sent to the x-ray room (aprox. 10 min. later). Obviously, the results of these two tests arrive at ICCU some time later. First, the physician are ready to analyse the chest x-ray (aprox. 15 min. after the patient is sent two the x-ray room). Finally (aprox. 30 min. after the blood sample was taken) the result of the blood analysis are returned to the physician. However, and taken into account that these results are referred to the time at the the blood sample and the chest x-ray were taken, their respective data have to be inserted into the system associated to that time. Thus, from the chest x-ray, the physician deduces that a **slight cardiomegaly** is present as well as a **vascular redistribution, interstitial-alveolar patterns, alveolar infiltrate in the median right lobe.** and a **uncertain pleural line in the right hemithorax**. The translation of all these manifestations is shown in table (16), with $d(t_\delta, t_\epsilon) = (3,5,9,11)$

$$\boxed{\begin{array}{c} cardiomegaly((present = TRUE), t_\epsilon) \\ vascular\_redistribution((present = TRUE), t_\epsilon) \\ CK((present = TRUE), (grade = \{normal, high\}), t_\epsilon) \\ instersticial\_alveolar\_pattern((present = TRUE), t_\epsilon) \\ alveolar\_infiltrate((present = TRUE), \\ (location = medium\_right\_lobe), t_\epsilon) \\ pleural\_line((present = TRUE), (location = right\_hemitorax), t_\epsilon) \end{array}} \qquad (16)$$

From the lab tests can be deduced that the patient suffers a **leukocytosis with a left deviation**, a **moderate hyperglycaemia**, a **high moderate levels of CK**, a **moderate hypoxemia** and a **slight alkalosys**. The corresponding translation can be seen in table (17), where $d(t_\delta, t_\zeta) = (6,8,12,14)$.

$$\boxed{\begin{array}{c} leukocytosis((present = TRUE), (deviation = left), t_\zeta) \\ hyperglycaemia((present = TRUE), (intensity = moderate), t_\zeta) \\ CK((present = TRUE), (grade = \{normal, high\}), t_\zeta) \\ hypoxemia((present = TRUE), (intensity = moderate), t_\zeta) \\ alkalosys((present = TRUE), (intensity = slight), t_\zeta) \end{array}} \qquad (17)$$

Once the escenario used in this example has been described, we are going to proceed with the explanation of the modus operandi of our diagnosis model. First of all, we have to say that diagnosis task carries out its functionality through the execution of several diagnosis cycles. These cycles are defined by the presence of new manifestations. In other words, a diagnosis cycle starts each time a new group of data are present. Therefore, the first diagnosis cycle starts with data package (11) (in order to make the example more simple, we have only described abnormal manifestation). Of course, the hypotheses discrimination task is not executed, since at the first cycle, $PD_{old} = \emptyset$. In this first cycle, all the temporal patterns shown in figure 10 are instantiated, because the manifestations in data package (11) can be covered by all the temporal patterns. Thus, with this information we can say that the patient may suffer all the deseases shown in figure 10. However, and despite the lack of information, thanks to the *FTCN* formalism, our diagnosis task can determine the approximate appearance time of every desease. Figure 12 shows how the approximate appearance time of the *Retrograde Cardiac Insufficiency* temporal pattern, RCI hereinafter, (constraint between the corresponding temporal pattern and t_0 in figure 12-A) is calculated from the temporal information included in the manifestations and the temporal pattern definition (figure 12-B).

The next task to be executed in the first cycle is the differentiate task. In this task, all the patterns are finally accepted since the current evidence is enough. One of the most important characteristic of the diagnosis model proposed here is related to how the consistency of the implied hypotheses is calculated. For example, in order to calculate the consistency of the *Acute Cardiac Insufficiency* instantiated pattern, the differentiate task tries to foresee the implied hypotheses *RCI* and *ACI* (*Anterograde Cardiac Insufficiency*). As these two hypotheses have their corresponding instantiated pattern, the task tries to calculate their respective consistency. This new consistency calculation is carried out by a recursive call in which the consistency of the manifestations associated to their instantiated temporal pattern are evaluated. In a conventional diagnosis process, these two instantiated pattern would have been ruled out since, for example, there is no evidence about the presence of ST_Changes (see *RCI* temporal pattern definition in figure 11. However, in our model these two instantiated patterns are kept because, taking into account the temporal dimension, ST_Changes may appear during the 20 minutes after the appearance of the *RCI* or *ACI*. Therefore, at this point, the differentiate task cannot rule out these hypotheses since the temporal window associated to the ST_Changes are not yet closed. The last step of the first cycle are the generation of the set of the discriminant parameters, PD_{old}. This set will be conformed by those manifestation belonging to the instantiated patterns for which no evidence has been received, for example, ST_Changes will be one of the discriminant parameters.

In the second cycle, the diagnosis task takes as input the manifestations of the data package (12). With this evidence, the diagnosis tasks reinforce the consistency of the instantiated temporal patterns and reduce the uncertainty

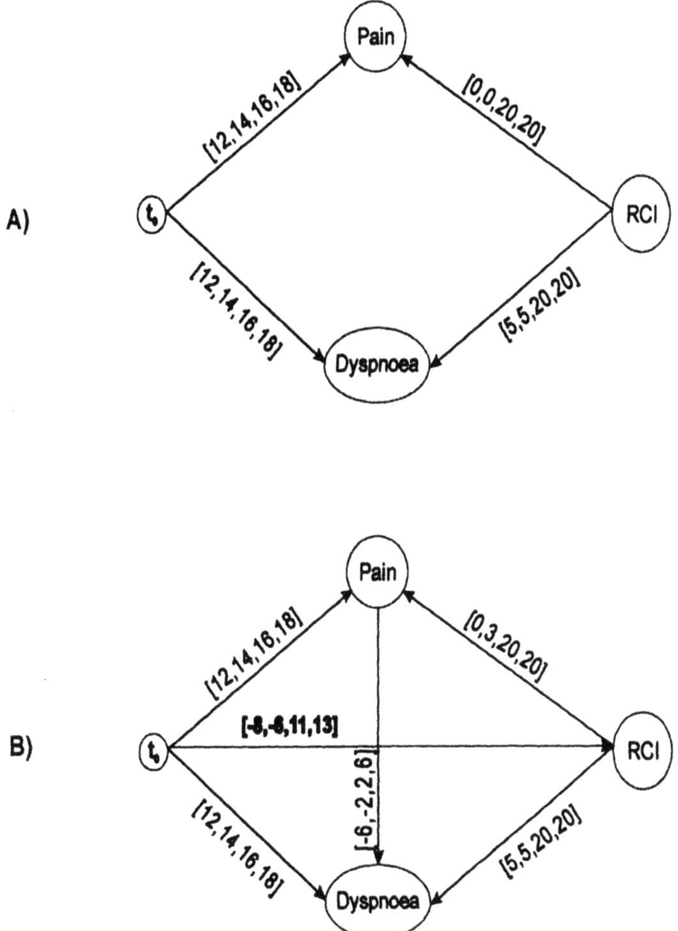

Fig. 12. Part of the generated *FCTN* showing the temporal fuzzy constraints between the instance of the *RCI* temporal pattern and some of its manifestations

of the appearance time of the corresponding diagnosis hypotheses (as a consequence of constraint propagation within the *FTCN* formalism). Another consequence of this cycle is the reduction of the set PD_{old} since some of the manifestations have appeared and, therefore, they have been introduced in the system.

The second cycle tries to explain the data package (13). As explained in Section 4, the discrimination task re-evaluate the consistency of the instantiated temporal patterns in the light of the new evidence. When the instantiated temporal pattern associated to the *Acute Isquemic Cardiopathy* will be selected for re-evaluation, the hypotheses discrimination task will try to anticipate the ST_Changes manifestation which will not be found. However, this time the temporal window associated to this manifestation is closed (the data package (13) are supposed to finish approximately at minute 21). Thus the temporal pattern associated to the *Acute Isquemic Cardiopathy*, and its corresponding implied hypotheses, can be ruled out. Once these temporal patterns are removed, the diagnosis task reinforces the consistency of the rest of the hypotheses, as new evidence are associated to them.

The rest of the cycles (data packages (14),(15),(16) and (17)) will only reinforce the consistency of the hypotheses that have been accepted (that is, those associated with pulmonary deseases). Figure (13) shows the hypotheses obtained by the diagnosis process and part of the *FTCN* generated in which some fuzzy temporal constraints among hypotheses are represented (of course, the complete *FTCN* will include all the manifestations and the fuzzy temporal constraints among them and the hypotheses). In the real patient record, the patient evolution (manifestations present two hours after the admission at ICCU) showed that he was suffering a *Pneumothorax*. Of course, if we had introduced evolution data into our diagnosis process, the diagnosis process would have ruled out the temporal patterns associated to *Pneumonia*. This example shows how our diagnosis process can be used as Decision Support System since, despite the lack of information, the diagnosis process is able to reach some diagnoses which may be useful to the physician. Of course, as new data are acquire from the patient the diagnosis will be more precise.

7 Conclusion, Related and Future Works

In this paper, a Model-Based Temporal Diagnostic Model is described. Temporal patterns are the key element of our model. These elements enable the definition of a model of abnormal behaviour of the system to be diagnosed (the patient) which captures all kinds of causal knowledge (as defined in [9]): pathophysiological knowledge (causal relations between pathophysiological states), evidential causal knowledge (causal relations between external manifestations and either pathophysiological or aetyological states) and diagnostic knowledge (relations between pathophysiological states and aetyological states). As can be deduced from previous sections, the diagnosis method proposed (without considering the temporal component) is similar to classical approaches to Model-Based Diagnosis (which can be analyzed more deeply in [4,19]) and it is especially similar to the so-called Cover and Differentiate [15,29]. However, we have introduced some modifications in order to cope with the requirements posed by the selected application domain (ICCU). These requirements are related to the continuous modus of operations, since the model is intended to be integrated in a intelligent monitoring system which has been designed to work during the patient's stay in the ICCU and to manage an asynchronous stream of events. In order to improve the performance of the basic Cover and Differentiate step, the Causal Network obtained as an

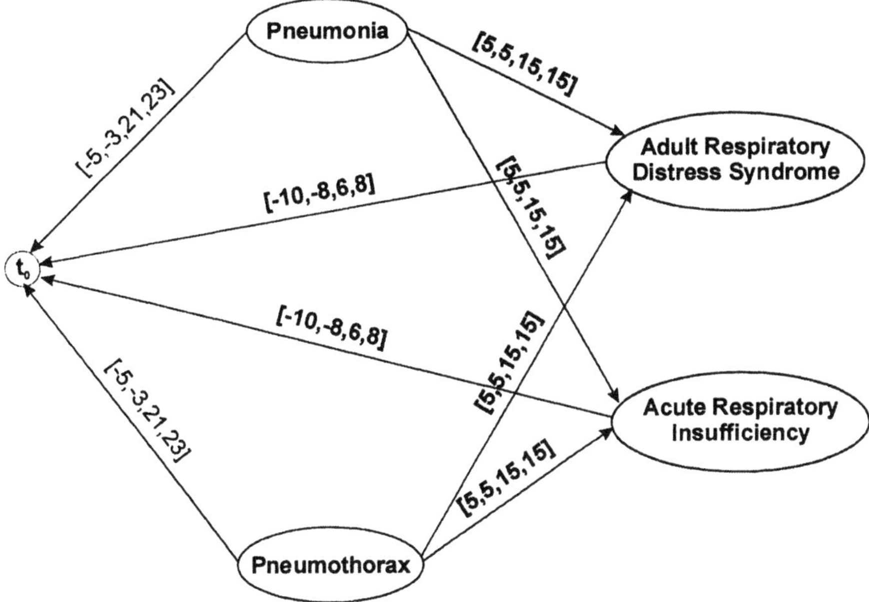

Fig. 13. Part of the generated *FCTN* showing the temporal fuzzy constraints among hypotheses generated by the diagnosis task

explanation is refined before the diagnosis process tries to explain the new manifestations. This refinement is performed by the Hypotheses Discrimination task and can modify the explanation (obtained in the previous diagnosis cycle) in the following ways:

- Some hypotheses may be rejected since they are inconsistent with new evidence detected from the beginning of the previous diagnosis cycle. This is a very important characteristic which allows us to assert retrospective information in the diagnosis process. Therefore, our diagnosis windows covers the manifestations observed from the origin of time to the moment the last diagnosis cycle starts. In other words, our diagnostic process builds up a **Historical Explanation** which tries to explain the patient's complete clinical record and associates temporal (fuzzy) labels to the hypotheses.
- Some hypotheses are reinforced since the new evidence confirms the hypotheses obtained in the last diagnostic cycle.

As indicated in previous sections, this process is driven by the discriminant hypotheses set (which is obtained by the Manifestation Detection Task with the help of the set PD_{new} of the last diagnosis cycle) and allows the Hypotheses Generation task to focus exclusively on a consistent explanation.

Apart from the above consideration, another important question is dealt with in this work: the so-called temporal dimension. Our model is based on the Fuzzy Temporal Constraint Network, *FCTN*, [3,2,22,5] which makes use of the possibility theory in order to represent the vagueness associated with the constraints defined between time points. In our approach, each constraint is defined as being a possibility distribution which defines the time elapsed between two time points. In order to adapt this formalism for temporal dimension management and representation to the abductive diagnosis model proposed here, a *FTCN*-based logic has been proposed, termed *FTCL* (Fuzzy Temporal Constraint logic) [7,6]. One of the most important characteristics of this formalism is that the vagueness inherent to the time location of symptoms, as they are acquired from the ICCU staff, can be modeled in a more natural way [10,31,32]. Another characteristic, considered important in other works such as [8,9,18], is that the *FTCN* associated with a temporal pattern specifies a partial order of events. This partial order defines different possible total orders. In this sense, it is noteworthy that this representation is more flexible than a representation based on totally ordered sequences and is more suitable for the medical domain, since not all patients present the manifestations in the same sequence. Therefore, a temporal pattern does not represent the typical sequence of manifestations, rather what is represented are the temporal constraints among these manifestations, which are imposed by cause-effect relations. This is the most important contribution of our approach, in contrast to those models which are not based on temporal constraints such as [12,9]. In [21] a temporal diagnosis model based on temporal constraints can be analyzed, but no fuzzy time representation is used.

The concept of temporal pattern is also defined in [14]. However, Dojat's model of temporal pattern only defines causal relations between diagnostic concepts and external manifestations and does not consider the pathophysiological knowledge, and therefore no causal relations between different pathophysiological states are defined. Another important difference with Dojat's model is that in our model, constraints between events are defined by fuzzy numbers (instead of time intervals) which, as we said before, facilitates the representation of the vagueness inherent to the time location of the manifestations.

Another important advantage of our diagnosis model is that the performance of the model has been improved by the use of Temporal Abstracted Manifestations. As can be deduced from the previous sections, our diagnosis model operates over qualitative significant values which are extracted from the biomedical signals. The temporal granurality of the abstracted manifestations is lower than those corresponding to the biomedical signal events since the former represents qualitative changes in the signals. This is important because while the patient's state is stable, new events are not generated so new diagnosis cycles are not started. The advantages of the temporal abstraction in the diagnosis process has also been stressed in other works such as [17,25,28,30]. Of course, a module implementing the temporal abstraction process must exist. In our case, the temporal abstraction mechanism is performed by a separate agent which is called *perception specialist* [16].

Future works related to this paper will include the development of a multi-agent architecture for the integration of the perception, diagnosis and treatment modules in order to provide an intelligent monitoring system (a first version of the proposed architecture can be analysed in [27,26]). Other open issues are the inclusion of some mechanisms which make it possible to integrate "maybe" type causal relations and to include contextual factors in the specification of the temporal patterns. The latter is a very promising feature since it will allow us to include those factors that can modify the interpretation of the pattern (such as the treatment applied, age, smoker or non-smoker,...). The diagnostic model described so far is under evaluation by the ICCU staff with real cases. Finally, we are trying to apply the proposed model to other domains beyond the medical one but of similar modeling characteristics.

References

1. J. J. Van Der AA. *Intelligent Alarms in Anaesthesia: a Real Time Expert System Application.* PhD thesis, Technical University of Eindhoven, 1990.
2. S. Barro, R. Marín, R. P. Otero, R. Ruíz, and J. Mira. On the handling of time in intelligent monitoring of CCU patients. In *Proceedings of the 14th Annual International Conference of the IEEE Engineering in Medicine and Biology Society*, 871–873, 1992.
3. S. Barro, R. Marín, J. Mira, and A. R. Patón. A model and a language for the fuzzy representation and handling of time. *Fuzzy Sets and Systems*, **61**, 153–175, 1994.
4. V. R. Benjamins. *Problem Solving Methods for Diagnosis.* PhD thesis, University of Amsterdam, 1993.
5. V. Brusoni, L. Console, P. Terenziani, and D. Theseider Dupré. A spectrum of definitions for temporal model-based diagnosis. *Artificial Intelligence*, **102**, 39–79, 1998.
6. M. A. Cárdenas. *A Constraint-Based Logic Model for Rerepresenting and Managing Temporal Information. (In Spanish).* PhD thesis, Universidad de Murcia, 1998.
7. M. A. Cárdenas, R. Marín, I. Navarrete, and M. Balsa. Fuzzy temporal constraint logic: A valid resolution principle. *Fuzzy Sets and Systems*, **117**(2), 231-250, 2000.
8. M. J. Chantler, G. M. Coghill, Q. Shen, and R. R. Leitch. Selecting tools and techniques for model-based diagnosis. *Artificial Intelligence in Engineering*, **12**, 81–98, 1998.
9. L. Console and P. Torasso. On co-operation between abductive and temporal reasoning in medical diagnosis. *Artificial Intelligence in Medicine*, **3**, 291–311, 1991.
10. L. Console, A. J. Rivolin, and P. Torraso. Fuzzy temporal reasoning on causal models. *International Journal of Intelligent Systems*, **6**, 107–133, 1991.

11. L. Console and P. Torraso. A spectrum of logical definitions of model-based diagnosis. In Walter Hamscher, Luca Console, and Johan de Kleer, editors, *Readings in Model-Based Diagnosis*, 78–88. Morgan Kauffmann Publisher, Inc., 1992.
12. L. Console, L. Protinale, and D. T. Dupré. Using compiled knowledge to guide focus abductive diagnosis. *IEEE Transactions on Knowledge and Data Engineering*, **8**(5), 690–706, 1996.
13. M. Dojat and C. Sayettat. Realistic model for temporal reasoning in real-time patient monitoring. *Applied Artificial Intelligence*, **10**, 121–143, 1996.
14. M. Dojat, N. Ramaux, and D. Fontaine. Scenario recognition for temporal reasoning in medical domains. *Artificial Intelligence in Medicine*, **14**, 139–155, 1999.
15. L. Eshelman. MOLE: A knowledge-acquisition tool for cover-and-differentiate systems. In S. Marcus, editor, *Automating Knowledge Acquisition for Expert Systems*, 37–80. Kluwer, Boston, 1988.
16. S. Fraga, P. Félix, M. Lama, E. Sánchez, and S. Barro. A proposal for a real time signal perception specialist. In *International Symposium on Engineering of Intelligent Systems EIS'98*, **3**, 261–267, 1998.
17. J. Gamper and W. Nejdl. Abstract temporal diagnosis in medical domains. *Artificial Intelligence in Medicine*, **10**(3), 1116–1122, 1997.
18. Ira J. Haimowitz and Isaac S. Kohane. Managing temporal worlds for medical trend diagnosis. *Artificial Intelligence in Medicine*, **8**, 299–321, 1996.
19. W. Hamscher, L. Console, and J. de Kleer. *Readings in Model-Based Diagnosis.* Morgan Kauffman, San Mateo, 1992.
20. W. J. Long. Evaluation of a new method for cardiovascular reasoning. *Journal of the American Medical Informatics Association*, **1**, 127–141, 1994.
21. W. Long. Temporal reasoning for diagnosis in causal probabilistic knowledge base. *Artificial Intelligence in Medicine*, **8**, 193–215, 1996.
22. R. Marín, S. Barro A. Bosch, and J. Mira. Modeling time representation from a fuzzy perspective. *Cybernetics and Systems*, **25**(2), 207–215, 1994.
23. R. Marín, M. Balsa M. A. Cárdenas, and J. L. Sánchez. Obtaining solutions in fuzzy constraint networks. *International Journal of Approximate Reasoning*, **3-4**, 261–288, 1996.
24. A. A. F. Van der Maas, A. H. M. Ter Hofstede, and P. F. de Vries Robbé. Formal description of temporal knowledge in case report. *Artificial Intelligence in Medicine*, **16**, 251–282, 1999.
25. W. Nejdl and J. Gamper. Harnessing the power of temporal abstractions in model-based diagnosis of dynamic systems. In *Proceedings of the 11th ECAI*, 667–671, Amsterdam, 1994.
26. J. T. Palma, R. Marín, J. L. Sánchez, and M. A. Cárdenas. A diagnosis task in an intelligent patient supervisory system. In *Proc. of the XV IFIP World Computer Congress-Information Technologies and Knowledge-based Systems IT&KNOWS'98*, 159–172, Vienna-Budapest, 1998.
27. J. T. Palma. *Applying Knowledge Engineering to Real-Time Knowledge Based Systems: A CommonKADS Extension* (in Spanish). PhD thesis, Universidad de Murcia, 1999.
28. T. Peng and J. Reggia. *Abductive Inference Methods for Diagnositic Problem Solving.* Springer-Verlag, Berlin, 1991.
29. A. T. Schreiber. *Pragmatics of the Knowledge Level.* PhD thesis, University of Amsterdam, 1992.

30. Y. Shahar and M. Musen. RÉSUMÉ: A temporal-abstraction system for patient monitoring. *Computers and Biomedical Research*, **26**, 255–273, 1993.
31. F. Steimann and K. P. Adlassing. Clinical monitoring with fuzzy automata. *Fuzzy Set and Systems*, **61**, 37–42, 1994.
32. F. Steimann and K. P. Adlassnig. A fuzzy medical data model. In *Proceedings of the 12th European Meeting on Cybernetics and Systems Research*, 271–278, Singapore, 1994. World Scientific.

A Fuzzy Model for Pattern Recognition in the Evolution of Patients

Paulo Félix[1], Senén Barro[1], Manuel Lama[1], Santiago Fraga[1], and Francisco Palacios[2]

[1] Departamento de Electrónica e Computación
Universidade de Santiago de Compostela
E-15706 Santiago de Compostela, SPAIN
[2] Hospital General Universitario de Elche
Alicante, SPAIN

1 Introduction

The solution to the problem of the interpretation of a particular system is approached on the basis of a search for relationship between its behaviour and certain signs that can be observed in an often complex or noisy environment, and which are identifiable with certain events and other regularities that can be grouped together under the general term, *pattern*. In recent years there has been growing interest in the representation and recognition of patterns in the evolution of a particular system, more specifically, in the development of models permitting their integration into information systems in which time plays a fundamental role.

We refer principally to approaches to the problem which take a structural perspective in pattern representation as a starting point; these require a segmentation of the input data, which later contrast with a small number of elements that define the pattern, in which the treatment of imprecision and uncertainty is tackled.

An initial group of proposals are based on the use of a qualitative language for pattern description: basically, sign-based languages. Amongst these proposals, that of Cheung and Stephanopoulos [4] is worthy of special mention. Their proposal is based on the representation of a given profile by means of triangular episodes. The application of this model in pattern recognition is dealt with in [2], using a decision tree-based inductive learning technique. The principal limitations arise from the representation model, which considers semantics that only captures absolutely precise or qualitative meaning.

Haimowitz and Kohane present a multivariable trend representation model (TrenDx) [14], which is applied as a prototype for the diagnosis of growth disorders in children, and for the detection of significant trends in haemodynamics and the analysis of the content of gasses in blood in Intensive Coronary Care Unit patients. The model attaches great importance to the representation of temporal information, and to the treatment of its uncertainty. This is resolved by using numerical ranges of values, and is based on the use of a package developed by Kohane (Temporal Utility Package), which supplies a representational language for the type of temporal expressions that are habitually found in clinical diagnosis problems. TrenDx offers the possibility of linking a constraint on the values of each variable to each temporal interval through the definition of a model of up to second degree polynomial regression, in which coefficients may correspond to qualitative values.

The fuzzy set theory has been a significant breakthrough in the representation of vague or imprecise knowledge, allowing the incorporation of a large number of nuances to this type of representation. One of the first proposals to make use of fuzzy sets was the one presented by Ligomenides. More than just a representational mode, with specific procedures, Ligomenides [16] proposes a model for the artificial acquisition of perceptive knowledge, which enables pattern recognition tasks to be carried out with a degree of flexibility that the author associates with human perceptive processes, using a fuzzy set-based similarity measure. His work builds on the *Formal Descriptive Scheme (FDS)* concept, a procedure that defines a similarity relation between a prototype and a pattern obtained in a sampling process. The signal is filtered and segmented into a series of sections that are based on the change in the curvature, according to the classic criterion for signs, with "strictly concave", "strictly convex" or "strictly linear" sections being obtained.

Drakopoulos has developed tFPR [6], a structural fuzzy pattern recognition system based on the sigmoidal representation of membership functions. The model segmentizes the signal upon which the detection is to be carried out; measurements are taken on each section of certain typical features such as curvature, slope, range, etc. These measurements are contrasted with the fuzzy description made for each section, and a local evaluation is obtained and is aggregated to those obtained for all the other sections, in order to obtain a global measurement of similarity. The innovative aspect is to be found in the modelling of the membership functions by means of sigmoidal functions, which are shown to minimise non-linear computations. In order to achieve this, it is accompanied by a simple low-level language for the description of the profile. The author himself ends up conceding that learning is the most convenient form of acquisition for this model.

Steimann has developed DIAMON-1, which is a monitor design system that incorporates various techniques for signal-symbol conversion [22]. Steimann proposes a fuzzy trend model which shows a linear computational cost with regard to the number of samples compared, owing to the simplicity of the model at a representational level: each one of the trends is reasoned on individually, thus the problem of working with sequences of trends is avoided. Steimann justifies this by considering that the segmentation of trends, although interesting from a theoretical point of view, is, in practice, unnecessary, since a single fuzzy trend is capable of covering a wide array of real evolutions. This is valid for certain cases of simple trends, which can be assimilated to simple fuzzy sections, although it is not true for those with more complex morphology.

Lowe *et al.* [17] present an extension of Steimann's ideas in which the representation of a fuzzy duration for each trend is introduced. This enables them to define a pattern that includes the representation of trends on different parameters in a tree-structure, in which the onset of each sub-pattern refers to the instant of the onset of its parent one. This proposal can be considered as a less expressive approach to the same goals that are pursued by the one presented here, however, with certain drawbacks: for instance, the lack of a study of the problem of choice in the segmentation, which hinders the obtention of measurements of global consistency in the matching of a single parameter. Furthermore, within a tree structure there is a loss of precision as its depth increases; the calculation of durations involves a fuzzy sum operation in which vagueness increases.

In this chapter we present the MFTP model, which generalizes a prior approximation to the representation of imprecise knowledge on the evolution of a single physical parameter, and which we called Fuzzy Temporal Profile (FTP) [9]. The FTP model is based on two fundamental ideas:

- *Linguistic acquisition of knowledge*, in a register as close as possible to that used by human experts in communicating their knowledge. We have developed an artificial language which allows the description of the evolution of a physical parameter, its projection in the terms that define the FTP model, and its integration into a more general model of reasoning and representation on temporal events [11].
- *Modelling of the vagueness and uncertainty that characterizes human knowledge*, i.e., we try to capture, as far as possible, the richness of nuances contained in descriptions made by the expert. In order to do so, the FTP model is based on the *constraint network* formalism and on the *fuzzy set theory*. The former supplies the representational structure that facilitates the computational projection of a linguistic description. The latter permits the manipulation of vagueness and uncertainty which are characteristic of the terms used in natural language.

The main qualitative leap that has been made since the first Fuzzy Temporal Profile model up until the Multivariable Fuzzy Temporal Profile model, which is described in the present work, stems from the necessity, in the problem of interpretation, of representing and reasoning on the association of behaviour patterns in the evolution of more than one parameter. Associating parameters is precisely the point of making *per se* irrelevant changes valuable due to their association with other changes in different parameters, which, in turn, are not sufficiently meaningful either.

In spite of the Multivariable Fuzzy Temporal Profile being proposed as a generic model, independent of a particular application domain, we have implemented it in an intelligent patient supervision system in Intensive Coronary

Care Units. There are a number of reasons why MFTPs constitute a highly useful tool in this domain: on one hand, the vagueness inherent in expert medical knowledge, which makes the availability of models that are capable of representing and reasoning on the basis of vague information necessary; on the other hand, the descriptive and verbalizable nature of this knowledge, which makes it possible to formalize it using a language with which physicians may express it in a manner that is similar to the one that they habitually use. Hence the MFTP model may serve as a tool for physiopathological research. The availability of knowledge acquisition tools will enable physicians to define complex temporal patterns of clear clinical significance, and to store the results of their matching with other real cases in a multi-patient database, for subsequent clinical studies.

In the first section of this proposal, we summarize the fundamental concepts of the Fuzzy Temporal Profile model, to then go on to define a Multivariable Temporal Profile. The following section deals briefly with the problem of minimizing the profile, in terms of analysing the consistency of the information which describes it. We then propose the practical application of the model to the task of pattern recognition. This is accompanied by an example from the field of medicine, at which our application is aimed. Lastly we give conclusions, and look towards certain possible extensions to the model.

2 Fuzzy Temporal Profile Model

2.1 Time

We consider time as being projected on a one-dimensional discrete axis $\tau = \{t_0, t_1, ..., t_i, ...\}$ [3]. Thus, given an i belonging to the set of natural numbers $\mathbb{N}$, t_i represents a *precise instant.* We assume that t_0 represents the temporal origin, before which the existence of any fact is not relevant for the problem under consideration. We consider a total order relation between the precise instants ($t_0 < t_1 < ... < t_i < ...$), and a uniform distance between them, in such a way that for every $i \in \mathbb{N}$, $t_{i+1} - t_i = \Delta t$, where Δt is a constant. Thus t_i represents a distance $i \times \Delta t$ to the time origin t_0. Δt represents the *discretization factor,* and its selection will normally coincide with the sampling period of the signal on which we are working.

2.2 Initial definitions

Taking Zadeh's extension principle as a starting point [24], we will now go on to introduce the concepts of *fuzzy value* and *fuzzy increase*, on which the bulk of the concepts of the model are based.

Definition 1. Given a discourse universe U (in our case, $\mathbb{R}$) we extend the concept of value to what we will call **fuzzy value c**, represented by a possibility distribution π_c over $\mathbb{R}$ [7]. In this way, given a precise value $v \in \mathbb{R}$,

$\pi_c(v) \in [0, 1]$ represents the possibility of **c** being precisely v. The extreme values 1 and 0, respectively, represent the absolute and null possibility of **c** being equal to v. By means of π_c we can define a fuzzy subset C of $\mathbb{R}$, which contains the possible values of **c**, assuming that C is a disjoint subset, in the sense that its elements represent mutually excluding alternatives for **c**. Considering μ_C as the membership function that is associated to C, we have

$$\forall v \in \mathbb{R},\ \pi_c(v) = \mu_C(v).$$

In general, membership functions and possibility distributions that are associated to the different concepts that we will define are used indistinctly, except where explicitly stated otherwise. We will always assume that π_c is *normalized*, i.e., $\exists v \in \mathbb{R},\ \pi_c(v) = 1$. We also assume that π_c is *unimodal*, i.e.: $\forall v, v', v'' \in \mathbb{R},\ v < v' < v'',\ \pi_c(v') \geq min\{\pi_c(v), \pi_c(v'')\}$.

In the temporal domain, the concept of fuzzy value will serve to represent that of *fuzzy date* [3].

Definition 2. We introduce the concept of **fuzzy increment** in order to represent amounts, such as, for instance, the difference between two values. A fuzzy increment D is represented by means of a normalized and unimodal possibility distribution π_D, which is defined, in general, over $\mathbb{R}$. In this way, given a $d \in \mathbb{R}, \pi_D(d) \in [0, 1]$ represents the possibility of D being precisely equal to d.

Given an ordered pair of fuzzy values (**a**,**e**), the *distance* between **a** and **e** is given by a fuzzy increment. This distance is represented by means of a possibility distribution $\pi_{D(a,e)}$:

$$\forall d \in \mathbb{R},\ \pi_{D(a,e)}(d) = \sup_{d=t-s} min\{\pi_a(s), \pi_e(t)\}$$

It has been shown [15] that if a and e correspond to unimodal and normalized distributions, $\pi_{D(a,e)}$ will also possess these properties.

In the temporal domain, the concept of fuzzy increment will serve to represent those of *duration* or *fuzzy temporal extension* between the fuzzy instances.

Definition 3. We define **fuzzy interval** by means of its maximum and minimum fuzzy values, and its extension, which is a fuzzy increment and represents the difference between the maximum and minimum values of the interval. $I_{(A,E,D)}$ denotes the interval delimited by the values A and E, with a distance between them D.

In order for the interval to be rational, it must necessarily have started before it can finish. For this reason, we assume that D, the fuzzy set that defines the possible values of the extension of the interval, will be unimodal and normalized, and its support will be included in the set of positive numbers:

$\forall m \in \mathbb{R},\ m \leq 0,\ \pi_D(m) = 0$. In this manner, in a constraint model such as the one that we propose, even though the distributions of A and E overlap, the constraint on the extension of the interval will reject any assignment to A of any instant that is the same as or posterior to E.

In the temporal domain, the fuzzy interval concept is used to represent *fuzzy temporal intervals*, which together with fuzzy instants and fuzzy durations, make up the conceptual entities with which we represent time in our model. All events that take place in time will have, in their representation, a temporal support formed by one of these entities.

2.3 Definition of the model

The initial aim is to represent an evolution profile relative to a physical variable $v(t)$, which takes real values in time. We have developed a model, which we have named *Fuzzy Temporal Profile* (FTP) [9], which operates through a fuzzy linear description of the evolution of the aforementioned variable. An FTP is a network of fuzzy constraints between a set of nodes, which perform the role of significant points.

Each significant point is defined as a pair of variables: one corresponding to the physical parameter and the other to time. The fuzzy profile constraints limit the fuzzy duration values, the fuzzy increase and the fuzzy slope between each pair of significant points.

We now go on to define the fundamental concepts of the model.

Definition 4. We define **significant point** associated with a variable $v(t)$, which we call X_i^v, as the pair formed by a variable of the domain V_i^v, and a temporal variable T_i^v.

$$X_i^v = < V_i^v, T_i^v >,$$

where V_i^v represents an unknown value of the physical parameter, and T_i^v represents an unknown time instant. In the absence of any constraints, the variables V_i^v and T_i^v may take any precise value v_i and t_i, respectively.

Definition 5. A unary constraint L_i^v on a temporal variable T_i^v is defined by means of a normalized and unimodal possibility distribution $\pi_{L_i}^v(t)$, whose discourse universe is the time axis τ.

$$\forall\, t \in \tau:\ \pi_{L_i}^v(t)\ \in\ [0,1],$$

so that given a precise time instant t_i, $\pi_{L_i}^v(t_i)$ represents the possibility that T_i^v takes precisely the value t_i.

The unary constraint L_i^v restricts the domain of values which may be assigned to T_i^v to those time instants t_i which satisfy $\pi_{L_i}^v(t_i) > 0$. The degree of possibility of t_i, $\pi_{L_i}^v(t_i)$ can be interpreted as a degree of preference in the assignment. The possibility distribution $\pi_{L_i}^v(t)$ associated to a unary constraint induces a fuzzy subset on the time axis, to which we give the same symbol as the constraint L_i^v. Formally, the distribution $\pi_{L_i}^v(t)$ corresponds to the possibility distribution of a fuzzy value, according to definition 1. Thus we can interpret a unary constraint L_i^v as the assignment of a fuzzy value, which we call *fuzzy instant*, to the variable T_i^v.

On the other hand, L_i^v could correspond, in the linguistic variable domain, to the assignment of a linguistic description l_i (for example, *"early in the morning"*), from the set $\mathcal{L} = \{l_1, l_2, ..., l_n\}$ of descriptions of values of the discourse universe τ. The development of the FTP model has led to the formulation of a language, described in [11], which enables the description of a profile to be projected onto a constraint network that is defined by means of possibility distributions.

Definition 6. A binary constraint L_{ij}^v on two temporal variables T_i^v and T_j^v is defined by means of a normalized and unimodal possibility distribution $\pi_{L_{ij}}^v$, whose discourse universe is $\mathbb{Z}$.

$$\forall\, l \in \mathbb{Z}: \ \pi_{L_{ij}}^v(l) \ \in \ [0,1].$$

Given a precise value l_{ij}, $\pi_{L_{ij}}^v(l_{ij})$ represents the possibility that the temporal distance between T_i^v and T_j^v takes precisely the value l_{ij}.

The constraint L_{ij}^v jointly restricts the possible value domains of the variables T_i^v and T_j^v. In the absence of other constraints, the assignments $T_i^v = t_i$ and $T_j^v = t_j$ are possible if $\pi_{L_{ij}}^v(t_j - t_i) > 0$ is satisfied. The possibility distribution $\pi_{L_{ij}}^v$ associated to a binary constraint, which we represent as L_{ij}^v, induces a fuzzy subset in the temporal distance domain. Formally, the distribution $\pi_{L_{ij}}^v$ corresponds to the possibility distribution of a fuzzy increase, according to definition 2. Thus, we may interpret a binary constraint L_{ij}^v as the assignment of a fuzzy increase, which we call *fuzzy duration*, to the distance between the variables T_i^v and T_j^v.

We have attempted to model those qualitative relations that appear in the bibliography. Thus, amongst instants we represent those of convex point algebra [23]: *before* ($\pi_{<0}$), *after* ($\pi_{>0}$) and *the same* ($\pi_{=0}$), and its disjunctive combinations: *before or the same* ($\pi_{\leq 0}$), *after or the same* ($\pi_{\geq 0}$) and the *universal constraint* ($\pi_{\mathcal{U}}$). We reject the representation of the relation *different* ($\pi_{\neq 0}$), since its possibility distribution is not unimodal. Furthermore, a representation based on fuzzy sets enables the model to capture the imprecision present in the quantitative relations between temporal events, and which can be found in expressions of the type *"approximately 5 minutes after"*.

With regard to the qualitative relations that we represent between an instant and an interval, these derive from applying the relations mentioned in the previous paragraph on the aforementioned instant, and on those making up the onset and the end of the interval. The qualitative relations that we represent between intervals are the primitive ones of Allen's interval algebra [1]. Figure 1 shows an example of how one of the temporal relations between intervals is projected onto the network.

$(T_i^{TEMP}, T_u^{TEMP}, \pi_{L_{iu}}^{TEMP})$::=(<interval-interval rel.>(T_a^{TAQ}, T_e^{TAQ}))=(LITTLE AFTER (T_a^{TAQ}, T_e^{TAQ}))

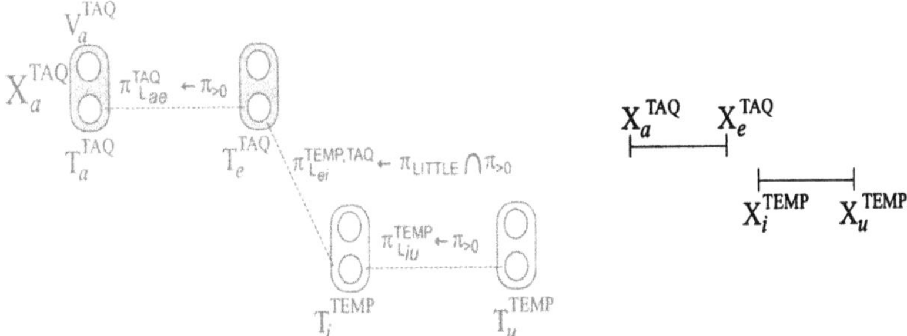

Fig. 1. Projection of the relation between temporal intervals 'A LITTLE AFTER' on the constraints of the model. 'TEMP' and 'TAQ' represent any two parameters. The upper part shows the rewriting rule [11] which corresponds to the specification of an interval in relation to another, previously-defined one. It is projected onto the constraint network by introducing two significant points X_i^{TEMP} and X_j^{TEMP}, along with the corresponding temporal constraints.

Definition 7. A unary constraint D_i^v on a variable of the domain V_i^v is defined, in a similar way to L_i^v, by means of a normalized and unimodal possibility distribution $\pi_{D_i}^v(v)$, whose discourse universe is $\mathbb{R}$.

$$\forall\, v \in \mathbb{R}:\ \pi_{D_i}^v(v)\ \in\ [0,1].$$

Formally, the distribution $\pi_{D_i}^v(v)$ corresponds to the possibility distribution of a fuzzy value. Thus we may interpret a unary constraint D_i^v as the assignment of a *fuzzy value* to the variable V_i^v.

Definition 8. A binary constraint D_{ij}^v on two variables of the domain V_i^v and V_j^v is defined, in a similar way to the constraint L_{ij}^v, by means of a normalized and unimodal possibility distribution $\pi_{D_{ij}}^v$, whose discourse universe is $\mathbb{R}$.

$$\forall\, d \in \mathbb{R}:\ \pi_{D_{ij}}^v(d)\ \in\ [0,1].$$

Formally, the distribution $\pi_{D_{ij}}^v$ corresponds to the possibility distribution of a fuzzy increase. Thus we may interpret a binary constraint D_{ij}^v as the assignment of a *fuzzy increase* to the distance between V_i^v and V_j^v.

We add an additional significant point $X_0^v =< L_0^v, D_0^v >$ to the model, which represents a precise origin for the time and values axes. An arbitrary value may be assigned to this point, but for the sake of simplicity, we assign it the value $L_0^v = 0, D_0^v = 0$. In this way, all unary constraints may be treated as binary constraints $L_{0i}^v = L_i^v, D_{0i}^v = D_i^v$.

It is supposed that all the significant points are different, and that they verify total temporal order, which impedes the assignment of two different values to the same instant. We only consider those significant points that are ordered by the relation $L_{ij}^v > 0$, since any constraint $L_{ij}^v < 0$ can be substituted by its symmetrical constraint L_{ji}^v, which is positive, and equivalent to the original one.

Definition 9. A quaternary constraint M_{ij}^v on two significant points X_i^v and X_j^v, is defined by means of a normalized and unimodal possibility distribution $\pi_{M_{ij}}^v$, whose discourse universe is $\mathbb{R}$.

$$\forall\, m \in \mathbb{R}: \ \pi_{M_{ij}}^v(m) \ \in \ [0,1].$$

Given a precise value m_{ij}, $\pi_{M_{ij}}^v(m_{ij})$ represents the possibility that the slope of the line that joins X_i^v and X_j^v be precisely m_{ij}.

The constraint M_{ij}^v jointly restricts the domains of V_i^v, V_j^v, T_i^v and T_j^v. In the absence of other constraints, the assignments $V_i^v = v_i$, $V_j^v = v_j$, $T_i^v = t_i$ and $T_j^v = t_j$ are possible if $\pi_{M_{ij}}^v((v_j - v_i)/(t_j - t_i)) > 0$ is satisfied. The possibility distribution $\pi_{M_{ij}}^v$ associated with a quaternary constraint induces a fuzzy subset in the slope domain, which we represent as M_{ij}^v. Formally, the distribution $\pi_{M_{ij}}^v$ corresponds to the possibility distribution of a fuzzy value. Thus we can interpret a constraint M_{ij}^v as the assignment of a fuzzy value, which we call *fuzzy slope*, to the line which joins X_i^v and X_j^v.

The elements defined up until this point enable us to make a representation of a profile from a set of signal events: certain significant points, and where the representation of a fact which spreads over a temporal interval is limited to the events corresponding to the extremes of this interval. This representation seems to be suitably adapted to the semantics of expressions such as *"... fifteen minutes later, the temperature is somewhat lower"*, in which experts show their possible ignorance as to the evolution of the temperature during these fifteen minutes, and in any case, their total lack of interest in what happened during this period. We will say that the meaning of these expressions corresponds to what we term *unconstrained evolution* [10] (see figure 2).

Nevertheless, natural language allows the expression of different descriptions of the manner in which the evolution between two points takes place [12], such as in the case of *"... throughout the following fifteen minutes the temperature rises moderately ten degrees"* or *"during the last two hours the temperature has been high"*. With the aim of incorporating the representation of the evolution between two significant points, we have modeled an expandable set of evolutions that are associated to the different semantics of the section between significant points, so that the compatibility between the descriptor of the section and a fragment of the temporal evolution of a physical variable can be calculated. This section descriptor is identified with a membership function that includes information on the change in the physical parameter (D_{ij}^v), and the rhythm of variation (M_{ij}^v) in the interval of

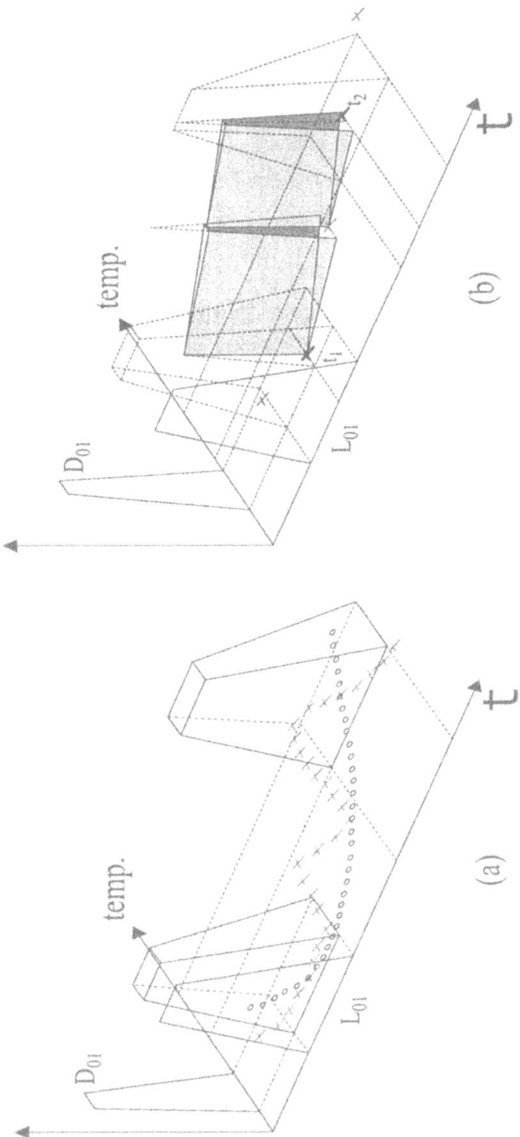

Fig. 2. Graphic example of the representation of two different semantics in the evolution of the section between two significant points. In (a) two different evolutions are shown that have the same degree of compatibility with the semantics of a sentence of the type "... *a little after, the temperature is much greater*"; (b) shows the descriptor of the semantics of a sentence of the type, "...*throughout the following minutes the temperature rises moderately...*".

duration (L_{ij}^v) (see figure 2). We thus define a further constraint, S_{ij}^v, which makes a descriptor of its evolution correspond to each section.

Thus we redefine the constraint between each two significant points:

Definition 10. A fuzzy constraint R_{ij}^v on two significant points X_i^v and X_j^v is a 4-tuple formed by a fuzzy duration L_{ij}^v, a fuzzy increase D_{ij}^v, a fuzzy slope M_{ij}^v and a semantic label S_{ij}^v.

$$R_{ij}^v =< L_{ij}^v, D_{ij}^v, M_{ij}^v, S_{ij}^v > .$$

Definition 11. We define a **Fuzzy Temporal Profile** (FTP) $\mathcal{N}^v = \{\mathcal{X}^v, \mathcal{R}^v\}$ on the parameter v, as a finite set of significant points $\mathcal{X}^v = \{X_0^v, X_1^v, \ldots, X_{N^v}^v\}$, and a finite set of constraints $\mathcal{R}^v = \{< L_{ij}^v, D_{ij}^v, M_{ij}^v, S_{ij}^v >, 0 \leq i,j \leq N^v\}$ defined on the variables which constitute these points.

An FTP may be represented by way of a directed graph (figure 3), in which the nodes correspond to significant points, and the arcs correspond to the constraints on the variables of the nodes which they join.

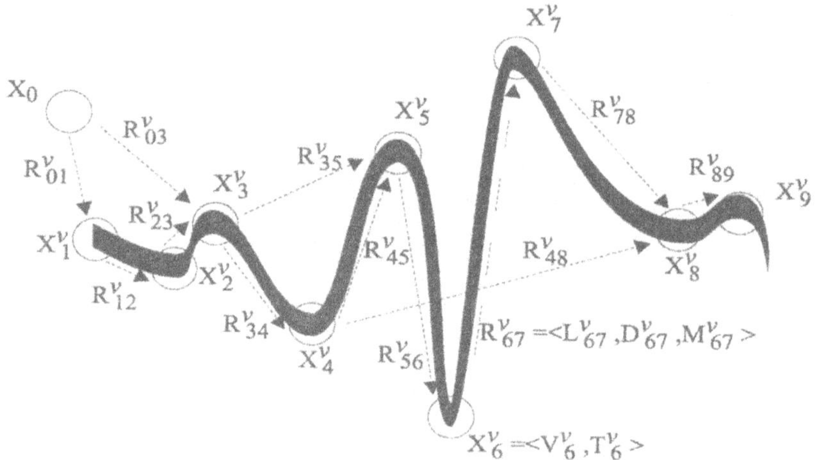

Fig. 3. An intuitive idea of an FTP and of a possible network that describes it.

3 Multivariable Fuzzy Temporal Profiles

The aim of the Fuzzy Temporal Profile model is the recognition of morphologies of special significance on a signal, taking a linguistic description of these morphologies as a starting point. In this sense it was proposed as a study of the semantics of those expressions that experts -and in particular, medical experts- employ to communicate and reason on the evolution of a physical parameter.

The FTP model that we have described has been included into an intelligent patient supervision system [13], the objective of which is to interpret the state and evolution of patients interned in Intensive Coronary Care Units. Although the model is useful in a number of cases, it is not so when multiple parameters interact in such a way that only certain combinations in the evolution of certain parameters supply evidence of critical situations. The anomalous evolution of a given parameter is frequently not as important as its relation with the context that is made up of the evolution of other parameters.

Thus it is necessary to extend the model in order to allow the representation, and subsequent recognition, of multivariable patterns. These patterns demonstrate a particular chronology of events defined by means of FTPs on different parameters, and which, together, have special clinical significance. Whilst experience has shown us the great interest that there is in the representation of temporal information amongst different signal events, this has not been the case with other possible relations, which may arise amongst these very events, such as value or rhythm variation relations. For this reason we have limited ourselves to modelling the MFTPs as a network of temporal relations between FTPs (figure 4).

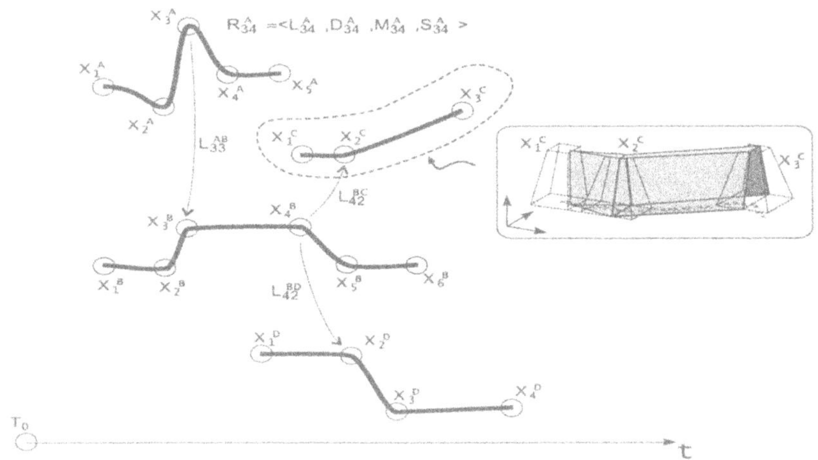

Fig. 4. Example of a multivariable fuzzy temporal profile

Thus we have added an additional constraint that defines a fuzzy temporal extension between significant points X_i^υ and X_j^ω, corresponding to different parameters υ and ω, amongst which there is a partial temporal order. This constraint enables us to establish temporal relations between the different profiles that are described for each parameter (e.g. *"the palpitations end a little before the end of the ischaemic episode"*).

Definition 12. A binary constraint $L_{ij}^{v\omega}$ on two temporal variables T_i^v and T_j^ω is defined by means of a normalized and unimodal possibility distribution $\pi_{L_{ij}}^{v\omega}$, whose discourse universe is $\mathbb{Z}$.

$$\forall\, l \in \mathbb{Z} : \pi_{L_{ij}}^{v\omega}(l) \in [0,1]$$

Given a precise value l_{ij}, $\pi_{L_{ij}}^{v\omega}(l_{ij})$ represents the possibility that the temporal distance between T_i^v and T_j^ω takes precisely the value l_{ij}.

Definition 13. We define a **Multivariable Fuzzy Temporal Profile** $\mathcal{M} = \{\mathcal{N}, \mathcal{L}\}$ as a finite set of fuzzy temporal profiles $\mathcal{N} = \{\mathcal{N}^1, \mathcal{N}^2, ..., \mathcal{N}^r\}$, and a finite set of constraints $\mathcal{L} = \{L_{ij}^{v\omega}, 1 \leq v, \omega \leq r,\ 0 \leq i \leq N^v,\ 0 \leq j \leq N^\omega\}$ that are defined between the significant points corresponding to different parameters.

4 Minimizing the MFTP

The definition of an MFTP will arise from the projection, in a set of constraints between significant points, of a linguistic description made by an expert, making use of the language introduced in [11], which on one hand, allows the description of the evolution of a physical parameter, and on the other, enables it to be integrated into a network of relations between temporal facts. Nevertheless, there are no guarantees that the description of a profile obtained in this manner will not contain redundant or inconsistent information.

Minimizing an MFTP involves eliminating from the domain of each variable those values that are incompatible with the constraints on that variable, in order to obtain an MFTP in which relations are defined in the most precise manner possible [20,18,19]. Therefore, the minimization process implies the elimination of redundant information from the network, as well as the detection of inconsistent information.

The general problem of minimizing an FTP is NP-complete [12]. Given that the definition of an MFTP carries out the integration of a set of FTPs by means of a network of fuzzy temporal constraints, its minimization also defines an NP-complete problem. For this reason a set of formal tools for the analysis of local levels of consistency for the information from the MFTP has been developed [9], eliminating redundant information and detecting the existence of inconsistencies, by way of computationally more efficient procedures. As this study is not primarily concerned with the general problem of MFTP minimization, we will limit ourselves to making brief reference to the obtention of *section* and *path consistency* [18,5] which, although they do not guarantee the general minimization of an MFTP, are of great usefulness in debugging the majority of information given in the linguistic description of the profile.

In order to achieve *section consistency*, we apply a corresponding procedure to the duration, increment and slope constraints which join two significant points X_i and X_j of a certain parameter v. The representation of these constraints $R_{ij}^v =< L_{ij}^v, D_{ij}^v, M_{ij}^v, S_{ij}^v >$ is inherently redundant. For example, L_{ij}^v and D_{ij}^v define an estimated slope, which thus transports information which is additional to that given by M_{ij}^v. By combining the three pieces of information, we can reduce the imprecision existing in the input values for L_{ij}^v, D_{ij}^v and M_{ij}^v, and obtain a consistent representation of the section R_{ij}^v.

We have developed procedures for the obtention of *path consistency* in the subnetworks of value: $\mathcal{N}_V^v = \{D_{ij}^v,\ 1 \leq v \leq r,\ 0 \leq i,j \leq N^v\}$ for each parameter, formed by the increment constraints; and in the temporal subnetwork $\mathcal{N}_T = \{L_{ij}^v, L_{hk}^{v\omega};\ 1 \leq v,\ \omega \leq r,\ 0 \leq i,j,h \leq N^v,\ 0 \leq k \leq N^\omega\}$, formed by all the duration constraints on the network; including those L_{ij}^v that are defined between the significant points of a single parameter, as well as those that are defined between significant points corresponding to different parameters. In the same manner as in the previous case, the aim is to make a set of constraints that are implicit in the description of the network explicit, corresponding, in this case, to the paths induced. For example, L_{ij}^v and $L_{jk}^{v\omega}$ define an approximate duration which transports, as such, information that is additional to that given by $L_{ik}^{v\omega}$. By combining all the paths induced on each one of the constraints we reduce imprecision in the information.

5 Matching of an MFTP with the Evolution of a System

Once a multivariable fuzzy temporal profile has been defined and minimized, its practical application consists of identifying its appearance during the real evolution of a system, by obtaining some measurement of compatibility between the evolution of the physical parameters that characterize the system and the description that is made of them in the MFTP. Henceforth, we will refer to this calculation as *matching*. The real evolution will generically be made up of a set $\mathcal{P}$ of a series of precise data $\mathcal{P} = \{P^1, P^2, ..., P^r\}$ obtained at different instants:

$$P^v = \{(v_{[1]}^v, t_{[1]}^v), ..., (v_{[m]}^v, t_{[m]}^v), ...\}$$

where $v_{[m]}^v$ is the precise value of the parameter $v(t)$ at the precise instant $t_{[m]}^v$.

Given that it is the contstraint network formalism that serves as a support for the MFTP model, the problem of matching is closely linked with that of signal segmentation in a set of sections, which are compared with the constraints that define the MFTP. In short, matching can be understood as a search for the form of segmentation which shows the greatest degree of consistency with the MFTP.

For the FTP model the segmentation of a fragment of signal is given by the choice of a set of as many precise instants ($\mathcal{T}^v = \{t_1^v, ..., t_{N^v}^v\}$) as there are significant points in the profile. For this segmentation a degree of consistency with a given profile is defined as follows:

Definition 14. The **degree of consistency** of the segmentation $\mathcal{T}^v = \{t_1^v, ..., t_{N^v}^v\}$ with the constraints of the profile FTP^v are given by:

$$\mu^{FTP^v}(\mathcal{T}^v) = \min_{0 \leq i,j \leq N^v} \{\mu_{ij}^R(t_i^v, t_j^v)\}$$

where μ_{ij}^R is the function that describes the section between the significant points X_i^v and X_j^v, in the calculation of which are involved the duration, increase and slope constraints, L_{ij}^v, D_{ij}^v and M_{ij}^v, respectively, and the shape of which depends fundamentally on the semantics S_{ij}^v that characterizes the section. The fuzzy set of the segmentations that are consistent with the profile is denoted by FTP^v.

The MFTP model allows temporal relations to be established between significant points that correspond to different parameters, due to which the definition of consistency changes.

Definition 15. The **degree of consistency** of the segmentation of a set of parameters $\mathcal{T}^\mathcal{P} = \{\mathcal{T}^1, ..., \mathcal{T}^r\}$ with the constraints of a given $MFTP$ is given by:

$$\mu^{MFTP}(\mathcal{T}^1, ..., \mathcal{T}^r) = \min\{ \min_{\substack{1 \leq v,w \leq r \\ 0 \leq h \leq N^v \\ 0 \leq k \leq N^w}} \{\pi_{L_{hk}}^{vw}(t_k^w - t_h^v)\}, \min_{\substack{0 \leq i,j \leq N^v \\ 1 \leq v \leq r}} \{\mu_{ij}^R(t_i^v, t_j^v)\}\}$$

$MFTP$ is the name given to the fuzzy set of segmentations that are consistent with the corresponding profile.

In order to resolve this calculation, we devise a tree search-based segmentation procedure, so that, following an ordered method, a significant amount of spurious assignments can be rejected, thereby reducing the computational cost of the procedure.

The search tree has as many levels as significant points, and it branches at the possible segmentations that are realized for each one of them. The first node of the tree represents the temporal origin, which has been set at $T_0 = 0$ for all parameters, and the leaves represent a complete segmentation carried out on all the parameters that are involved. Thus we will incrementally construct a solution for the MFTP, by means of successive choices for the significant points of the profile, with the degree of consistency being calculated in a partial manner. In order to do this, we follow the typical *first in depth* search method [21]. In order to delimit the sufficiently satisfactory solutions, we consider a lower limit c_{inf} that prunes all those branches for which consistency exceeding the set limit cannot be obtained [8].

Given that the search starts from an *a priori* order of the segmentation for each parameter, for the sake of simplicity in the resulting expressions, we take the temporal order of the significant points itself, covering the list of parameters as and when they appear in $\mathcal{P}$, although later on it will be seen that it is generally more efficient to follow a different strategy.

At each step for the obtention of the global consistency between the evolution of the system and the MFTP, we expand a k-tuple $(t_0^v, t_1^v, ..., t_k^v)$ of segmentation points in the evolution of the parameter v to the following significant point X_{k+1}^v. If there is a $t_{[m]}^v \in P^v$ so that the consistency of the segmentation is greater than c_{inf}, we take $t_{[m]}^v$ as a valid segmentation point for X_{k+1}^v. If no instant satisfying the prior condition is found, we go back to the segmentation of the previous significant point, X_k^v. When a global segmentation $(\mathcal{T}^0, ..., \mathcal{T}^r)$ with a consistency greater than c_{inf} is found, this will be considered the current optimal solution. In order to accede as rapidly as possible to the best possible solutions, we then update $c_{\text{inf}} = \mu^{MFTP}(\mathcal{T}^0, ..., \mathcal{T}^r)$ and we go back in search of a better solution.

In figure 5 we present a simplified version of the segmentation algorithm. For each significant point, a list A_i^v is constructed in which the possible instants on which segmentation is to be carried out are stored. The algorithm is recursive and resolves the segmentation and the handling of failures in a single procedure, by returning to the previous significant point.

```
procedure SEGMENTATION(i^v,min,max);
begin
      maxx=min;
      if (i^v = N^v) then
       if (v = r) then return(max)
       else v = v + 1;
      A_i^v ← {t_i^v = t^v[m] : μ^MFTP(T^1, T^2, ..., t_1^v, ..., t_i^v) ≥min};
      while(A_i^v ≠ ∅) do
       begin
        take and erase a t^v[m] of A_i^v;
        maxx=μ^MFTP(T^1, T^2, ..., t_1^v, ..., t_i^v);
        maxx=min{max,SEGMENTATION(i^v+1,min,maxx)};
       end;
      return(maxx);
end;
```

Fig. 5. Segmentation procedure.

The resolution of the matching problem with this algorithm is highly inefficient, due to which it is essential to propose a matching strategy that exploits knowledge already available on the problem. We formulate this strategy in two different environments: on one hand, in the *domain*, through the search for heuristics that may speed up the recognition of profiles on each one of the parameters, based on the properties of their typical evolutions; on the other hand, in the *model*, in which the properties of the MFTP to be detected in the different levels of abstraction in which they may be defined are studied.

5.1 Heuristics in the domain scope

Due to the high computational cost of the segmentation process on each parameter, we employ heuristics to increase the efficiency of this process, based, as has previously been mentioned, on the properties of the signals with which the matching is carried out.

In this sense, we consider the search on each signal for those features of the profile that stand out especially given the characteristics of the signal: a section, or a group of sections, or the value of a given significant point (see figure 6). We use the constraints that define these features as a starting point in the segmentation process, which, to a great degree, enables us to prune the search tree.

At the level of the different signals being handled, we order the segmentation so that we first tackle those signals demonstrating the highest probability of successful matching: good noise-signal ratio, outstanding knowledge of their significant features, etc.

5.2 Heuristics in the scope of the model

As has already been stated, we can improve the efficiency of the matching algorithms by studying the structural properties of the MFTP. We can consider the definition of an MFTP on multiple levels of abstraction, each one of which includes the aggregation of elements from lower levels of abstraction. The highest level considers an MFTP as a pattern of manifestations, each one of which corresponds to a fact of special clinical importance, and which is represented by a sub-profile of the original one. At the lowest level, we find the definition of the different FTPs on each one of the parameters.

On this MFTP structure, the increase in efficiency in the matching is given by the *aggregation of compatibility into the calculation* and by the *order in the segmentation*, which are closely related.

The aggregation of compatibility into the calculation is the result of translating the structure of levels of abstraction in the MFTP into the matching process, which defines a *profile recognition task*. Each level of abstraction describes its own objects, which combine in different ways to form objects with a temporal granularity that is lower than in the following level. Thus an FTP corresponding to a simple manifestation may form part of different MFTPs. This leads to the matching of each object mentioned being carried out independently from the rest, in the end including all the objects with the

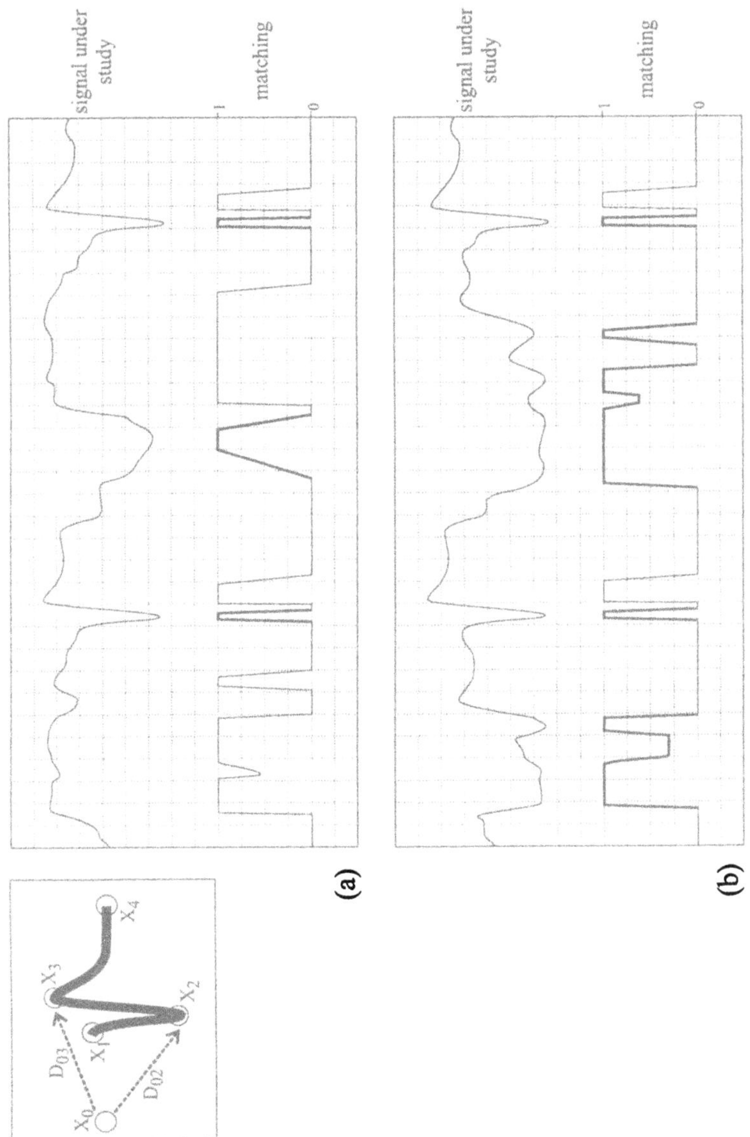

Fig. 6. In this example the detection of the profile appearing at top left is undertaken. The compatibility between the two signals with different behaviour patterns is shown. In (a) the compatibility of each signal sample with the fuzzy values corresponding to the constraints D_{02} (thick line) and D_{03} (thin line) is shown. It can be seen how the former is a better beginning for the segmentation process. Whereas, (b) shows a signal in which the opposite is true: the better starting point for the detection is X_3.

constraints that bind them, which are normally temporal constraints that define a partial order between the objects. We thus reject an optimal global calculation of consistency, since failure in the detection of an object would oblige us to revise the matching with the previously recognized objects. In short, there is a fragmentation of the matching process that is associated to the structure of an MFTP, in which there is a search for the local maxima in the detection of each one of the objects that make it up.

In each level of abstraction, the order in the segmentation is fundamental to resolve the problem of choice which is posed by the matching problem. In lower levels of abstraction this is formulated as an order which initially implements the segmentation for those significant points that are modelled by means of more precise constraints, beginning with temporal constraints. A description of an FTP which has temporal references to the origin, such as *"at approximately 15:00 temperature is normal"*, or to previously identified events, such as *"a little after the onset of the infarct"*, generally enables the profile to be located faster than if there is no temporal reference given ($\pi^{v}_{L_{0i}} = \pi^{vw}_{L_{ih}} = \pi_{\mathcal{U}}$, $1 \leq i \leq N^{v}$); in the latter case, the entire signal will, in principle, need to be covered by the matching process.

In the highest levels of abstraction the order in the segmentation will be linked, firstly, to the selection of those objects that are modelled by means of simpler topologies [12], in order to obtain, as rapidly as possible, the greatest possible amount of evidence.

5.3 Sub-optimal approaches

Here we propose a tree search-based segmentation procedure (which, in theory, is highly complex in computational terms) for implementing the optimal segmentation of the signals being monitored. The aim is to translate the maximum expressiveness allowed by the representation of profiles into a segmentation procedure by means of the MFTP model. This solution is a starting point, from which to restrict the expressiveness of the model and the quality of the profile recognition process, with the resulting increase in the efficiency of the recognition task. The idea is, on one hand, to simplify network topology and, on the other, to maximise the fulfillment of the local criteria that determine the segmentation, to the detriment of an optimum global fulfillment. Thus it is at the other end of the strategy that is employed here that we can place the typical algorithm; this is of linear computational complexity with regard to the number of samples that are processed, and consists of carrying out the segmentation of a signal by maximising its membership with respect to each two neighbouring sections.

6 Integration of the MFTP Model into a Patient Supervision System

As has already been mentioned, we have started with the implementation of the MFTP model in a patient supervision system in Intensive Coronary Care Units. This system employs a blackboard architecture, in which a heterogeneous set of specialists co-operate in carrying out the monitoring-diagnosis-treatment cycle. The monitoring consists of verifying whether there is any discrepancy between the expected values and the ones that are observed. Thus the cycle starts with the monitoring task, which generates discrepancies. The diagnosis task assumes that they correspond to a certain physiopathological problem and attempts to find an explanation for the abnormal behaviour that has been detected. The explanation that is obtained is made up of a set of states that are internal to the system, and which may play the role of causal factors in the detected discrepancies. Finally, the treatment task proposes a remedy for correcting the discrepancies, and returning the patient to a normal state.

As has already been seen, the MFTP is a representation of a set of temporal relations between facts described on the evolution of different parameters. Each one of these facts constitutes a manifestation that is implicated, on the basis of one or more hypotheses, in patient's evolution. Furthermore, the MFTP model allows the task of observing this evidence to be structured, through the application of temporal abstraction processes on the set of parameters that are linked to the manifestations that are involved. Hence we include the representation of temporal facts by means of the MFTP model in a diagnostic reasoning scheme in which the temporal relations between the different elements play a fundamental role.

We now go on to give an example of the representation of an evolutionary pattern using the MFTP mode. Here we are concerned with what is referred to in the medical domain as *'acute strain-induced ischaemia'*, and the evolution of two parameters is described: on one hand, the 'ST level'; and on the other, a compound parameter: the double product 'heart rate' by 'systolic blood pressure' ($HR \times BPs$).

Linguistically, the acute strain-induced ischaemia can be described in the following manner: *"The acute strain-induced ischaemia starts with a rise in the double product HR×BPs, until increasing to, approximately, 10% over its basal value, during a period of between 5 and 60 seconds. A short time later, the ST falls to at least 0.01mV. The double product continues rising slightly and subsequently starts to fall until reaching 10% of its basal value. The ST remains below 0.01mV until between 10 and 20 seconds later. The double product returns to the base-line between half a minute and two minutes after the onset of the ischaemia, and the ST returns to basal levels a little later."*

The figure shows a representation given by the MFTP of the strain-induced ischaemia, and an example of its matching.

7 Discussion and Future Work

In this chapter we have presented a model for the representation and recognition of patterns on multiple parameters. The MFTP model is based on a linguistic acquisition of information and, as such, highlights the treatment of vagueness and uncertainty that are inherent in natural language [11].

The MFTP model is a solution that is based on the construction of a constraint network in which information is represented using the fuzzy set theory. This solution provides the versatility of constraint networks, which is needed for analyzing information -study of its consistency-, as well as the capability of the fuzzy set theory for handling imprecision and uncertainty.

The application of the MFTP model is carried out by means of a set of algorithms which allows the development of a signal pattern recognition tool. Even though, theoretically, these algorithms are of a high computational complexity, in practice, the inclusion of suitable heuristics has proved to be useful. Nevertheless, the use of these algorithms is not advisable for those applications that require real-time information processing. In this sense, and although the development of certain sub-optimal (though very efficient) algorithms is immediate, in the future we will concentrate on the study of new network topologies and new matching algorithms, which, being more efficient than the one presented here, will not adversely affect the quality of the solution that is found.

A model of these characteristics responds well to the needs of a domain such as medicine, in which a large proportion of knowledge is of a descriptive nature, in particular in the supervision of patients in an ICCU, where a large number of parameters are monitored in order to obtain the best possible interpretation of the state and evolution of the patient.

The model needs to continue in its developmental phase in order to be totally integrated into a signal perception specialist system for the supervision of patients in an ICCU. This integration will determine the evolution of the model, fundamentally with regard to its expressiveness and efficiency.

8 Acknowledgments

This work was funded by the Xunta de Galicia and the Ministerio de Educación y Cultura through research projects PGIDT99PXI20601B and 1FD97-0183, respectively.

References

1. Allen, J. (1984) Towards a general theory of action and time. Artificial Intelligence. **23**, 123–154.
2. Bakshi, B. R., Stephanopoulos, G. (1994) Representation of process trends-Part IV: Induction of real-time patterns from operating data for diagnosis and supervisory control. Computers Chemical Engineering, **18**(4), 303–332.

3. Barro, S., Marín, R., Mira, J., Patón, A. (1994) A model and a language for the fuzzy representation and handling of time. Fuzzy Sets and Systems, **61**, 153–175.
4. Cheung, J. T. Y., Stephanopoulos, G. (1990) Representation of process trends-Part I: A formal representation framework. Computers Chemical Engineering, **14**(4/5), 495–510.
5. Dechter, R., Meiri, I., Pearl, J. (1991) Temporal constraint networks. Artificial Intelligence, **49**, 61–95.
6. Drakopoulos, J. A., Hayes-Roth, B. (1998) tFPR: A fuzzy and structural pattern recognition system of multi-variate time-dependent pattern classes based on sigmoidal functions. Fuzzy Sets and Systems, **99**, 57–72.
7. Dubois, D., Prade, H. (1989) Processing fuzzy temporal knowledge. IEEE Transactions of Systems, Man and Cybernetics, **19**(4), 729–744.
8. Dubois, D., Fargier, H., Prade, H. (1996) Possibility theory in constraint satisfaction problems: handling priority, preference and uncertainty. Applied Intelligence, **6**, 287–309.
9. Félix, P., Barro, S., Marín, R., Taboada, M. J., Engel, A. (1995) Patrones temporales borrosos en la supervisión de pacientes. Actas del V congreso español sobre Tecnologías y Lógica Fuzzy, 321–326.
10. Félix, P., Fraga, S., Marín, R., Barro, S. (1999) Trend detection based on a fuzzy temporal profile model. Artificial Intelligence on Engineering, **13**(4), 341–349.
11. Félix, P., Fraga, S., Marín, R., Barro, S. (1999) Linguistic representation of fuzzy temporal profiles. International Journal of Uncertainty, Fuzziness and Knowledge-Based Systems, **7**(3), 243–256.
12. Félix, P. (1999) Perfiles Temporales Borrosos: Un modelo para la representación y reconocimiento de patrones sobre señal, Tesis Doctoral. Universidade de Santiago de Compostela. (In Spanish).
13. Fraga, S., Félix, P., Marín, R., Barro, S. (1998) A proposal for a real time signal perception specialist. International ICSC Symposium on Engineering of Intelligent Systems, EIS'98, 261–267.
14. Haimowitz, I. J., Le, P. P., Kohane, I. S. (1995) Clinical monitoring using regresion-based trend templates. Artificial Intelligence inMedicine, **7**, 473–496.
15. Kaufmann, A., Gupta, M. M. (1985) Introduction to fuzzy arithmetic. Van Nostrand Reinhold.
16. Ligomenides, P. A. (1988) Real-time capture of experiential knowledge. IEEE Transactions on Systems, Man, and Cybernetics, **18**(4), 542–551.
17. Lowe, A., Harrison, M. J., Jones, R. W. (1999) Diagnostic monitoring in anaesthesia using fuzzy trend templates for matching temporal patterns. Artificial Intelligence in Medicine, **16**, 183–199.
18. Mackworth, A. (1977) Consistency in networks of relations. Artificial Intelligence, **8**, 99–118.
19. Marín, R., Barro, S., Bosch, A., Mira, J. (1994) Modeling the representation of time from a fuzzy perspective. Cybernetics and Systems: an International Journal, **25**(2), 217–231.
20. Montanari, U. (1974) Networks of constraints: fundamental properties and applications to picture processing. Information Science, **7**, 95–132.
21. Russell, S. J., Norvig, P. (1996) Artificial Intelligence: A modern approach. Prentice-Hall.
22. Steimann, F. (1996) The interpretation of time-varying data with DIAMON-1. Artificial Intelligence in Medicine, **8**, 343–357.

23. Vilain, M., Kautz, H. (1986) Constraint propagation algorithms for temporal reasoning. Proceedings of the AAAI'86, 377–382.
24. Zadeh, L. A. (1975) The concept of a linguistic variable and its application to approximate reasoning (Part 1). Information Science, **8**, 199–249.

Mass Assignment Methods for Medical Classification Diagnosis

Jim F. Baldwin, Carla Hill and Christiane Ponsan

Department of Engineering Mathematics
University of Bristol
Queens Building
University Walk
Bristol BS8 1TH, UK
E mail: {Jim.Baldwin, Carla.Hill, C.Ponsan}@bris.ac.uk

1. Introduction

Nowadays, in areas such as medicine, many real-world classification problems rely heavily on large collections of data that are not understandable to human users. Therefore, there is a need for transparent models to represent such databases. In this chapter, we present two methods for learning classification rules which aim at being simplistic and transparent in nature. Both methods use fuzzy sets to describe the universes of discourse since their fuzzy boundaries allow a realistic representation of neighbouring concepts. As a consequence, interpolation effects as well as data compression are obtained in the learned models. Moreover, the fuzzy sets can be labelled with words which allows the inferred rules to be interpreted linguistically. In order to generate these rules, probability distributions need to be extracted from fuzzy sets, which is feasible using the fundamental results of mass assignment theory [2].

The first method, namely the mass assignment FOIL (MA-FOIL), generates classification rules which are based upon features that are powerful in describing the classes. These rules are either *Fril rules* or *Fril extended rules* which are implemented in the Artificial Intelligence programming language Fril. The advantages in using these *conditionalised* rules come from the fact that we can handle uncertainty by instantiating variables with fuzzy sets and by having the consequent (head of the rule) following from the antecedent (body of the rule) with a probabilitic value or interval. Since the original features might not be ideal, a genetic programming algorithm [6] creates new additional features as algebraic combinations of the original features. The fitness function aims at providing a high discrimination between the classes. For this purpose it basically evaluates the point semantic unification [1] between fuzzy sets formed on the feature universes which represent the various classes.

Similarly to FOIL [8,9], we repeat to generate branches for each class separately which, translated into Fril rules, explain a part of the given examples for the considered class. The concepts that are added to a branch are selected according to a weight expressing their importance for this class. The algorithm terminates when all examples are covered and the resulting branches for each class are combined in a Fril extended rule.

In the second method, we introduce a ***semantic discrimination analysis*** to select the best subsets of *n* features amongst the original ones for distinguishing the classes. By forming subsets of features, this approach aims at conserving the original features while exploiting their eventual correlations. The discrimination of subsets rests on an evaluation function that is known as the *semantic unification* [1] between the fuzzy sets generated for all classes with respect to the subset under consideration. Initially, all subsets containing a small number of features are evaluated; those which are retained are used to form subsets of a larger number of features. Finally, classification rules are formed on the selected subsets of features.

Both methods have been carried out on the Wisconsin Breast Cancer database [10,11] gathering the records of breast mass diagnoses. The selected features obtained with both methods are displayed along with the classification performances given by the learned rules with respect to these features. Comparison with results obtained by *Principal Component Analysis* to find the best features is given at the end of this chapter.

2. Theoretical Background

Before describing the methods we recall some theoretical results that are relevant to both cases. The implementation of these is ensured by an Artificial Intelligence logic programming language, Fril [4,5], which extends the logic programming language Prolog by allowing fuzzy sets as fundamental objects and associating degrees of truth with clauses.

2.1. Enough Mass Assignment Theory

We explain the basic ideas and enough detail of the mass assignment theory to understand this paper.

First consider a non-fuzzy situation. You are told that the fair dice is even. Even corresponds to the crisp set {2, 4, 6}. The elements 2, 4, 6 have membership of 1 in the set even and the elements 1, 3, 5 have membership 0. You therefore know that the possibility of the dice having a value 2 is 1 and the same for dice values 4 and 6. The possibility for 1, 3, and 5 are all 0. The probability distribution for the dice values is not fully known. You do know that the probability of 1, 3 and 5 are all 0. You also know that the probability of the dice value being 2 or 4 or 6 is 1. We therefore know the probability distribution of the power set of the dice values, namely

$$Pr(\{2, 4, 6\}) = 1$$

This distribution over the power set we call the mass assignment. There is a family of distributions over the dice values corresponding to this mass assignment. We can distribute the probabilities amongst the elements 2, 4, and 6 in any way such that they sum to 1. We can use the prior distribution of the dice to give a unique distribution over the dice values from the mass assignment. Since it is a fair dice we can distribute the mass of 1 evenly amongst the elements {2, 4, 6} to provide the distribution

$$Pr(2 \mid even) = Pr(4 \mid even) = Pr(6 \mid even) = 1/3.$$

This is an entropy argument. If the dice is not fair then we use the prior to distribute the mass in the same proportions as the prior. The resulting distribution we will call the least prejudiced distribution.

Given this distribution we can determine the probability of any set of dice values given an even dice. For example

$$Pr(\{2, 4\} \mid even) = 2/3$$

We call this point value semantic unification.

If we replace the crisp set "even" with a fuzzy set "small" say, we should only have to modify our understanding slightly to allow for memberships which can take any value in the range [0, 1].

To see this more clearly imagine a voting situation in which each member of a representative group of voters is asked to accept or reject that a given element belongs to the set even. The voting acceptances would be as follows

1	**2** **voters**	**3**	**4**	**5**	**6**	**7**	**8**	**9**	**10**
2	2	2	2	2	2	2	2	2	2
4	4	4	4	4	4	4	4	4	4
6	6	6	6	6	6	6	6	6	6

In order to modify what we have done for crisp sets to the case for fuzzy sets we must provide a semantics for the concept of a fuzzy set. If the voters are told that the dice value is small, then there will be doubts whether to accept some elements.

We still require acceptance or rejection. The voters in the group will have different thresholds for acceptance. Suppose the voting is as follows

1	**2**	**3**	**4**	**5**	**6**	**7**	**8**	**9**	**10**
	voters								
1	1	1	1	1	1	1	1	1	1
2	2	2	2	2	2	2	2		
3	3	3	3	3	3				

then we will say that the fuzzy set small is

$$\text{small} = 1 / 1 + 2 / 0.8 + 3 / 0.6$$

where we use the notation element / membership of fuzzy set.

The membership of a given element x in the fuzzy set is the proportion of persons who accept that element.

In the above voting, 2 voters accept {1}, 2 voters accept {1, 2} and 6 voters accept {1, 2, 3}. This corresponds to a mass assignment

$$\text{MA small} = \{1\} : 0.2,\ \{1, 2\} : 0.2,\ \{1, 2, 3\} : 0.6$$

which is a probability distribution over the power set of dice values.

The starting point of mass assignment theory is the same as random set theory and the Dempster Shafer theory.

If we require a unique distribution over the dice values then we will distribute the masses associated with each set in the mass assignment amongst the elements of the corresponding set according to the prior. For example, voter 1 when told the dice is small would accept that the dice value could be 1 or 2 or 3 and would say these occur with equal probability since the dice is fair.

The least prejudiced distribution would then correspond to

$$\text{lpd}_{small} = \quad 1 : 0.2 + 0.2/2 + 0.6/3 = 0.5, \quad 2 : 0.2/2 + 0.6/3 = 0.3, \quad 3 : 0.6/3 = 0.2$$

giving

$$\Pr(1 \mid \text{small}) = 0.5,\ \Pr(2 \mid \text{small}) = 0.3,\ \Pr(3 \mid \text{small}) = 0.2$$

The entropy argument is now localised to the individual sets rather than the set of elements as a whole.

The corresponding point value semantic unification will use the least prejudiced distribution to provide a probability for any fuzzy set defined over the dice values when given the value is small. Suppose we wish to know

Pr(medium | small)

where the fuzzy set medium is defined as

Medium = 2 / 0.3 + 3 / 1 + 4 / 1 + 5 / 0.3

Using the voting model to interpret this fuzzy set the mass assignment for medium is

MA medium = {3. 4} : 0.7, {2, 3, 4, 5} : 0.3

Then we will write

Pr(medium | small) = 0.7 Pr({3 or 4 | small)
+ 0.3 Pr({2 or 3 or 4 or 5} | small)
= 0.7(0.2 + 0) + 0.3(0.3 + 0.2) = 0.29

The mass assignment interpretation theory approach to fuzzy sets provides a totally different approach to fuzzy inference. It basically accepts the concept of a fuzzy set, interprets the fuzzy set using the voting model and relates inference to probability theory. This has the advantage that there is no conflict between the two types of uncertainties Fril is a logic programming type language with both probabilistic and fuzzy uncertainties allowed. The rules are conditionalised with probabilities and variables of predicates can be instantiated to fuzzy sets. Rules of inference are from probability theory. We use point semantic unification to provide the conditional probabilities of fuzzy sets in the rules when given fuzzy sets as data.

The advantage of using fuzzy sets as compared with crisp sets is that we obtain greater compression and greater accuracy. Using fuzzy sets allows for less rules to be used and interpolation effect arising from the overlapping fuzzy sets.

2.2. Fuzzy Partition

The human perception of the surrounding world requires vague concepts to cope with the large amount of information that is available. Fuzzy sets are mathematical objects which can be used to represent imprecise concepts such as those present in human language. For instance the concept of *height* can be described with a set of fuzzy labels {very short, short, medium, tall, very tall} partitioning the universe [0, 2m] of heights (see Figure 1).

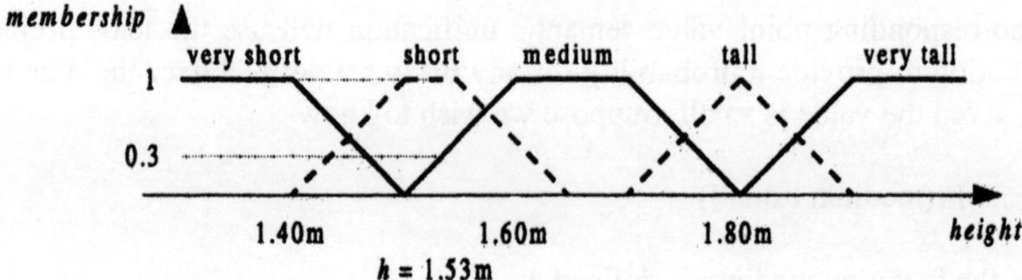

Figure 1: Fuzzy partition of height universe

The height h = 1.53m of a person can be linguistically expressed as the following fuzzy set:

$$h = \text{short} / 1 + \text{medium} / 0.3$$

defined on the discrete universe of labels for "height". The fuzzy set h means that the person is 'short' with a membership degree of 1 and 'medium' with a membership degree of 0.3. The fundamental results of mass assignment theory [2] allow us to convert the above fuzzy set into a probability distribution, namely the *least prejudiced distribution* (lpd). Therefore the least prejudiced probability representation in this case is given by:

$$\text{lpd}_h : \text{short} : 0.85 , \text{medium} : 0.15$$

Similarly to the fuzzy set h, this distribution is defined on the discrete universe of labels for "height". The values 0.85 and 0.15 express the probabilities of "short" and "medium" given the height is h, (Pr(short|h) and Pr(medium|h)), respectively.

Using fuzzy sets, rather than crisp sets, to partition the universes allows an element to belong to two neighbouring concepts, thereby favouring interpolation to take place. Moreover, such fuzzy partitions constitute a succinct means of representation, which results in data compression. Since fuzzy sets can be labelled with words, the learned model can always be interpreted linguistically in order to be more understandable.

2.3. Point Semantic Unification

The point semantic unification measures the degree of "match" between two fuzzy sets **f** and **g** provided they are defined on the same universe. By performing the conditioning operation between the mass assignments of **f** and **g** [1], the point semantic unification evaluates the conditional probability of **f** given **g**. This value, Pr(**f**|**g**), is representative of the discrimination between the two fuzzy sets; the lower the conditional probability, the better the discrimination.

Figure 2 gives an illustration of the "match" between 2 fuzzy sets. The point semantic unification gives the following values:

Pr(about_3|about_7) = 0.03
Pr(about_3|about_4) = 0.49

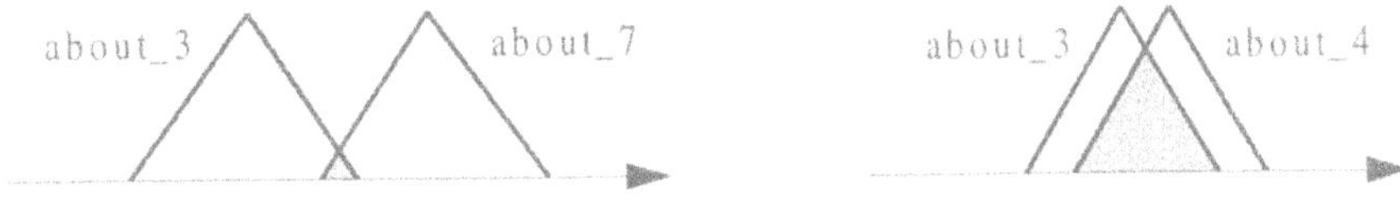

Figure 2: Point semantic unification of fuzzy sets

These values reveals that the distinction between the fuzzy sets "about_3" and "about_7" is greater than between the fuzzy sets "about_3" and "about_4". In the following methods, the point semantic unification is fundamental for distinguishing between fuzzy sets representing different classes.

2.4. Fril Extended Rules for Knowledge Representation

The learned models, in their final format, are represented by a Fril extended rule [4] associated with each class. For example the following rule uses fuzzy sets to categorise the size of a person X:

((Size of X is *large*)(general(
    ((Height of X is *medium*)(Weight of X is *heavy*))
    ((Height of X is *tall*)(Weight of X is *average*))
    ((Height of X is *very tall*)(Weight of X is *average*))
((0.7)(0.8)(1))) : ((1 1)(0 0))

This rule indicates that the probability for the head or consequent "Size of X is *large*" given the first body rule "Height of X is *medium* and Weight of X is *heavy*", $Pr(h|b_1)$, is 0.7. Similarly, the probabilities for the head given the second body rule, $Pr(h|b_2)$, and for the head given the third body rule, $Pr(h|b_3)$, are 0.8 and 1 respectively. These factors are obtained from the data at hand, using a specific calculus based on mass assignment theory. The support pair ((1 1)(0 0)) at the end of the rule represents an equivalence, in which case we can use Jeffrey's rule to calculate the probability for the combined body or antecedent and simply transmit it to the head.

Therefore, the probability for the head for a particular instance is

$$\Pr(h) = \sum_{i=1}^{3} \Pr(h \mid b_i) \Pr'(b_i) = 0.7 \Pr'(b_1) + 0.8 \Pr'(b_2) + 1 \Pr'(b_3)$$

where the probabilities $\Pr'(b_i)$ are calculated for this specific instance using the point semantic unification.

In classification problems, a Fril extended rule is formed for each class to infer class probabilities for unknown cases where the highest probability determines the class.

3. MA-FOIL

In order to model a problem domain MA-FOIL induces classification rules from a given database. Decision trees consisting of one branch only are built iteratively for each class. Such a branch, translated into a Fril rule, explains a part of the examples given for a specific class. When all examples for a class are covered we form a Fril extended rule consisting of the single branches. Using the Fril extended rules inferred for the different classes we can then classify unknown cases.

In order to compress our model and improve its performance new features for distinguishing between the classes are provided by a genetic programming algorithm [6]. Its fitness function is mainly a discrimination function computed by the point semantic unification operation originated in mass assignment theory [2].

3.1. Creation of New Features via Genetic Programming

In order to learn a good model for a given classification problem it is desirable to find attributes or features which contain a high level of information about the classes and their differences. The given features are not always the most powerful features for this purpose. Sometimes it is helpful to create new features which can then be used to describe the problem in a much easier manner than before. Hence a bigger compression and a better understanding as well as a better performance of the inferred model can be achieved. We developed a genetic programming algorithm which operates in an algebraic means in order to generate such new features. The resulting solution designates features which perform, considered separately, the highest discrimination between the classes.

An easy example for simplifying the learned model by creating a new feature is given below:

Example 1:

Lets assume we have given data points in the regular grid $[0,1]^2$ with classifications profit and loss, see Figure 3, and we want to learn rules for these classes dependent on income and outgoing.

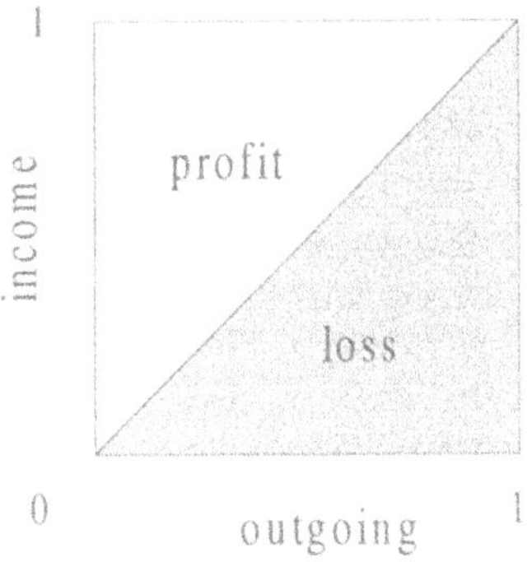

Figure 3: Profit example

Given the original features income and outgoing we can put 2 totally overlapping fuzzy labels on the universes and then infer some rules containing these concepts. But obviously the whole problem is much easier to describe if we create a new feature, namely 'income – outgoing' with 2 labels positive and negative.

The rules for both cases are shown below:

Rules profit with original features:

((profit)(general (
    ((outgoing is small)(income is large))
    ((outgoing is small)(income is small))
    ((income is large)(outgoing is large)))
((0.86) (0.53) (0.53)))):((1 1)(0 0))

((loss)(general (
    ((outgoing is large)(income is small))
    ((outgoing is large)(income is large))
    ((income is small)(outgoing is small)))
((0.83) (0.47) (0.47)))):((1 1)(0 0))

Rules profit with new feature:

((profit)(general (
    ((income – ougoing is positive)))
((1)))):((1 1)(0 0))
((loss)(general (
    ((income – outgoing is negative)))
((1)))):((1 1)(0 0))

Even though 'income – outgoing' is a combined feature it is very easy to understand, the number of clauses decreased dramatically, and the performance of the rules is much higher, indeed it now delivers 100% correctness.

Genetic Programming [6] provides a way to search the fittest solution for a problem. It is based upon the idea of the survival of the fittest found in evolution theory. At the beginning of the process an initial population is randomly generated where individuals are composed of functions and terminals appropriate to the problem domain. In our case 500 individuals are generated as algebraic combinations of the original attributes by using the operators +, - , * , / . The depth limit of the generated features is restricted to 6.

In order to generate a new generation we have to select individuals from the current population which then serve as parents for the individuals in the next population. This selections takes place proportional to a fitness function to assure the survival and creation of good individuals where the fitness function is chosen according to the considered problem domain. Our goal is to receive attributes that are good discriminators between the classes. Therefore the chosen fitness function consists mainly of a discrimination function. In order to keep the features fairly understandable we also included a dimension function which makes sure that short features are preferred to long ones if the discrimination is the same

$$\text{Fitness}(\text{Att}) = w_{discr} * \text{Discrimination}(\text{Att}) + w_{dim} * \text{Dimension}(\text{Att})$$

where w_{discr} and w_{dim} add up to 1. Preferable the weight w_{discr} lies in the interval [0.7,1], while w_{dim} lies in [0,0.3].

Discrimination:

The point semantic unification [1] provides an easy method to calculate a value describing the discrimination ability of an attribute relative to the classes. For this purpose we have to form fuzzy sets on the attribute universe where each fuzzy set represents a class in question. We achieve this simply by plotting the membership degree of a data point p_i for a specific class C_k to the membership degree of the attribute value v_i, calculated for this data point, for the fuzzy set representing this class on the attribute universe, $(\mathbf{F}_{Ck})_{Att}$.

$$\mu_{(\mathbf{F}_{C_k})_{Att}}(v_i) := \mu_{C_k}(p_i)$$

If the same value is received from more than one data point we take the average membership degree for this value. More explicitly,

$$(\mathbf{F}_{C_k})_{Att} = \sum_{v_i} v_i / \bar{\mu}_{(\mathbf{F}_{C_k})_{Att}}(v_i)$$

where $\bar{\mu}_{(\mathbf{F}_{C_k})_{Att}}(v_i)$ is the average membership for v_i

Example 2:

Take for instance the small database shown in Table 1 consisting of 9 data points. The x- and y-value as well as the class value are given.

Table 1 : Database for forming fuzzy sets

Index	x	y	class
1	1	1	good
2	1	2	good
3	1	3	bad
4	2	1	bad
5	2	2	bad
6	2	3	bad
7	3	1	bad
8	3	2	good
9	3	3	good

Let us now assume the genetic programming algorithm generated a new attribute, namely x+y. In Table 2 one can see the calculated values for this new feature and the membership degrees for both classes. In this case we have two class labels 'good' and 'bad' which can be represented as two discrete fuzzy sets, namely good/1 and bad/1. Hence a data point labelled good has a membership degree $\mu_{good}=1$ in the fuzzy set good/1 and a membership degree $\mu_{bad}=0$ in the fuzzy set bad/1.

Table 2: New attribute values and class membership degrees

Index	x+y	μ_{good}	μ_{bad}
1	2	1	0
2	3	1	0
3	4	0	1
4	3	0	1
5	4	0	1
6	5	0	1
7	4	0	1
8	5	1	0
9	6	1	0

As one can see, the values 3, 4 and 5 occur more often with different membership degrees for the class labels. Table 3 now shows the resulting average membership degrees we use to form the two discrete fuzzy sets, $(\mathbf{F}_{good})_{x+y}$ and $(\mathbf{F}_{bad})_{x+y}$, on the universe of x+y, which represent the classes good and bad respectively. An illustration of these is given in Figure 4.

Table 3: Average membership

x+y	number	average μ_{good}	average μ_{bad}
2	1	1	0
3	2	1/2	1/2
4	3	0	1
5	2	1/2	1/2
6	1	1	0

The reason for taking the average membership degree for a specific attribute value is that we want to take the information from each data point leading to that value into account to the same degree. All these data points are treated with the same importance. If we would take the maximum degree just a few or one data point delivers the resulting membership degree which is a poorer representation of the present situation.

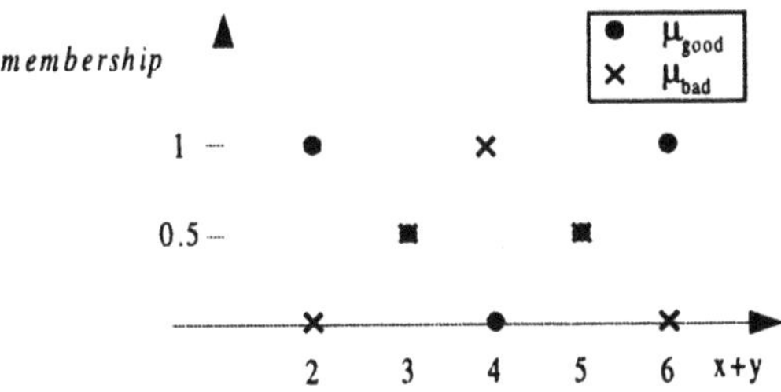

Figure 4: Fuzzy partition of height universe

If the universe of the considered attribute is continuous we connect the calculated membership degrees to continuous fuzzy sets. The so formed the fuzzy sets are then normalised.

When dealing with large databases and complicated features it can happen that the formed fuzzy sets oscillate a lot. Keeping fuzzy that of this kind would reduce the transparency of the inferred model to an enormous amount. It also decreases the generalisation abilities of the considered attribute when presented with unseen cases. In order to avoid this disadvantages keep the process as simple as possible and provide a reasonable generalisation we involved a smoothing option for the fuzzy sets. If the gap between two peaks on the output space is smaller than the length of the universe multiplied by a smoothing parameter, we join these peaks together to one peak. The smoothing parameter depends on the interest of the user for transparency as well as on the generalisation ability. With respect to the later the parameter can be optimised by comparing the results for different parameters achieved for a training and a control set.

We can now use the point semantic unification provided by mass assignment theory to match the resulting fuzzy sets representing the different classes. The discrimination for an attribute Att is calculated as:

$$\text{Discrimination(Att)} = \max_{i \neq j} \quad \{1 - \Pr((\mathbf{F}_{C_i})_{\text{Att}} \mid (\mathbf{F}_{C_j})_{\text{Att}})\}$$

and delivers values in the interval [0,1]. The lower the match between the fuzzy sets, the higher the discrimination and the better the feature. The maximum over the different directions corresponds to the view that an attribute is important even if it is just a good discriminator between two of the classes. It does not have to discriminate well between all given classes. This is of course just the case if we consider problems with more than two possible classifications. This attitude corresponds to our rule inducing algorithm MA-FOIL which can use different attributes to describe different classes. Not each attribute has the same importance for each class.

Dimension:

If the features become too complex we are not able to understand or interpret them any more. Hence we included a dimension function which associates high values with short features and low values with long features, i.e. long features are punished. This value is calculated as the membership degree of the depth of the considered attribute in the fuzzy set shown in Figure 5.

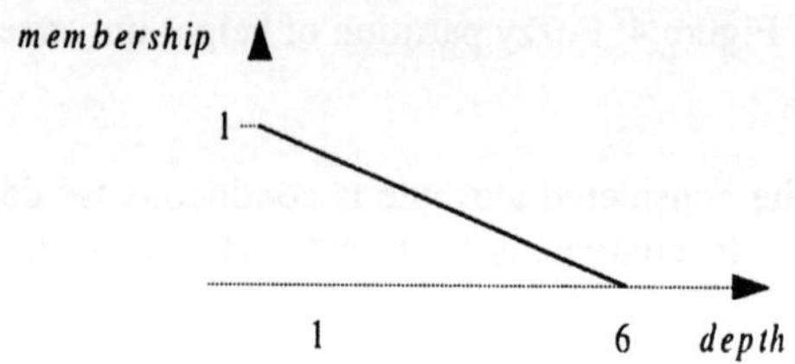

Figure 5: Dimension function

Hence the values for the dimension function lie also in the interval [0,1].

After selecting the parents from the current generation proportional to the above described fitness function we can now obtain a new generation by using the reproduction and crossover operators. The reproduction operator operates on only one individual in the current population and produces only one individual/offspring in the next generation. The selected parent is copied, without alteration, from the current population into the new population. The crossover operation creates variation in the population by producing new offspring that consists of parts taken from each parent. Once two individuals are selected a point/node in each individual is chosen randomly (independently) using a uniform distribution, to be the crossover point for that individual. These individual points/nodes correspond to the root of the exchange tree fragments and their locations to the insertion points. The first offspring is produced by deleting the crossover tree fragment of the first parent and then inserting the crossover tree fragment of the second parent at the crossover point of the first parent. The second offspring is produced in a similar manner. The depth limit for producing new offspring is restricted to 12.

The process of selecting parents and producing a new generation is repeated 51 times. At the end of the last iteration the best-so-far solution and the best solutions from the last generation are designated as solutions. These new features are then used as background knowledge when inferring the rules that build a model for the problem domain. Together with the fuzzy sets on their universes the new features are transferred to the rule extraction algorithm.

3.2. Rule Extraction with MA-FOIL

Given a classification problem, our goal is to learn a model for this problem which consists of Fril rules describing each class. MA-FOIL now infers rules from the given examples and some additional background knowledge.

In order to get the most advantages from the original, simpler, features and the new features found by the genetic programming algorithm as good discriminators between the classes, we just add the new features together with the fuzzy sets on their universes as background knowledge to the knowledge base. We even hope to find combinations of features, connected by 'and', which describe the classes more successfully than the original or the new features on their own. For the original features fuzzy sets on their universes are formed in the same way than described above, where the smoothing parameter must be chosen to be the same as in the genetic programming algorithm. In the following the fuzzy sets on the feature spaces are treated as labels or concepts.

There already exists a decision tree algorithm for classification problems which includes uncertainties, namely MA-ID3 [5]. This algorithm deals with all examples at one time and induces complex decision trees which explain all classes using the same branches and hence the same concepts. The only differences are different supports for different classes at the end of a branch. But it is possible that distinct concepts have a different impact for describing various classes. Hence we wish to use different concepts for the description of each class. This results in shorter and less rules which makes the inferred model easier to understand and increases its transparency.

Example 3:

Lets assume we want to describe a database which can be illustrated with Figure 6.

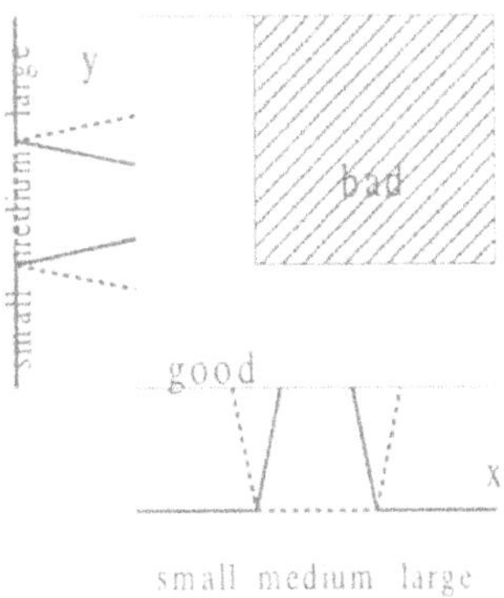

Figure 6: Illustration of MA-FOIL idea

MA-ID3 finds a decision tree consisting of 9 branches in order to describe all data. For each class a Fril extended rule is formed consisting of these 9 branches and the respective supports for this class.

But as one can easily verify, not all this branches are needed to describe good or bad data points.

Here we are aiming for two branches describing 'good' and four branches describing 'bad', namely

good:	x is small	bad:	x is medium and y is medium
	y is small		x is medium and y is large
			x is large and y is medium
			x is large and y is large

In order to receive different branches for the various classes we have to find a description for each class separately. Also we want to achieve a collection of single branches in opposite to complex trees in order to be able to begin a new branch with a different attribute and hence to reduce the complexity of the model.

The idea to built branches iteratively that, translated into clauses 'head if body', explain a part of the given examples originates in the inductive logic programming algorithm FOIL [8,9]. Here we deal with a two valued logic and crisp concepts, which results in a yes or no decision for examples to belong to a concept. Given are examples for a target concept and some background knowledge consisting of attributes that can be used to describe the target concept. FOIL searches from general to specific, i.e. when building a branch it starts with the most general clause (the head or target relation is true) and then specifies by adding literals/concepts to the body of the clause. The selection of such a concept is based upon the information gain or entropy. FOIL stops adding literals to the body when no more negative examples are covered by the built branch (consistency). With the remaining positive examples and all negative examples it repeats to build branches in the same manner as before. When all positive examples are explained (completeness), the algorithm terminates and the learned branches build the description of the examples.

Including uncertainties in form of fuzzy sets and probabilities requires to change this idea in a few aspects. First of all we do not have crisp concepts but in our case the concepts are fuzzy sets on the attribute universes. Hence we do not have positive and negative examples for a target concept, but the data points belong to different class labels with membership degrees between zero and one. This is also true for all given attributes. Therefore we cannot run the algorithm by distinguishing between the two values yes and no, but we run it by using probabilities. For this purpose all attribute values x_i of a data point $\langle x_1,\ldots,x_n\rangle$ are represented as fuzzy sets on the labels or concepts, $\mathbf{f_{ij}}$, on the attribute universes:

$$x_i = \sum_{j=1}^{m} \mathbf{f}_{ij} / \mu_{\mathbf{f}_{ij}}(x_i)$$

where $\mu_{\mathbf{f}_{ij}}(x_i)$ is the membership degree of x_i in $\mathbf{f}_{ij}$

Using mass assignment theory [2], this fuzzy set is then converted into a least prejudiced probability distribution:

$$\mathrm{lpd}_{x_i}: \quad \mathbf{f}_{i1} : \mathrm{lpd}_{x_i}(\mathbf{f}_{i1}), \quad \mathbf{f}_{i2} : \mathrm{lpd}_{x_i}(\mathbf{f}_{i2}), \quad \ldots \quad \mathbf{f}_{im} : \mathrm{lpd}_{x_i}(\mathbf{f}_{im})$$

We also attach a support S to the end of every branch which is evaluated using a specific calculus based on mass assignment theory.

A branch can then be translated into a Fril rule:

((head)(body)):S

and we can interpret this as the conditional probability Pr(head|body)=S.

Since we want to find descriptions for each class independently MA-FOIL repeats the rule finding part for each class separately. Considering a specific class C_k we just take the data points into account which belong to this class with a positive membership degree. Similar to FOIL, branches which explain a part of the examples are generated iteratively until all examples are explained. When building a branch we start with the most general rule $((C_k)) : (0\ 1)$, which expresses that the probability for class C_k lies in the interval [0,1], and then specify by adding concepts to the body of the rule. Omitting the other classes we cannot use the entropy any longer to select concepts which should be added to a branch. Hence a weight for the selecting purpose was introduced which describes the importance a concept has in respect to the considered data points. It compares the sum of the probabilities that the data points lie in the branch (including the new concept) as well as in the considered class. Because we do not have negative examples which indicate when we should stop adding literals to a branch, there is a need for another stopping criterion. If the support attached at the end of a branch exceeds a predefined threshold, i.e. the probability for the class under consideration is big enough, we stop adding literals to the body of the rule. The next branch is then built with the remaining proportions of the given examples, i.e. we subtract the explained part of the examples form our local training set. The remaining probability of a data point p for the class C_k, which is still to be explained, is therefore calculated as:

$$\mathrm{Pr}_{rest,p}(C_k) = \mathrm{Pr}_{old,p}(C_k) - \mathrm{Pr}_p(\mathrm{branch}) * \mathrm{lpd}_p(C_k)$$

These updated probabilities build the local training set for generating the next branch.

Like FOIL we stop building branches for a class when all examples for this class are explained, i.e. $Pr_{rest,p}(C_k) = 0$ for all p.
Because we are dealing with uncertainties in the rules and the examples belong to the concepts with certain degrees between zero and 1, we cannot connect the branches learned for a class as easy as in pure logic where an 'or' connection is chosen. In our case a Fril extended rule connects the single branches and is used to classify unknown cases.

An overall illustration of the rule extraction is given below.

Algorithm for rule extraction with MA-FOIL:

- Represent attribute values as fuzzy sets on the labels on the attribute universes
- Convert fuzzy set representations into least prejudiced probability distributions
- Repeat for all classes C_k, k=1,...,n:

1. Build local training set consisting of data points with $lpd(C_k)>0$
2. Built branch that explain part of the examples:
   a) Start with most general rule $((C_k)):(0\ 1)$
   b) Calculate weights of importance for all possible concepts
   c) Add concept with highest weight to the branch and calculate support S
   d) Stop if S big enough or no attributes left;
      Else discard used attribute and go to ii)
3. Update local training set
4. Stop if all examples are explained
   Else go to 2.
5. Combine all learned branches in a Fril extended rule for class C_k
6. Increase k to k+1, i.e. consider next class, and go to 1.

4. Semantic Discrimination Analysis for Feature Selection

In order to reduce the dimensionality of large databases, feature selection methods have often been used to discard redundant and irrelevant features before the machine learning stage. In this section, we introduce *a semantic discrimination analysis* to select the best subsets of n ($n < N$) features for distinguishing target concepts.

The method relies on the semantic unification of multidimensional fuzzy sets that are representative of each class and that are formed with the cross product space approach. Once these subsets have been selected, Fril extended rules can be generated with respect to these, capturing thereby the correlations between the features constituting the subsets.

4.1. Cross Product Space Approach

The cross product space approach provides an algorithm for extracting multidimensional fuzzy sets, i.e. Cartesian granule fuzzy sets, from numerical data using the theory of mass assignments [2]. In this section, we describe the method in parallel with a illustrative example.

Consider a database defined on n features F_i , $i \in \{1,\ldots,n\}$, where each vector $x = \langle x_1,\ldots,x_n \rangle$ present in the database belongs to one of the classes C_k , $k \in \{1,\ldots,K\}$. First a Cartesian granule space is built for each class C_k. For this purpose, the universes Ω_i of features F_i are partitioned with the fuzzy partitions P_i as previously explained (see Section 2.1). Then, the Cartesian granule space is the discrete universe drawn from the cross product of the fuzzy sets constituting each partition P_i. Hence a Cartesian granule is defined as the concatenation of n individual fuzzy sets, each one of them coming from a partition P_i.

The number of Cartesian granules in the Cartesian granule space depends on the number of features (n) and the granularity of the partitions P_i, i.e. the number of fuzzy sets present in the partitions. Consequently, if the partitions P_i are composed of m_i fuzzy sets, $i \in \{1,\ldots,n\}$, then there will be $D = m_1 \times m_2 \times \ldots \times m_n$ Cartesian granules in the Cartesian granule space built on the n features.

Example:

Suppose that we are given a database of individuals' *height* and *weight*. Their sizes are then classified as "small", "medium" or "large". The universes of the features *height* and *weight* are partitioned by the partitions P_1 = {very short, short, medium, tall, very tall} and P_2 = {light, average, heavy} respectively, as represented in Figure 7.

The Cartesian granule space would then consist of $D = 3 \times 5 = 15$ Cartesian granules. At the intersection of any fuzzy sets, such as *average* and *short* from each partition of the universes of *height* and *weight*, a Cartesian granule such as "*average* $\times$ *short*" can be found.

When a vector $x = \langle x_1,\ldots,x_n\rangle$ of class C_k is considered, its components x_i can be linguistically expressed with the fuzzy sets $\mathbf{f}_{ij}$, $j = \{1,\ldots,m\}$ which partition the universes of the features F_i. More explicitly,

$$x_i = \sum_{j=1}^{m} \mathbf{f}_{ij} / \mu_{\mathbf{f}_{ij}}(x_i)$$

where $\mu_{\mathbf{f}_{ij}}(x_i)$ *is the membership value of* x_i *in* $\mathbf{f}_{ij}$

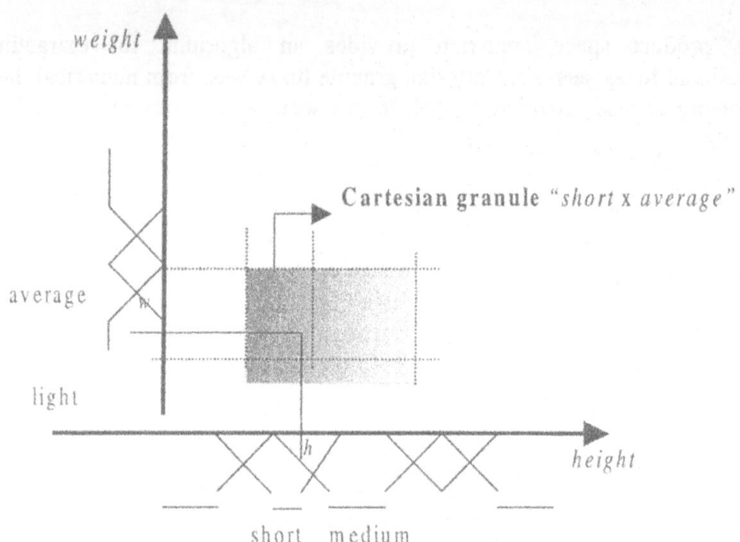

Figure 7: An example of a partially drawn Cartesian granule space built on the features *height* and *weight.*

As previously seen, this fuzzy set can be converted into a probability distribution (*lpd*) which attributes a probability to every $\mathbf{f}_{ij}$, $j = \{1,\ldots,m\}$, given the value x_i:

$$lpd_{x_i}: \quad \mathbf{f}_{i1} : lpd_{x_i}(\mathbf{f}_{i1}), \quad \mathbf{f}_{i2} : lpd_{x_i}(\mathbf{f}_{i2}), \quad \ldots \quad \mathbf{f}_{im} : lpd_{x_i}(\mathbf{f}_{im})$$

In our example, consider an individual x whose height and weight are h=1.53m and w=58 Kg respectively (see Figure 7). Then, the components h and w can be linguistically expressed as follows:

h = short/1 + medium/0.3
w = light/0.4 + average/0.6

Both fuzzy sets can be converted into two least probability distributions, lpd_h and lpd_w respectively, by working on mass assignments [2]. These probability distributions are discrete since they are defined on the fuzzy sets partitioning the universes of *height* and *weight.*

Therefore:

$$\mathrm{lpd_h(short)} = 0.85 \quad \mathrm{lpd_h(medium)} = 0.15$$
$$\mathrm{lpd_w(light)} = 0.4 \quad \mathrm{lpd_w(average)} = 0.6$$

At this point, we introduce a *counting procedure*, based on mass assignment theory [2], which is adapted to fuzzy partitions in order to deal with the information brought by the individual x whose size is "small". As a result, in the Cartesian granule space associated with class "small", the Cartesian granules "*short*× *light*", "*short*× *average*", "*medium*× *light*" and "*medium*× *average*" would be affected by the data records of x as follows:

- The Cartesian granule "*short*× *light*" would receive the value of $0.85 * 0.4 = 0.34$
- The Cartesian granule "*short*× *average*" would receive the value of $0.85*0.6 = 0.51$
- The Cartesian granule "*medium*× *light*" would receive the value of $0.15 * 0.4 = 0.06$
- The Cartesian granule "*medium*× *average*" would receive the value of $0.15 * 0.6 = 0.09$

As illustrated in Figure 7 by the grey scale, the Cartesian granules "*short*× *light*" and "*short*× *average*" are more affected by the values of h and w than the other Cartesian granules. If crisp sets were used to partition the universes of discourse, then only one Cartesian granule would be affected, eradicating thereby all interpolation effects. When another individual of class "small" is considered, the same counting procedure applies, the results of which are added to the previous amounts associated with each Cartesian granule. Thus a data point affects more than one Cartesian granule due to the counting procedure and the use of fuzzy sets instead of crisp sets for partitioning the universes. This has a direct consequence regarding the smoothness in the representation of the data under consideration. By gathering all the information brought by individual cases belonging to a same class in one Cartesian granule space defined by a few Cartesian granules, data compression is also taking place.

After considering all vectors of class C_k present in the database, we obtain a discrete frequency distribution over the Cartesian granule space. This frequency distribution can be turned into a discrete probability distribution should we divide the values associated with each Cartesian granule by the total number of vectors belonging to class C_k. Regarding this probability distribution as the *least prejudiced distribution*, we can extract a discrete fuzzy set for class C_k, denoted here by $(\mathbf{F}_{Ck})_{Sn}$, defined on the cross product space of the *n* features (forming the subset S_n) under consideration. In the above example, the fuzzy set $(\mathbf{F}_{small})_{S2}$ with S2 being the subset {*height, weight*} would have for members the Cartesian granules "*short× light*", "*short× average*" , "*medium × light*" , "*medium× average*", "*tall × heavy*", etc.

4.2. Semantic Discrimination Analysis

Using the point semantic unification, the conditional probabilities $Pr(\mathbf{F}_{Ck}| \mathbf{F}_{Ck'})_{Sn}$ and $Pr(\mathbf{F}_{Ck'}| \mathbf{F}_{Ck})_{Sn}$ can be evaluated for the fuzzy sets $(\mathbf{F}_{Ck})_{Sn}$ and $(\mathbf{F}_{Ck'})_{Sn}$, $k=\{1,\ldots,K\}$, $k'=\{1,\ldots,K\}$ with $k\neq k'$.

Then the value $(p_k)_{Sn}$ is calculated as follows:

$$(p_k)_{S_n} = \frac{1}{K-1} \sum_{k'=1,k'\neq k}^{K} \Pr(\mathbf{F}_{C_k} | \mathbf{F}_{C_{k'}})_{S_n}$$

This value is used to determine the ability of the subset S_n to distinguish the class C_k from the other classes. Consequently, the subsets S_n for which $(p_k)_{Sn}$ are small, contain the *n* features according to which the data points belonging to class C_k can be distinguished from the data points belonging to other classes. Similarly, if $(p_{k'})_{Sn}$ is relatively small, then the subset S_n is also a subset to consider in order to find the data points belonging to class $C_{k'}$.

4.3.Selection of the Best n-feature Subsets for Class C_k

The subsets of *n* features amongst the *N* original fields are selected through a procedure that is detailed in the following. Initially, the subsets contain one feature ($i=1$) and they become subsets of 2 features after one cycle of the flow diagram (see Figure 8).

The process is repeated for all $i=\{1,\ldots,n\}$, if *n* features are wanted in the final subsets. For all subsets S_i containing *i* features, the fuzzy sets $(\mathbf{F}_{Ck})_{Si}$ are generated. By evaluating the $(p_k)_{Si}$, the best *i-feature* subsets S_i' are selected for class C_k. Subsets of $i+m$ features ($m = 1,\ldots,i$) are formed by taking the union of S_i' with one another. For example, the union of the subsets {*Att1 Att2 Att3*} and {*Att1 Att3 Att4*} would produce the subset {*Att1 Att2 Att3 Att4*}. Amongst the newly formed subsets, those possessing $i+1$ features becomes the new S_i in the flow diagram (see Figure 8). On the other hand, those possessing $i+m$ features, $m = \{2,\ldots,i\}$, are retained for the cycle in which the subsets of $i+m$ features are to be selected. The selection of the best subsets S_i' out of the subsets S_i is done according to two criteria: (i) the value $(p_k)_{Si}$ must be relatively small, and (ii) it is also desirable to retain as many different features as possible in the selected subsets.

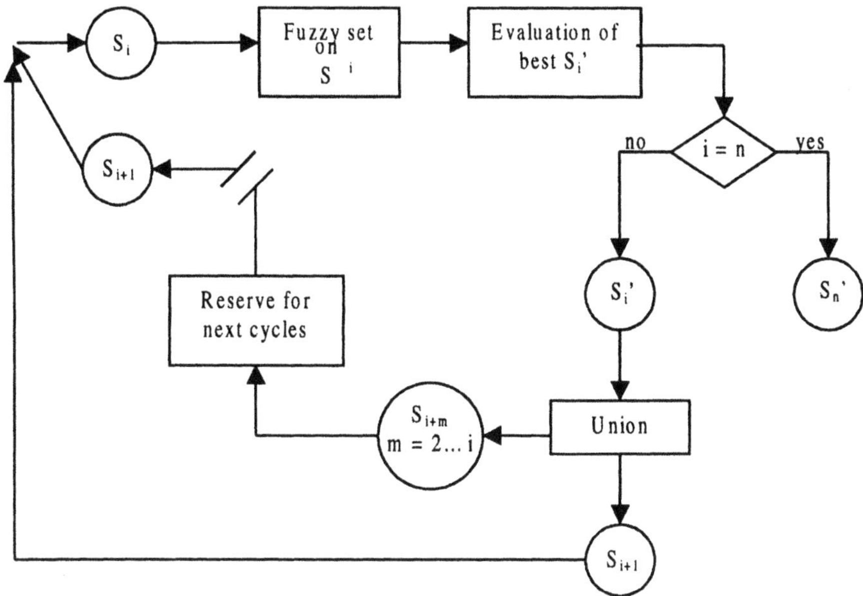

Figure 8: Flow diagram representing the selection of subsets of n features

4.4. Forming Fril Extended Rules on the Selected Subsets

After selecting the best subsets for classifying the data, these can be used to generate classification rules. Here, such rules are Fril extended rules acting as linguistic interpretation of a Cartesian granule space built on the selected subsets. There is one Fril extended rule for every class present in the database, where each clause in the body of the rule expresses linguistically a Cartesian granule. In the above example, the format of such a rule would be for class "small" as follows:

((Size of X is *small*)(general(
  ((Height of X is *short*)(Weight of X is *light*))
  ((Height of X is *short*)(Weight of X is *average*))
  ...
  ((Height of X is *tall*)(Weight of X is *light*))
  ((0.8)(0.7)...(0.4))) : ((1 1)(0 0))

The probabilities at the bottom of the rule indicates the relevance of each Cartesian granule as expressed by the clauses in the body of the rule. Here, we mention briefly how these probabilities are extracted from the data. In section 4.1, we explained how to build a Cartesian granule space on n features for a particular class C_k. With the counting procedure repeated for all the elements belonging to C_k, followed by a normalisation procedure, the Cartesian granules (CG_d, $d=1,\ldots,D$) are associated with a probability, $\Pr(CG_d|C_k)$. In other words, the process of building a discrete probability distribution on the Cartesian granule space for C_k relies on the fact that we know the class of each element in the training set. However, in the Fril extended rule formed for class C_k , the conditional probabilities that are required are $\Pr(C_k|CG_d)$, with $d=1,\ldots,D$. That is why Bayes' theorem is introduced here:

$$\Pr(C_k \mid CG_d) = \frac{\Pr(CG_d \mid C_k) \times \Pr(C_k)}{\Pr(CG_d)}$$

Furthermore, the theorem of total probabilities allows us to write that

$$\Pr(CG_d) = \sum_{k=1}^{K} \Pr(CG_d \mid C_k) \times \Pr(C_k)$$

It is therefore possible to obtain the conditional probabilities governing the Fril extended rules generated for each class present in the database. When an element of unknown class is presented, its data records are matched with the rules in order to infer a probability for each class. The higher probability determines the class the element belongs to.

5. The Wisconsin Breast Cancer Database

In medicine, increasingly advanced technological means of measurement help to retrieve large amounts of information from living organs. For instance, breast cells can now be analysed with high precision regarding their shape and texture. In the 1980s, Dr. Wolberg desired to accurately diagnose breast masses based solely on the analysis of a Fine Needle Aspiration (FNA). He identified 9 visually assessed characteristics of an FNA sample which he considered relevant to diagnosis. Good classification performances based on these characteristics can be obtained [7]: with a training dataset twice the size of the test set, Bennett and Mangasarian obtained 97% and 97.4% of well classified diagnoses on the training and test sets respectively.

Later the Wisconsin Breast Cancer database [10,11] was formed by gathering 569 digitized images of fine needle aspirates of breast masses. In this database, each image represents a group of cell nuclei described by 10 real-valued parameters. Since the mean, standard error and largest (i.e. the mean of the three largest values) of these parameters were computed for every image, a database consisting of 30 features was generated and we decided to number the features from 1 to 30 (see Table 4). Amongst the diagnoses present in the database, 357 were benign and 212 were malignant. The database was divided into a training set and a test set of 400 and 169 cases respectively such that the proportion of benign and malignant cases is the same in both sets.

Table 4: The 30 parameters describing an image of a fine needle aspirate of a breast mass.

Feature	Mean	Standard error	Largest
Radius	1	11	21
Texture	2	12	22
Perimeter	3	13	23
Area	4	14	24
Smoothness	5	15	25
Compactness	6	16	26
Concavity	7	17	27
Concave points	8	18	28
Symmetry	9	19	29
Fractal dimension	10	20	30

Table 5: Results of classification on the Wisconsin Breast Cancer database

Method	Features in use	Training set	Test set
MA-FOIL	Best created features	88.8%	82.8%
MA-FOIL	Created and original features	98.8%	91.1%
FER on Subsets	{8,22,23}	97.3%	92.9%
FER on Subsets	{14,24,28}	95.6%	94.1%
PCA	First 3 components	92.8%	91.7%

6. Results and Discussion

In this section the results of classification obtained with the above described methods on the Wisconsin Breast Cancer database are presented in Table 5. To restrict the complexity of the learned models, the depth of the Fril extended rules (FER) is limited to three concepts per body rule.

The MA-FOIL algorithms, applied to this database, finds four new features for which the fitness function delivers high values. Generally these are products of two original features and therefore easy to understand. When these features are used to extract the rules four branches are built for each class, "benign" and "malignant" exploiting all features. The results of classification achieved with these rules are displayed in the first row of Table 5.

Adding the created features to the original features results in three branches for describing the class "benign", while six branches are needed for the class "malignant". In the learned rules eleven of the original features are used in addition to the created features. This leads to a neat improvement in the results of classification as shown in second row of Table 5.

Genetic programming enlarges the choice of features for the rule extracting technique by creating new ones, which often leads to better results. In some cases the genetic programming algorithm even produces the ideal feature which can be used on its own to describe the database.

The semantic discrimination analysis allowed us to select the best 3-feature subsets to categorise the "benign" and "malignant" diagnoses present in the Wisconsin Breast Cancer database. The best subset found for class "benign" consists of features numbered 8, 22 and 23 according to Table.4 while the best subset found for class "malignant" consists of features numbered 14, 24 and 28. This method does not generate new features but aims at finding features that are correlated in such a fashion that they significantly contribute in the categorisation of a diagnosis. From the expert point of view, the semantic discrimination analysis can help to identify patterns that were hidden in the original data. When Fril extended rules are built on the selected subsets of features, the curse of dimensionality problem, which occurs when too many features are used, is avoided. The classification performances that are achieved with such rules are displayed in the third and fourth rows of Table 5.

For comparison, the Principal Component Analysis was also applied to the Wisconsin Breast Cancer database to find the best three features capturing the variance in the data. These features are linear combinations of the original features and are generally much more complicated than those produced by the genetic programming algorithm used in MA-FOIL. In addition to being more transparent, the models built on the features found by the mass assignment methods give comparable, if not better, results of classification than those obtained with the model built on the principal components.

MA-FOIL produces very simple rules with very few branches, but they contain more features than the rules formed after semantic discrimination analysis. On the other hand the latter rules built on the selected subset of features contain more body rules than those produced by MA-FOIL. Since the results of classification are similarly satisfactory in both cases, the expert is left with the choice of either very simple rules or rules based on very few attributes.

References

[1] Baldwin JF (1987) Support Logic Programming. In: A.I. *et al* (eds) Fuzzy Sets – Theory and Applications. Reidel, Dordrecht-Boston, pp 133-151

[2] Baldwin JF (1991) A Theory of Mass Assignments for Artificial Intelligence. Lecture Notes in Artificial Intelligence 833:22-34

[5] Baldwin JF, Martin TP, Pilsworth BW (1988) Fril Manual. Fril Systems Ltd., Bristol, BS8 1QX, UK

[3] Baldwin JF, Martin TP, Pilsworth BW (1995) Fril – Fuzzy and Evidential Reasoning in Artificial Intelligence. Research Studies Press Ltd

[4] Baldwin JF, Lawry J, Martin TP (1998) Mass Assignment Based Induction of Decision Trees on Words. In: Proceedings IPMU, Paris, France, pp 524-531

[7] Koza JR (1998) Genetic Programming, On the Programming of Computers by Means of Natural Selection. A Bradford Book, The MIT Press

[6] Mangasarian OL, Bennett KP (1989) Robust Linear Programming Discrimination of Two Linearly Inseparable Sets.Optimization Methods and Software 1:23-34

[8] Quinlan JR (1990) Learning logical definitions from relations. Machine Learning, 5(3):239-266

[9] Quinlan JR, Cameron-Jones RM (1995) Induction of Logic Programs: Foil and Related Systems. New Generation Computing, Special Issue on ILP 13:287-312

[10]Wolberg WH, Tanner MS, Loh WY (1988) Diagnosis Schemes for Fine Needle Aspirates of Breast Masses. Analytical and Quantitative Cytology and Histology 10:225-228

[11]Wolberg WH, Street WN, Heisey DM, Mangasarian OL (1995) Computer-derived Nuclear Features Distinguish Malignant from Benign Breat Cytology. Human Pathology 26:792-796

Acquisition of Fuzzy Association Rules from Medical Data

Miguel Delgado, Daniel Sánchez, and Maria-Amparo Vila

Department of Computer Science and Artificial Intelligence
University of Granada
Avda. Andalucía 38
18071 Granada, Spain

1 Introduction

Association rules are one of the best studied models for knowledge acquisition in the field of Data Mining. Many papers regarding algorithms, measures and related problems can be found in the literature. A brief summary of the main works (to our knowledge) in this area can be found in the references of this paper.

During the last years there has been an increasing interest in finding association rules among values of quantitative attributes in relational databases [21,28], as this kind of attributes are rather frequent. Quantitative values introduce several problems in the process of mining association rules, such as an increment in the complexity of the algorithms [22]. Approaches for solving the problem are based on clustering the values in order to reduce the granularity. The first algorithms [21,28] perform a partition of the domain of the quantitative attributes, and then they find association rules among the intervals. However, crisp clusters introduce some problems related to the sharp boundaries between them.

Recently a new approach, fuzzy association rules, has arisen as the best solution for this problem [3,8]. In this approach, the granularity is reduced by means of a set of linguistic labels represented by fuzzy sets over the domain of the attribute. These rules are more comprehensible for humans, as they are based on the same linguistic terms we use in conversation and reasoning. In this paper we propose new measures of the accuracy and importance of fuzzy association rules, and we show they are appropriate for the acquisition of knowledge in large medical databases. The paper is organized as follows. In section 2 we introduce the concepts related to association rules in relational databases, and we describe the problem of finding quantitative association rules. Section 3 is devoted to the definition of fuzzy association rule. In section 4 we describe our new measures of accuracy and usefulness. In section 5 we show the experiments we have performed on large medical databases. Finally, section 6 contains our conclusions and future research avenues in this area.

2 Association Rules

Association rules were introduced in the field of Data Mining by Agrawal, Imielinsky and Swami in [1]. These rules relate the presence of sets of items (called "itemsets") in transactions, each transaction being a set of items. Association rules were first studied in market basket data, where each basket is a transaction containing the set of items bought by a client. One example of such rules is "everybody that buy bread buy milk", usually noted as $bread \Rightarrow milk$. This rule relate the presence of bread with the presence of milk in a market basket. However, the concepts of item and transaction can be considered as abstract concepts, that can be identified with distinct objects depending on the kind of associations we are looking for in data. An application of this idea to the discovery of functional dependencies with exceptions (usually called approximate dependencies) has been proposed in [5].

When mining rules from data it is important to measure both the accuracy and the usefulness of the rules, that is to say, the accomplishment degree and the amount of data supporting the rule respectively. The usual measures of accuracy and usefulness of association rules are called *confidence* and *support* respectively, and they are based on the concept of support of an itemset, defined as the percentage of transactions containing the itemset. Let I be a set of items, let T be a set of transactions containing items of I, and let $I_1, I_2 \subseteq I$ with $I_1 \cap I_2 = \emptyset$. We note the support of an itemset I_k as $supp(I_k)$. Then, the support of the association rule $I_1 \Rightarrow I_2$ is

$$Supp(I_1 \Rightarrow I_2) = supp(I_1 \cup I_2) \tag{1}$$

and its confidence is

$$Conf(I_1 \Rightarrow I_2) = \frac{supp(I_1 \cup I_2)}{supp(I_1)} \tag{2}$$

An association rule is considered to be interesting when both its support and its confidence are greater than two user-defined thresholds called *minsupp* and *minconf* respectively. In that case, the rule is said to be an *strong rule*.

Finding such strong association rules is known as the *Boolean Association Rules Problem* (BARP). Algorithms designed to perform this task work usually in two steps. In a first step a set of itemsets with support above *minsupp* is obtained by exploring the lattice of the itemsets with respect to set inclusion. Such itemsets are called *large itemsets* or *frequent itemsets* in the literature. In the second step, starting from the large itemsets and their support, a set of association rules and their confidence is obtained, and the strong rules are reported as the final result. The first step, finding large itemsets, is the most computationally expensive because of the big amount of itemsets it must deal with. This fact has motivated the development of new algorithms in order to improve the efficiency of the search with respect to previous ones. All of them use the support to bound the search in the lattice of the itemsets, thus reducing the searching time. Some "classical" algorithms are *AIS* [1], *Apriori* and *AprioriTid* [2], *SETM* [7], *OCD* [11] and *DHP* [13]. In subsequent years, other approaches for designing more efficient algorithms have been proposed, see for example [9,14,15,17,18,24,23,27].

2.1 Association Rules in Relational Databases

We begin this section introducing some of the basic concepts of relational databases. A more detailed description can be found for example in [10]. Roughly speaking, a relational database is a collection of data structured in tables, also called relations. Every relation contains the description of a set of objects of the same type. For every relation, each column is an attribute used in the description, while each row, also called tuple, contains the description of one object. Each attribute A takes values in an associated domain $Dom(A)$. The cell defined by a tuple t and a column A contains the value of the attribute A for the object described in the tuple t, usually noted as $t[A]$. A set of attributes is called a *relational scheme.* A relation is said to be an instance of a relational scheme.

Association rules in relational databases relate the presence of values of some attributes with values of some other attributes in the same tuple. More formally, let $ER = \{(A_1, \ldots, A_m)\}$ be a relational scheme and let r be an instance of ER.

Definition 1. We introduce the set of items associated to ER to be

$$I^{ER} = \{\langle A_j, a\rangle \text{ such that } a \in Dom(A_j)\ \forall j \in \{1, \ldots, m\}\} \tag{3}$$

Definition 2. We introduce the transaction $\tau^t \subseteq I^{ER}$ associated to a tuple $t \in r$ to be

$$\tau^t = \{\ \langle A_j, t[A_j]\rangle \mid j \in \{1, \ldots, m\}\ \} \tag{4}$$

Definition 3. We introduce the set of transactions associated to a relation r to be

$$T^r = \{\tau^t \mid t \in r\} \tag{5}$$

Example 1. To illustrate these definitions, let us consider the relation in table 1. The transaction τ^{t_1} associated to tuple t_1 contains the set of items $\{\langle \#ID, 1\rangle, \langle Year, 1991\rangle, \langle Course, 3\rangle\}$, the transaction τ^{t_2} associated to tuple t_2 contains the set of items $\{\langle \#ID, 2\rangle, \langle Year, 1991\rangle, \langle Course, 4\rangle\}$, and so on.

Transactions can be represented as columns in a table where the rows are labeled with items. The set of transactions for the relation of table 1

Table 1. Some data about 8 students

	#ID	Year	Course
t_1	1	1991	3
t_2	2	1991	4
t_3	3	1991	4
t_4	4	1991	4
t_5	5	1990	4
t_6	6	1990	3
t_7	7	1990	3
t_8	8	1990	2

is represented in table 2. One "0" in the cell for column t_k and row i tell us that the item i is not in the transaction t_k. On the contrary, one "1" points out that the item is in the transaction. Looking table 2 by columns, we see the usual definition of a transaction as a subset of items. Looking at this representation by rows, an item can be seen as a subset of the set of transactions. This lead us to another definition.

Table 2. Transactions for the relation of table 1

	τ^{t_1}	τ^{t_2}	τ^{t_3}	τ^{t_4}	τ^{t_5}	τ^{t_6}	τ^{t_7}	τ^{t_8}
$\langle \#ID, 1\rangle$	1	0	0	0	0	0	0	0
$\langle \#ID, 2\rangle$	0	1	0	0	0	0	0	0
$\langle \#ID, 3\rangle$	0	0	1	0	0	0	0	0
$\langle \#ID, 4\rangle$	0	0	0	1	0	0	0	0
$\langle \#ID, 5\rangle$	0	0	0	0	1	0	0	0
$\langle \#ID, 6\rangle$	0	0	0	0	0	1	0	0
$\langle \#ID, 7\rangle$	0	0	0	0	0	0	1	0
$\langle \#ID, 8\rangle$	0	0	0	0	0	0	0	1
$\langle Year, 1990\rangle$	0	0	0	0	1	1	1	1
$\langle Year, 1991\rangle$	1	1	1	1	0	0	0	0
$\langle Course, 2\rangle$	0	0	0	0	0	0	0	1
$\langle Course, 3\rangle$	1	0	0	0	0	1	1	0
$\langle Course, 4\rangle$	0	1	1	1	1	0	0	0

Definition 4. We introduce the representation of an itemset I based on the set of transactions T^r to be

$$\Gamma_I^r = \{\tau \in T^r \mid I \subseteq \tau\} \tag{6}$$

Example 2. From the set of transactions of table 2 it follows among others that

$$\Gamma^r_{\{\langle Year,1990\rangle\}} = \{\tau^{t_5}, \tau^{t_6}, \tau^{t_7}, \tau^{t_8}\}$$
$$\Gamma^r_{\{\langle Year,1990\rangle,\langle Course,3\rangle\}} = \{\tau^{t_6}, \tau^{t_7}\}$$

All the transactions in an instance of a relational scheme (i.e. in a relation) have the same number of items, and that is the number of attributes in the relational scheme. This is a special characteristic of transactions in relational databases (transactions in the abstract sense are not restricted to have the same number of items in general). In addition, for every attribute there is one and only one item in every transaction such that the attribute appears in the pair that define the item. Both properties can be appreciated when looking at table 2.

2.2 The Problem of the Granularity

In the context of relational databases, finding strong association rules leads to several problems related to the granularity of the attributes. Attributes described with high granularity (i.e. many precise values) provide a large number of items. As the complexity of the search increases exponentially with the number of items, a large number of items needs a lot of time and space to be analyzed. As another consequence, the support of the items is expected to be low, and hence the support of the rules involving such items is also expected to be low, so it is very difficult to find large itemsets and strong rules. The following example is described in [16].

Example 3. Working with a relation containing data about sanitary emergencies attended at the University Hospital of Granada, we found that the most frequent hour of entrance in the urgency service (22:45) was present in only 11 tuples of 81368, so the support of the item $\langle EHour, 22:45\rangle$ was $11/81368 = 1.351E^{-4}$. Therefore, we could not find any strong rule involving items associated to the hour of entrance.

This is not the last problem. Though a strong rule could be found, this rule would have a poor semantic content. In the previous example, even if the support of the item $\langle EHour, 22:45\rangle$ were high enough, a rule of the form, for example, $\langle EHour, 22:45\rangle \Rightarrow \langle Diagnostic, "Broken\ bone"\rangle$ has a poor semantic content because it tell us nothing about what happens one minute before or after 22:45.

This problem has been solved by clustering (either manual or automatically) the values of the domains with high granularity. The set of clusters is then considered to be the new domain of the attribute, and hence its granularity is reduced. In this scenario, the set of items associated to the attribute is the set of pairs $\langle attribute, cluster\rangle$, and the support of an item is the percentage of tuples where the value of the attribute is in the cluster. In the last example, instead of 86400 values of EHOUR (taking into account hour, minute and second), we would have only 24 (clustering together every value of EHOUR with the same hour), or even less (clustering together values corresponding to morning, afternoon, and night). Therefore, the number of items is reduced and the support of each item is increased, so the algorithms are more efficient and also we can find strong rules. Moreover, these rules have a better semantic content (think for example of a rule of the form $\langle EHour, Afternoon\rangle \Rightarrow \langle Diagnostic, "Broken\ bone"\rangle$ with respect to the rule $\langle EHour, 22:45\rangle \Rightarrow \langle Diagnostic, "Broken\ bone"\rangle$).

2.3 Quantitative Association Rules

The way the values of an attribute with high granularity are clustered depends on the type of the values. When the values are ordered (for example, numerical values) it is usual to group them to form intervals. The attributes with numerical domains are called *quantitative*, and the task of finding rules that relate items of the form $\langle Attribute, Interval\rangle$ with other items is called the *Quantitative Association Rules Problem* (QARP).

There are two main approaches in the literature to solve the QARP. The first one is to cluster the values of the attribute during the search for large itemsets. An example is the algorithm proposed in [21]. This algorithm splits the set of values in a set of intervals of the same (small) size, and if the support of two intervals is small, they are joined together. A *maxsupp* value is used to avoid joining together too many intervals. Another paper that follows this approach is [12], where new measures of usefulness/importance are proposed in order to obtain a better partition of the domain of quantitative attributes.

The second approach to solve the QARP is to cluster the values before the search. An algorithm that follows this approach is proposed in [28]. In this work, the clustering is performed automatically by taking the values with maximum support as centroids of the clusters, and using the support for the clustering. Another algorithm is introduced in [25], where predefined labeled partitions (called "domain concept hierarchies" in [25]), defined subjectively by the user, are used to group attribute values into higher level concepts. An example of such subjective partitions is shown in figure (1). The interval of values 0-5 is labeled "infant", the interval 6-12 "youngster", and so on.

As can be seen in figure 1, the domain of attributes with high granularity is partitioned into intervals with sharp boundaries, but in turn this leads to several problems. One of such problems is related to the meaning of the clusters. It is usual to identify clusters with meaningful concepts for a better understanding of the associations among them. It is the case of the partition of figure 1, where each interval is labeled according to its meaning. But in many occasions, the concepts we use are imprecise and cannot be suited by intervals. For example, the boundary between the concepts "middle age" and "oldster" should not be sharp, as it is not clear that a 60 years old is a middle aged but not an oldster person, and a 61 years old is an oldster but not a middle aged one. The boundaries between these concepts, as well as between every pair of consecutive intervals in figure 1, should not be sharp but imprecise, so an ordinary partition is not the best way to represent them. Another problem related to the boundaries, described in [8,21], is that items $\langle Attribute, Interval\rangle$ with low support could be large by adding to the interval some values near the boundaries. Hence, the support of the intervals of

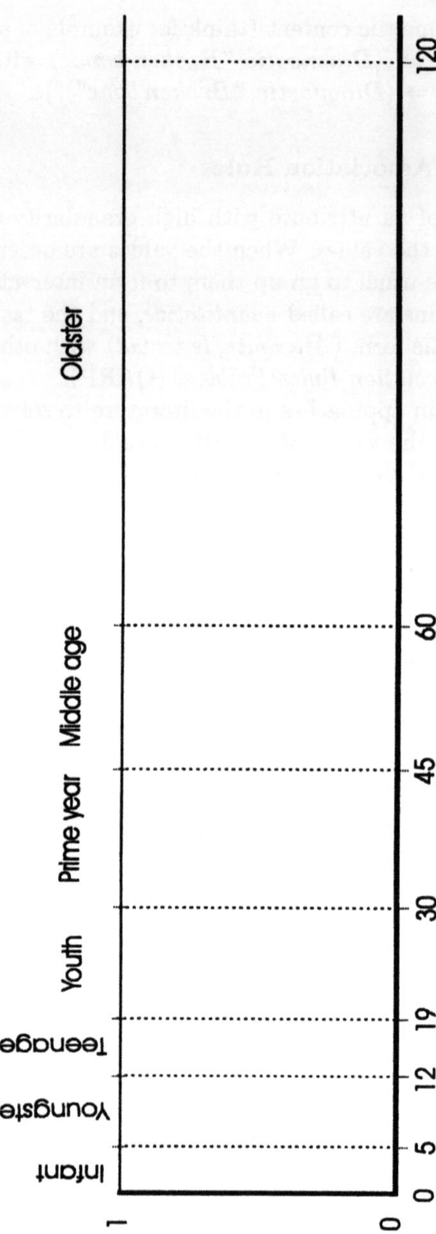

Fig. 1. Ordinary partition of the domain "Age" (years) as described in [25]

crisp partitions can be very sensitive to small moves of the boundaries. This last problem can be concealed by using algorithms for clustering the values in terms of their support, but it could happen that no meaningful concept matched the clusters so obtained. In the next section we will talk of a recently proposed solution to the QARP, based on the theory of fuzzy sets.

3 Fuzzy Association Rules

The theory of fuzzy sets provides an important tool to solve the problem just discussed. Performing a fuzzy clustering of the domains allow us to obtain good representations of imprecise concepts. For example, an alternative representation of concepts related to the age, proposed in [16], is shown in figure 2. Although they are not exactly the same concepts of figure 1, this is not the key point of the discussion. What we want to show is that fuzzy sets (in this example, trapezoid fuzzy sets) are more appropriate that crisp intervals in order to represent linguistic concepts about age employed in the natural language. The concepts of figure 1 can also be easily fuzzified.

In figure 2 it can be seen that the representation by means of fuzzy sets is more suitable. For example, a 60 years old person is considered to be old (it is in the boundary of the core of the label "old"), but a 59 years old one is also considered to be old with a high degree (though lesser than the 60 years old one), a 58 aged person is also old but with a lesser degree that the 59 aged one, and so on. Thus, the transition between "being old" and "not being old" is not sharp but gradual between 60 and 50. So, the boundaries between fuzzy clusters are not sharp but smooth (as they should be). In addition, and because of this, items of the form $\langle Attribute, Label \rangle$ are less sensitive to small moves of the boundaries.

In this approach, rules that associate items of the form $\langle Attribute, Label \rangle$, where the label has an internal representation as a fuzzy set over the domain of the attribute, are called *fuzzy association rules*. Items of the form just described are called *fuzzy items*. Transactions involving fuzzy items are called *fuzzy transactions*. In the following we shall formalize these ideas. Let $ER = \{(A_1, \ldots, A_m)\}$ be a relational scheme and let r be an instance of ER. Let $Dom(A_j)$ be the domain of the attribute A_j for every $j \in \{1, \ldots, n\}$. Let $Et(A_j) = \{L_1^{A_j}, \ldots, L_{c_j}^{A_j}\}$ be a set of linguistic labels for the attribute A_j, such that each label has associated a representation by means of a fuzzy set (we use the same notation for the label and the membership function)

$$L_k^{A_j} : Dom(A_j) \to [0, 1]$$

It is clear that both a value and an interval of values are special cases of fuzzy sets over the domain of an attribute, that can be labeled with the value and the interval respectively. Hence, we can assume without losing generality that every attribute takes values from a set of linguistic labels represented

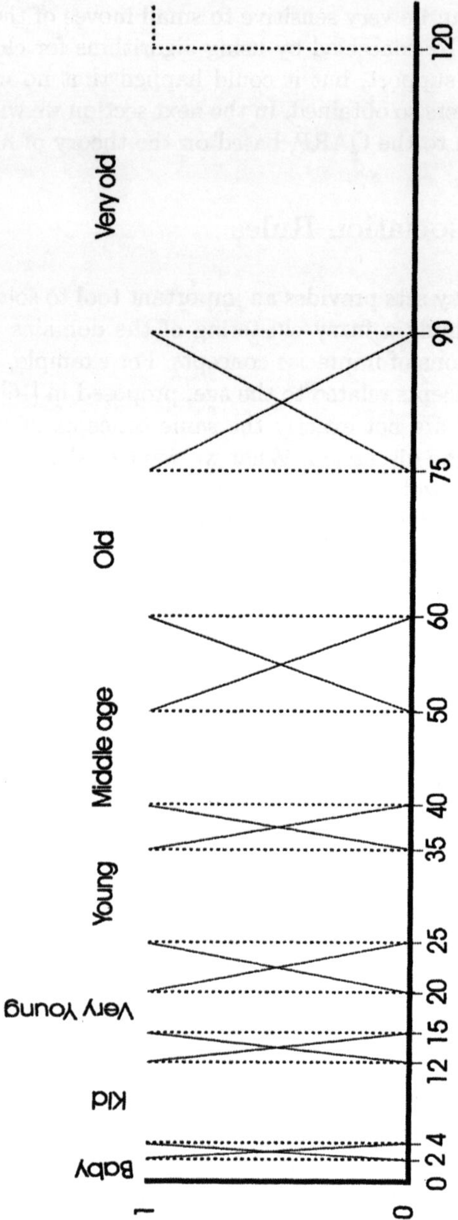

Fig. 2. Fuzzy labels for "Age" as described in [16]

by fuzzy sets. We shall note as L the (crisp) set of all the labels, that is to say

$$L = \bigcup_{j \in \{1,\ldots,m\}} Et(A_j) \tag{7}$$

Definition 5. We introduce the (crisp) set of fuzzy items with labels in L associated to ER to be

$$I_L^{ER} = \{\langle A_j, L_k^{A_j}\rangle \mid A_j \in ER \text{ and } k \in \{1,\ldots,c_j\}\ \forall j \in \{1,\ldots,m\}\} \tag{8}$$

We shall note by $atr(i)$ and $lab(i)$ the attribute and the label respectively of an item i, i.e.

$$atr\left(\langle A_j, L_k^{A_j}\rangle\right) = A_j$$
$$lab\left(\langle A_j, L_k^{A_j}\rangle\right) = L_k^{A_j}$$

Definition 6. We introduce a *fuzzy itemset* I_L to be any (crisp) subset of I_L^{ER} verifying $atr(i_L) \neq atr(j_L)$ for every $i_L, j_L \in I_L$.

Definition 7. Let r be an instance of ER and let $t \in r$ be a tuple. We introduce the fuzzy transaction associated to t with items in I_L^{ER} to be the fuzzy subset

$$\tilde{\tau}_L^t : I_L^{ER} \to [0,1]$$

such that

$$\tilde{\tau}_L^t\left(\langle A_j, L_k^{A_j}\rangle\right) = L_k^{A_j}(t[A_j]) \tag{9}$$

Definition 8. We introduce the (crisp) set of fuzzy transactions with items in I_L^{ER} associated to an instance r of ER, T_L^r, to be

$$T_L^r = \{\tilde{\tau}_L^t \mid t \in r\} \tag{10}$$

Definition 9. We introduce the representation of a fuzzy itemset with only one fuzzy item, $\{i_L\} = \{\langle A_j, L_k^{A_j}\rangle\}$, based on a set of fuzzy transactions T_L^r to be a fuzzy subset

$$\tilde{\Gamma}_{\{i_L\}}^r : T_L^r \to [0,1]$$

such that for every $t \in r$

$$\tilde{\Gamma}_{\{i_L\}}^r\left(\tilde{\tau}_L^t\right) = \tilde{\tau}_L^t(i_L) = L_k^{A_j}(t[A_j]) \tag{11}$$

Definition 10. We introduce the representation of a fuzzy itemset with more than one item I_L, based on a set of fuzzy transactions T_L^r to be a fuzzy subset

$$\tilde{\Gamma}_{I_L}^r : T_L^r \to [0,1]$$

such that for every $t \in r$

$$\tilde{\Gamma}_{I_L}^r\left(\tilde{\tau}_L^t\right) = \bigcap_{i_L \in I_L} \tilde{\Gamma}_{\{i_L\}}^r\left(\tilde{\tau}_L^t\right) = \bigcap_{i_L \in I_L} \tilde{\tau}_L^t(i_L) \tag{12}$$

We shall use the t-norm minimum to perform the intersection in equation 12.

Definition 11. Fuzzy association rule. We introduce a fuzzy association rule with labels in L in an instance r of ER to be a link of the form

$$I_L \Rightarrow J_L$$

verifying the following three properties:

1. $I_L, J_L \subseteq I_L^{ER}$
2. $I_L \cap J_L = \emptyset$
3. $atr\,(i_L) \neq atr\,(j_L) \quad \forall\, i_L, j_L \in I_L \cup J_L$

We shall name I_L and J_L *antecedent* and *consequent* of the rule, respectively. By the third property, both antecedent and consequent are fuzzy itemsets. Moreover, their union is also a fuzzy itemset.

Proposition 1. *An ordinary association rule in a relational database is an special case of fuzzy association rule.*

Proof. Trivial, as an ordinary value can be regarded as an special case of linguistic label.

Example 4. Let r be the relation of table 3, containing the age and hour of birth of six people. The relation r is an instance of the scheme $ER = \{Age, Hour\}$.

	Age	Hour
t_1	60	20:15
t_2	80	23:45
t_3	22	15:30
t_4	55	01:00
t_5	3	19:30
t_6	18	06:51

Table 3. Age and hour of birth of six people

The domains of both age (years) and hour (minutes) have a high granularity. In order to reduce the granularity we are going to use fuzzy labels. For the age we shall use the set of labels *Et*(*Age*)={Baby, Kid, Very young, Young, Middle age, Old, Very old} of figure 2.

Figure 3 shows the definition of the set of labels *Et*(*Hour*) = {Early morning, Morning, Noon, Afternoon, Night} for the attribute Hour, as described in [16]. Noon has not the usual meaning of "around twelve o'clock", but "between morning and afternoon".
Then it follows that

$$L = Et(Age) \cup Et(Hour)$$

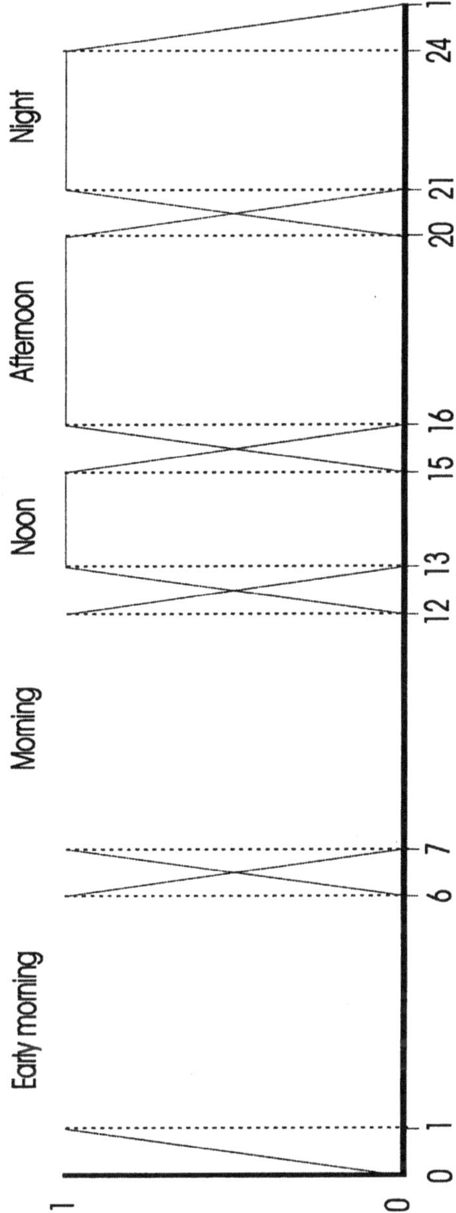

Fig. 3. Fuzzy labels for "Hour" as described in [16]

and $I_L^{ER} = \{\langle Age, Baby\rangle, \langle Age, Kid\rangle, \langle Age, Very\ young\rangle, \langle Age, Young\rangle, \langle Age, Middle\ age\rangle, \langle Age, Old\rangle, \langle Age, Very\ Old\rangle, \langle Hour, Early\ morning\rangle, \langle Hour, Morning\rangle, \langle Hour, Noon\rangle, \langle Hour, Afternoon\rangle, \langle Hour, Night\rangle\}$.

The set of fuzzy transactions with items in I_L^{ER} associated to r is

$$T_L^r = \{\tilde{\tau}_L^{t_1}, \tilde{\tau}_L^{t_2}, \tilde{\tau}_L^{t_3}, \tilde{\tau}_L^{t_4}, \tilde{\tau}_L^{t_5}, \tilde{\tau}_L^{t_6}\}$$

The columns of table 4 are the definition of the fuzzy transactions of T_L^r as fuzzy subsets of I_L^{ER}. For instance

$$\tilde{\tau}_L^{t_1} = \{1/_{\langle Age, Old\rangle} + 0.75/_{\langle Hour, Afternoon\rangle} + 0.25/_{\langle Hour, Night\rangle}\}$$
$$\tilde{\tau}_L^{t_3} = \{0.6/_{\langle Age, Very\ young\rangle} + 0.4/_{\langle Age, Young\rangle} + 0.5/_{\langle Hour, Noon\rangle} + 0.5/_{\langle Hour, Afternoon\rangle}\}$$

Table 4. Fuzzy transactions with items in I_L^{ER} for the relation of table 3

	$\tilde{\tau}_L^{t_1}$	$\tilde{\tau}_L^{t_2}$	$\tilde{\tau}_L^{t_3}$	$\tilde{\tau}_L^{t_4}$	$\tilde{\tau}_L^{t_5}$	$\tilde{\tau}_L^{t_6}$
$\langle Age, Baby\rangle$	0	0	0	0	0.5	0
$\langle Age, Kid\rangle$	0	0	0	0	0.5	0
$\langle Age, Very\ young\rangle$	0	0	0.6	0	0	1
$\langle Age, Young\rangle$	0	0	0.4	0	0	0
$\langle Age, Middle\ age\rangle$	0	0	0	0.5	0	0
$\langle Age, Old\rangle$	1	0.67	0	0.5	0	0
$\langle Age, Very\ old\rangle$	0	0.33	0	0	0	0
$\langle Hour, Early\ morning\rangle$	0	0	0	1	0	0.85
$\langle Hour, Morning\rangle$	0	0	0	0	0	0.15
$\langle Hour, Noon\rangle$	0	0	0.5	0	0	0
$\langle Hour, Afternoon\rangle$	0.75	0	0.5	0	1	0
$\langle Hour, Night\rangle$	0.25	1	0	0	0	0

The membership values follow from definition 7, for instance

$$\tilde{\tau}_L^{t_1}(\langle Age, Old\rangle) = Old(t_1[Age]) = Old(60) = 1$$

Also, in table 4 the row for item i_L contains the fuzzy set $\tilde{\Gamma}^r_{\{i_L\}}$. For instance

$$\tilde{\Gamma}^r_{\{\langle Age, Old\rangle\}} = \{1/\tilde{\tau}_L^{t_1} + 0.67/\tilde{\tau}_L^{t_2} + 0.5/\tilde{\tau}_L^{t_4}\}$$
$$\tilde{\Gamma}^r_{\{\langle Hour, Night\rangle\}} = \{0.25/\tilde{\tau}_L^{t_1} + 1/\tilde{\tau}_L^{t_2}\}$$

Descriptions of itemsets with more than one fuzzy item are, for instance

$$\tilde{\Gamma}^r_{\{\langle Age, Old\rangle, \langle Hour, Night\rangle\}} = \{0.25/\tilde{\tau}_L^{t_1} + 0.67/\tilde{\tau}_L^{t_2}\}$$
$$\tilde{\Gamma}^r_{\{\langle Age, Kid\rangle, \langle Hour, Afternoon\rangle\}} = \{0.5/\tilde{\tau}_L^{t_5}\}$$

Some rules involving fuzzy items in I_L^{ER} are:

$$\langle Age, Old\rangle \Rightarrow \langle Hour, Afternoon\rangle$$
$$\langle Hour, Afternoon\rangle \Rightarrow \langle Age, Baby\rangle$$

The problem that arises now is how to measure the accuracy and usefulness of fuzzy association rules. We shall discuss about that problem in the next section.

4 Accuracy and Usefulness of Fuzzy Association Rules

In this section we are going to introduce our new approach for measuring the accuracy and usefulness of Fuzzy Association Rules. We shall begin by generalizing the ordinary measures of support and confidence of association rules. Next we shall discuss briefly on the problems of these classical measures, and we shall introduce new measures based on the support and confidence. The last subsection is devoted to some related works.

4.1 Generalizing Support and Confidence

Because of the presence of imprecision affecting fuzzy association rules, we shall use quantified sentences [26] in order to generalize the support and confidence. Quantified sentences are statements of the form "Q of D are A" where Q is a linguistic quantifier [26] such as "Most" and "Almost all", and D and A are fuzzy sets defined on the same reference set, usually called X, that we assume to be finite. An example is "*All young* people are *intelligent*". The evaluation of a quantified sentence is a value in $[0,1]$ that measures the compatibility between the quantifier and the percentage of elements of D that are in A. In [6] we introduce a set of properties to be verified by any good method of evaluation, and several evaluation methods are discussed on the basis of those properties. Also in [6] a new method with better properties than existing ones, called GD, is introduced. We shall use GD in our work. The evaluation of a quantified sentence by means of GD is defined as

$$GD_Q(A/D) = \sum_{\alpha_i \in \Delta(A/D)} (\alpha_i - \alpha_{i+1})\, Q\left(\frac{|(A\cap D)_{\alpha_i}|}{|D_{\alpha_i}|}\right) \qquad (13)$$

where $\Delta(A/D) = \Lambda(A\cap D) \cup \Lambda(D)$, $\Lambda(F)$ being the level set of F, and $\Delta(A/D) = \{\alpha_1, \dots, \alpha_p\}$ with $1 = \alpha_1 > \alpha_2 > \cdots > \alpha_{p+1} = 0$. The set D is assumed to be normalized. If not, D is normalized and the normalization factor is applied to $A \cap D$.

Definition 12. We introduce the support of a fuzzy itemset I_L on the set of transactions T_L^r to be the evaluation, by means of the method GD, of the quantified sentence

$$M \text{ of } T_L^r \text{ are } \tilde{\Gamma}_{I_L}^r \qquad (14)$$

where M is the fuzzy relative quantifier, usually called *Most*, defined as

$$M(x) = x \;\; \forall x \in [0,1] \tag{15}$$

Example 5. Table 5 contains the support of four fuzzy itemsets described in example 4 in the relation of table 3:

Definition 13. We introduce the support of the fuzzy association rule

$$I_L \Rightarrow J_L$$

on the set of transactions T_L^r to be the evaluation, by means of the method *GD*, of the quantified sentence

$$M \text{ of } T_L^r \text{ are } \tilde{\Gamma}_{I_L}^r \cap \tilde{\Gamma}_{J_L}^r \tag{16}$$

where M is the fuzzy quantifier of equation 15.

Table 5. Support of four fuzzy itemsets described in example 4

Itemset	supp
$\{\langle Age, Old\rangle\}$	0.361
$\{\langle Hour, Night\rangle\}$	0.208
$\{\langle Age, Old\rangle, \langle Hour, Night\rangle\}$	0.153
$\{\langle Age, Kid\rangle, \langle Hour, Afternoon\rangle\}$	0.083

Definition 14. We introduce the confidence of the fuzzy association rule

$$I_L \Rightarrow J_L$$

on the set of transactions T_L^r to be the evaluation, by means of the method *GD*, of the quantified sentence

$$M \text{ of } \tilde{\Gamma}_{I_L}^r \text{ are } \tilde{\Gamma}_{J_L}^r \tag{17}$$

where M is the fuzzy quantifier of equation 15.

Example 6. Table 6 contains the support and confidence of some fuzzy association rules described in example 4 that hold in the relation of table 3.

Proposition 2. *If I is an ordinary (crisp) itemset, then its support as obtained by definition 12 is the ordinary support of I.*

Proof. The method *GD* verifies that, if A and D are crisp then

$$GD_M(A/D) = \frac{|A \cap D|}{|D|}$$

Table 6. Support and confidence of two fuzzy association rules described in example 4

Rule	Supp	Conf
$\langle Age, Old\rangle \Rightarrow \langle Hour, Afternoon\rangle$	0.125	0.331
$\langle Hour, Afternoon\rangle \Rightarrow \langle Age, Baby\rangle$	0.083	0.166

(see [6]). Hence

$$GD_M(\Gamma_I^r/T^r) = \frac{|\Gamma_I^r \cap T^r|}{|T^r|} = \frac{|\Gamma_I^r|}{|T^r|} = supp(I)$$

given that $|\Gamma_I^r|$ is the number of transactions containing the itemset I.

Proposition 3. *If I and J are ordinary (crisp) itemsets, then the support of the association rule $I \Rightarrow J$, obtained by definition 13, is the ordinary support of an association rule $I \Rightarrow J$ as defined in equation 1.*

Proof. By the mentioned properties of GD

$$GD_M(\Gamma_J^r \cap \Gamma_I^r) = \frac{|\Gamma_J^r \cap \Gamma_I^r|}{|T^r|} = supp(I \cup J)$$

because $\Gamma_J^r \cap \Gamma_I^r$ is the representation (set of transactions containing the itemset) of $I \cup J$.

Proposition 4. *If I and J are ordinary (crisp) itemsets, then the confidence of the association rule $I \Rightarrow J$, obtained by definition 13, is the ordinary confidence of an association rule $I \Rightarrow J$ as defined in equation 1.*

Proof. By the mentioned properties of GD

$$GD_M(\Gamma_J^r/\Gamma_I^r) = \frac{|\Gamma_J^r \cap \Gamma_I^r|}{|\Gamma_I^r|} = \frac{\frac{|\Gamma_J^r \cap \Gamma_I^r|}{|T^r|}}{\frac{|\Gamma_I^r|}{|T^r|}} = \frac{supp(I \cup J)}{supp(I)} = Conf(I \Rightarrow J)$$

Hence, finding fuzzy association rules using the measures of support and confidence as introduced in definitions 13 and 14 is a generalization of the BARP in relational databases. This is only true for the quantifier M. As our intention was to generalize the ordinary definitions of support and confidence, we have not tested other quantifiers.

4.2 New Measures Based on the Support and Confidence

The ordinary measures of support and confidence are in fact probability measures, the former being the probability that both antecedent and consequent are in a transaction, and the latter being the probability that the consequent is in a transaction where the antecedent is (i.e. conditional probability). Confidence has been shown to be inadequate for measuring the accuracy of association rules, see [4,16,20]. Some of its problems are:

- Confidence is not able to detect statistical independence between antecedent and consequent of an association rule, because statistical independence holds when

$$supp(I \cup J) = supp(I)supp(J) \tag{18}$$

and confidence of an association rule $I \Rightarrow J$ only takes into account $supp(I \cup J)$ and $supp(I)$.
- Because of the same reason confidence is not able to detect negative dependence between antecedent and consequent (i.e. the presence of the antecedent is associated to the absence of the consequent in a transaction). Negative dependence holds when

$$supp(I \cup J) < supp(I)supp(J) \tag{19}$$

- Conditional probability is not an intuitive measure, and hence it is difficult for an user to choose semantically meaningful values of *minconf*, and even to judge if a given confidence is good. This is a well-known problem in knowledge engineering, where it is known that in practice, experts tend to give conditional probabilities values under the real ones.

Another problem arises from the use of the support for measuring the usefulness of the rules. Support is usually considered to be good when it is above *minsupp*, but in fact association rules with very high support can be false, or at least doubtful, as has been shown in [4,16]. The problem is that if an association rule has high support then the consequent has high support (it is in most of the transactions) and hence any itemset seems to be a good predictor of the presence of the consequent in a transaction. An example described in [4] is the rule "Past military duty in the U.S. Army ⇒ No service in Vietnam", that holds in the U.S. CENSUS database with very high support and confidence. It seems to be clear that knowing that a person has served in the U.S. Army should increase our believe that he/she has served in Vietnam, but the rule tell us just the contrary. The problem is the high support (over 95%) of the item "No service in Vietnam" in the CENSUS database. Another example has been described in [16]. In a database with information about surgical operations, the item $\langle Prosthesis, No \rangle$ (no prosthesis has been implanted in the surgical operation) has a very high support, and hence any other item seems to be a good predictor of the absence of prosthesis in the operation, though in fact there is no relation among them.

Because of the problems of confidence and support, the amount of strong rules obtained from a database would be larger than it should. In some experiments performed in [16] over large medical databases, the number of strong rules obtained using support and confidence has been shown to be above the real number of strong rules by a factor of 20 and even more (considering only rules with one single item in the consequent). To fill this gap, we have proposed in [16] the use of other approaches to measure the accuracy and usefulness of fuzzy association rules. These are *certainty factors* [19] and *very strong rules.*

Definition 15. Given two itemsets I and J we name certainty factor of $I \Rightarrow J$ to the value

$$CF(I \Rightarrow J) = \frac{(Conf(I \Rightarrow J)) - supp(J)}{1 - supp(J)} \tag{20}$$

if $Conf(I \Rightarrow J) > supp(J)$, and

$$CF(I \Rightarrow J) = \frac{(Conf(I \Rightarrow J)) - supp(J)}{supp(J)} \tag{21}$$

if $Conf(I \Rightarrow J) \leq supp(J)$, assuming by agreement that if $supp(J) = 1$ then $CF(I \Rightarrow J) = 1$ and if $supp(J) = 0$ then $CF(I \Rightarrow J) = -1$.

The certainty factor is a measure of *increment* of our believe, taking values in $[-1, 1]$. Positive certainty factors measure the decrement of our believe against the consequent, given the antecedent is true. Shortliffe and Buchanan [19] show that it is easier for human experts to estimate certainty factors than to estimate conditional probabilities. Also, certainty factors verify the following properties [16]:

Property 1. Statistical independence between two itemsets I and J holds if and only if $CF(I \Rightarrow J) = 0$

Property 2. Negative dependence between two itemsets I and J holds if and only if $CF(I \Rightarrow J) < 0$

Property 3. $Conf(I \Rightarrow J) = 1$ if and only if $CF(I \Rightarrow J) = 1$

In addition, any existing algorithm for mining association rules can be easily modified to obtain the certainty factor for an association rule, because it is based on the confidence of the rule and the support of the consequent, and both are available in the second step of the process. An experimental comparison between confidence and certainty factor has been performed in [16], and the number of rules obtained has been reduced in all the experiments over large medical databases and the CENSUS database by using certainty factors. Hence, certainty factors solve the problems of the confidence. We shall use them in our work for measuring the accuracy of the rules, and from now on we shall say that an association rule is strong if its support and certainty factor are above *minsupp* and a threshold *minCF* respectively.

Definition 16. An association rule $I \Rightarrow J$ is said to be *very strong* if both $I \Rightarrow J$ and $\neg J \Rightarrow \neg I$ are strong rules.

With this definition, if an association rule $I \Rightarrow J$ has a very high support, the support of the rule $\neg J \Rightarrow \neg I$ will be very low, so the latter won't be a strong rule and hence the former won't be a very strong rule. Hence, we are avoiding the problem of association rules with very high support. Moreover, finding very strong association rules doesn't increase the complexity of the process despite the algorithm, because of the following proposition [16]

Proposition 5. *An association rule $I \Rightarrow J$ is very strong if and only if*

- *$I \Rightarrow J$ is a strong rule, and*
- $1 - supp(I) - supp(J) + supp(I \cup J) > minsupp$

The second condition can be easily checked in the second step of any existing algorithm, because at that point the support of antecedent, consequent and rule are available.

4.3 Related Work

Other approaches for mining fuzzy association rules can be found in [3,8]. In [3] two new measures called *adjusted difference* and *weight of evidence* are used in order to measure the importance and accuracy of fuzzy association rules. A rule is considered to be important when its adjusted difference is greater than 1.96 (the 95 percentiles of the normal distribution). The algorithm proposed in [3], called F-APACS, provide every important rule and its weight of evidence. It can be pointed out that

- One of the main advantages of F-APACS is that the user does not need to supply any threshold. Also, a mechanism for inferring quantitative values from the rules is provided.
- On the other hand, the adjusted difference is not provided to the user, so that all important rules would seem to be equally important.
- Opposite to the support, the adjusted difference is not shown to be adequate for bounding the search for important itemsets (in the sense of the adjusted difference). In any case, F-APACS does not use the adjusted difference for that purpose. Because of that, F-APACS seems to be restricted to finding rules with only one item in the antecedent and one item in the consequent. Otherwise, as the search is exhaustive, the algorithm would be too complex when the number of items were high.
- The adjusted difference is symmetric. Hence, if the rule $I \Rightarrow J$ is considered to be interesting, also $J \Rightarrow I$ is. This is not true in general. Hence, as the weight of evidence is not considered in order to choice important rules, the user could be provided with many important rules (in the sense of the adjusted difference) but with low accuracy.
- The formulation of the adjusted difference and weight of evidence, as shown in [3], is not very intuitive for a user who is not used to work with statistics (though only the latter is going to be provided with the rule).

The weight of evidence takes values in $[-\infty, \infty]$, so it is not easy to give an interpretation of the values in order to say if the gain of information is high or low.

Another proposal, closer to ours, is shown in [8]. In this work, usefulness of itemsets and rules is measured by means of a new measure called *significance factor*. The accuracy of a fuzzy association rule is called *certainty factor*, but the formulation and semantics are different from that of Shortliffe and Buchanan [19], followed by us in definition 15. Two ways for calculating the certainty factor are described in [8], though only one is to be used at a time. The first one is based on significance, in the same way that confidence is based on support. The second one obtains a measure of correlation between antecedent and consequent, based on statistics but slightly different from ordinary correlation. We can point out that

- It is easy to show that significance and certainty factor (only the version based on significance) are generalizations of the usual measures of support and confidence of association rules, as is the case of our measures of support and confidence. In this sense, they are expected to have the problems we have discussed in previous sections.
- Using correlation seems to be more adequate in order to obtain the value of the certainty factor. Its value ranges from -1 to 1. Positive values point out that antecedent and consequent are related. The bigger the correlation, the more related they are.

5 Experiments

We have performed several experiments on medical databases obtained from the Universitary Hospital of Granada. These databases contains data about urgency services and surgical operations. The relation URGENCY contains 81368 tuples about services attended between the 28th Oct 1997 and the 11th Oct 1998. The relation OPERATIONS contains 15766 tuples about surgical operations performed between the 26th Aug 1997 and the 1st Sep 1998.

5.1 Algorithm

One of the advantages of our measures of support and certainty factor is that it is not difficult to modify the existing algorithms in order to obtain them. The main modification in step 1 (finding large itemsets) is that we store the support of every α-cut minus the support of the strong α-cut of the same level, for every fuzzy itemset. We have used a fixed number of 100 α-cuts, so that for every itemset I_L we have an array v_{I_L} with 100 elements. This way, if $\tilde{\Gamma}^r_{\{i_L\}}(\tilde{\tau}^t_L) = \alpha$ then we add 1 to $v_{I_L}(100\alpha)$. Once the database has been scaned and v_{I_L} has been filled, the support of I_L (as defined in definition 12) is obtained from v_{I_L} by means of the algorithm of figure 4 in time $O(1)$. This modification does not increase time complexity of any existing algorithm for finding association rules.

1. $j \leftarrow 100$
   $supp \leftarrow 0$
2. While $j > 0$
   (a) $supp \leftarrow supp + (j * v_{I_L}[j])$
   (b) $j \leftarrow j - 1$
3. $supp \leftarrow supp/(100 * |r|)$

Fig. 4. Algorithm for obtaining the support of a fuzzy itemset I_L

In the second step of the algorithm, the confidence (as defined in definition 14) is obtained by means of the algorithm of figure 5 in time $O(1)$. Once the confidence of the rule has been obtained, and using the support of the rule and the consequent obtained in step 1, it is easy to obtain the certainty factor (by means of expressions in definition 15) and then checking if the rule is very strong (proposition 5), both in time $O(1)$.

1. $j \leftarrow 100$
   $conf \leftarrow 0$
   $max_\alpha \leftarrow 100$
   $acum_{I_L} \leftarrow 0$
   $acum_{I_L \cup \{i_L\}} \leftarrow 0$
2. {Obtain the maximum membership degree to $\tilde{\Gamma}^r_{\{i_L\}}$ }
   While ($max_\alpha > 0$) and ($v_{I_L}(max_\alpha) = 0$)
   (a) $max_\alpha \leftarrow max_\alpha - 1$
3. While $j > 0$
   (a) {Normalization }
       $alpha \leftarrow (j * max_\alpha)/100$
   (b) $acum_{I_L \cup \{i_L\}} \leftarrow acum_{I_L \cup \{i_L\}} + v_{I_L \cup \{i_L\}}(alpha)$
   (c) $acum_{I_L} \leftarrow acum_{I_L} + v_{I_L}(alpha)$
   (d) $conf \leftarrow conf + (acum_{I_L \cup \{i_L\}}/acum_{I_L})$
   (e) $j \leftarrow j - 1$
4. $conf \leftarrow conf/100$

Fig. 5. Algorithm for obtaining the confidence of a fuzzy association rule of the form $I_L \Rightarrow \{i_L\}$

We are not concerned in this work with designing faster algorithms than existing. Moreover, as the modifications we have introduced do not increase time complexity of existing algorithms (though we need more space in order to store the α-cuts of every fuzzy itemset), we only need to modify the faster one. In order to check the usefulness of our measures for fuzzy association rules, we have applied this modifications to the more basic version of an algorithm for finding association rules. The results are described in the next section.

5.2 Some experimental results

Some very strong association rules we have obtained in the relation OPERATIONS are shown in table 7.

Table 7. Very strong fuzzy association rules in relation OPERATIONS

#Rule	Rule	Supp	C.Factor
1	$\langle HStart, Noon\rangle \Rightarrow \langle HEnd, Noon\rangle$	0.13	0.91
2	$\langle Age, Baby\rangle \Rightarrow \langle Anesthesia, General\rangle$	0.01	0.9
3	$\langle Age, Kid\rangle \Rightarrow \langle Anesthesia, General\rangle$	0.06	0.77
4	$\langle Age, Baby\rangle \Rightarrow \langle HStart, Morning\rangle$	0.01	0.66
5	$\langle Age, Kid\rangle \Rightarrow \langle HStart, Morning\rangle$	0.05	0.48

Rule #1 has a very high certainty factor of 0.91 and it is interesting because the fuzzy interval for $Noon$ is small. The rest of the rules tell us that babies and kids are usually operated with general anesthetics (certainty factors 0.9 and 0.77) and that their operations start in the morning (certainty factors 0.66 and 0.48 respectively). No other age is so strongly related to a value of $HStart$.

With respect to the relation URGENCY, some very strong rules are shown in table 8.

Table 8. Very strong fuzzy association rules in relation URGENCY

#Rule	Rule	Supp	C.Factor
1	$\langle Attendance, Plaster\rangle \Rightarrow \langle HEntrance, Afternoon\rangle$	0.02	0.48
2	$\langle HEntrance, Morning\rangle \Rightarrow \langle Attendance, Observation\rangle$	0.12	0.43

In addition, we have verified that considering only support and confidence lead us to obtain more rules that we should. An example is the rule $\langle Age, Middle\ age\rangle \Rightarrow \langle Suspended, Yes\rangle$, with support 0.34 and confidence 0.92. This rule is strong for any value of *minsupp* and *minconf* under 0.34 and 0.92 respectively. However, as the support of the item $\langle Suspended, Yes\rangle$ is 0.92, this rule is not very strong at level 0.1. The certainty factor of this rule is 0.01, so antecedent and consequent are almost independent. Hence, this rule is unimportant. The same case arise with any other age, so when using only support and confidence, any age seems to be a good predictor that the operation is not going to be suspended. Using certainty factors and searching for very strong rules allow us to ensure that the rules obtained are really important associations among items.

We have also obtained some results that confirm that rules obtained from important rules by interchanging antecedent and consequent would not be important, whatever the measure of accuracy we use. As an example, the rule $\langle Anesthesia, General \rangle \Rightarrow \langle Age, Baby \rangle$, obtained from rule #2 of table 7, has certainty factor 0.01 and confidence 0.02, while rule #2 has certainty factor 0.91 and confidence 0.95. Hence, using the adjusted difference in [3] as the only criterion for reporting fuzzy association rules seems not to be sufficient.

6 Conclusions and Future Research

We have proposed new measures of accuracy and usefulness for fuzzy association rules that allow us to obtain only really important rules in relational databases. With our approach, the number of rules is reduced significatively, but no important rule is lost. We have shown the adequacy of our approach from both the theoretical and the practical point of view. Also, we have proposed a methodology for adapting the existing efficient algorithms to perform the task of finding fuzzy association rules, without increasing their time complexity. Once we have shown that our approach keep us from finding many uninteresting rules, what remains open is using the rules we discover in practice. Another future research avenue will be to study the use of fuzzy hierarchies in order to obtain fuzzy association rules at several levels in the taxonomy.

References

1. R. Agrawal, T. Imielinski and A. Swami (1993) Mining Association Rules Between Sets of Items in Large Databases, Proc. of 1993 ACM SIGMOD Conference, pp. 207-216.
2. R. Agrawal and R. Srikant (1994) Fast Algorithms for Mining Association Rules, Proc. of 20th VLDB Conference, pp. 478-499.
3. W.H. Au and K.C.C. Chan (1998) An Effective Algorithm for Discovering Fuzzy Rules in Relational Databases, Proc. IEEE Int'l Conf. on Fuzzy Systems, Vol. II, pp. 1314-1319.
4. S. Brin, R. Motwani, J.D. Ullman and S. Tsur (1997) Dynamic Itemset Counting and Implication Rules for Market Basket Data, SIGMOD Record, 26, 255-264.
5. M. Delgado, M.J. Martín-Bautista, D. Sánchez and M.A. Vila (2000) Mining Strong Approximate Dependencies from Relational Databases, Proceedings of IPMU'2000 (forthcoming).
6. M. Delgado, D. Sánchez and M.A. Vila (2000) Fuzzy Cardinality Based Evaluation of Quantified Sentences, International Journal of Approximate Reasoning, 23, pp. 23-66.

7. M. Houtsma and A. Swami (1995) Set-Oriented Mining for Association Rules in Relational Databases, Proc. of 11th International Conference on Data Engineering, pp. 25-33.
8. C.-M. Kuok, A. Fu and M.H. Wong (1998) Mining Fuzzy Association Rules in Databases, SIGMOD Record, 27, No 1, 41-46.
9. K.L. Lee, G.L. Lee and A.L.P. Chen (1999) Efficient Graph-Based Algorithm for Discovering and Maintaining Knowledge in Large Databases, Proc. of PAKDD-99, Third Pacific-Asia Conference on Knowledge Discovery and Data Mining, pp. 409-419.
10. D. Maier (1983) The Theory of Relational Databases, Computer Science Press.
11. H. Mannila, H. Toivonen and I. Verkamo (1994) Efficient Algorithms for Discovering Association Rules, Proc, AAAI Workshop on Knowledge Discovery in Databases, pp. 181-192.
12. R.J. Miller and Y. Yang (1997) Association Rules over Interval Data, Proc. of ACM-SIGMOD Int. Conf. on Management of Data, pp. 452-461.
13. J.-S. Park, M.-S. Chen and P.S. Yu (1995) An Effective Hash Based Algorithm for Mining Association Rules, SIGMOD Record, 24, 175-186.
14. N. Pasquier, Y. Bastide, R. Taouil and L. Lakhal (1999) Efficient Mining of Association Rules Using Closed Itemset Lattices, Information Systems, 24, 25-46
15. K. Rajamani, A. Cox, B. Iyer and A. Chadha (1999) Efficient Mining for Association Rules with Relational Database Systems, Proc IDEAS'99, Int. Database Engineering and Applications Symposium, pp. 148-155.
16. D. Sanchez (1999) Adquisición de Relaciones Entre Atributos En Bases de Datos Relacionales, Ph.D. Thesis, Department of Computer Science and Artificial Intelligence, University of Granada.
17. A. Savarese, E. Omiecinski and S. Navathe (1995) An Efficient Algorithm for Mining Association Rules in Large Databases, Proc. of 21th VLDB Conference, pp. 432-444.
18. L. Shen, H. Shen and L. Cheng (1999) New Algorithms For Efficient Mining of Association Rules, Information Sciences, 118, 251-268.
19. E.H. Shortliffe and B.G. Buchanan (1975) A Model of Inexact Reasoning in Medicine, Mathematical Biosciences, 23, 351-379.
20. C. Silverstein, S. Brin and R. Motwani (1998) Beyond Market Baskets: Generalizing Association Rules to Dependence Rules, Data Mining and Knowledge Discovery, 2, 39-68.
21. R. Srikant and R. Agrawal (1996) Mining Quantitative Association Rules in Large Relational Tables, Proc. of ACM SIGMOD Int'l. Conf. Management Data, pp. 1-12.
22. J. Wijsen and R. Meersman (1998) On the Complexity of Mining Quantitative Association Rules, Data Mining and Knowledge Discovery, vol. 2, 263-281.
23. M. Wojciechowski and M. Zakrzewicz (1998) Item Set Materializing for Fast Mining of Association Rules, in Advances in Databases and Information Systems. Proceedings of the Second East European Symposium, ADBIS'98, pp. 284-295.
24. S.-Y. Wur and Y.H. Leu (1999) An Effective Boolean Algorithm for Mining Association Rules in Large Databases, Proc. of 6th Int. Conf. on Advanced Systems for Advanced Applications, pp. 179-186.
25. S.-J. Yen and A.L.P. Chen (1996) The Analysis of Relationships in Databases for Rule Derivation, Journal of Intelligent Information System, 7, 235-259.

26. L.A. Zadeh (1983) A Computational Approach to Fuzzy Quantifiers in Natural Languages, Computing and Mathematics with Applications, 9, 149-184.
27. M.J. Zaki, S. Parthasarathy, M. Ogihara and W. Li (1997) New Algorithms for Fast Discovery of Association Rules, Proc. of Third Int. Conf. On Knowledge Discovery and Data Mining, pp. 283-286.
28. Z. Zhang and Y. Lu and B. Zhang (1997) An Effective Partitioning-Combining Algorithm for Discovering Quantitative Association Rules, in H. Lu and H. Motoda and H. Liu (Eds.): KDD: Techniques and Applications, World Scientific, pp. 241-251.